Psychiatric Genetics
Applications in Clinical Practice

Edited by

Jordan W. Smoller, M.D., Sc.D.
Beth Rosen Sheidley, M.S., C.G.C.
Ming T. Tsuang, M.D., Ph.D., D.Sc.

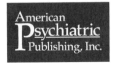

American
Psychiatric
Publishing, Inc.

Washington, DC
London, England

Copyright © 2008 American Psychiatric Publishing, Inc.
ALL RIGHTS RESERVED

Manufactured in the United States of America on acid-free paper
12 11 10 09 08   5 4 3 2 1
First Edition

Typeset in Adobe's Univers and Baskerville.

American Psychiatric Publishing, Inc.
1000 Wilson Boulevard
Arlington, VA 22209-3901
www.appi.org

Library of Congress Cataloging-in-Publication Data
Psychiatric genetics : applications in clinical practice / edited by Jordan W. Smoller, Beth Rosen Sheidley, Ming T. Tsuang.—1st ed.
    p. ; cm.
    Includes bibliographical references and index.
    ISBN 978-1-58562-206-1 (alk. paper)
    1. Mental illness—Genetic aspects. 2. Genetic counseling—
Psychological aspects. I. Smoller, Jordan W., 1961– II. Sheidley, Beth
Rosen, 1968– III. Tsuang, Ming T., 1931–
    [DNLM: 1. Mental Disorders—genetics. 2. Genetic Counseling—
psychology. 3. Mental Disorders—epidemiology. WM 140 P97417 2008]
    RC455.4.G4P783 2008
    616.89′042–dc22

                                                    2007044464

British Library Cataloguing in Publication Data
A CIP record is available from the British Library.

For Alexis–J.W.S.

For Nathaniel, Ella, and Benjamin–B.R.S.

For Snow–M.T.T.

Contents

Part 1:
General Principles

1 Psychiatric Genetics: A Primer 3
Stephen J. Glatt, Ph.D., Stephen V. Faraone, Ph.D., and
Ming T. Tsuang, M.D., Ph.D., D.Sc.

2 Principles of Genetic Counseling 27
Holly L. Peay, M.S., C.G.C., and
Beth Rosen Sheidley, M.S., C.G.C.

3 Risk Communication:
Simple Tools to Foster Understanding 47
Stephanie Kurzenhäuser, Ph.D., Dipl.Psych., and
Anja Dieckmann, Ph.D., Dipl.Psych.

Part 2:
Genetics of Specific Disorders

Part 3: Special Topics

Contributors

Paul S. Appelbaum, M.D.
Division of Law, Ethics, and Psychiatry, Department of Psychiatry, College of Physicians and Surgeons, Columbia University, New York, New York

Anne S. Bassett, M.D., F.R.C.P.C.
Clinical Genetics Research Program, Centre for Addiction and Mental Health; Department of Psychiatry, University of Toronto, Toronto, Ontario, Canada

Deborah Blacker, M.D., Sc.D.
Massachusetts General Hospital/Harvard Medical School; Harvard School of Public Health, Boston, Massachusetts

Eva W.C. Chow, M.D., M.P.H., F.R.C.P.C.
Clinical Genetics Service and Clinical Genetics Research Program, Centre for Addiction and Mental Health, Toronto, Ontario, Canada; Department of Psychiatry, University of Toronto, Toronto, Ontario, Canada

Lee S. Cohen, M.D.
Massachusetts General Hospital, Boston, Massachusetts

Anja Dieckmann, Ph.D., Dipl.Psych.
Max Planck Institute for Human Development, Berlin, Germany

Stephen V. Faraone, Ph.D.
Department of Psychiatry and Behavioral Sciences and Medical Genetics Research Center, SUNY Upstate Medical University, Syracuse, New York

Christine T. Finn, M.D.
Department of Psychiatry, Massachusetts General Hospital; Harvard Partners Center for Genetics and Genomics, Boston, Massachusetts

Stephen J. Glatt, Ph.D.
Department of Psychiatry and Behavioral Sciences and Medical Genetics Research Center, SUNY Upstate Medical University, Syracuse, New York

Kathleen A. Hodgkinson, M.Sc., Ph.D. Candidate
Clinical Genetics Research Program, Centre for Addiction and Mental Health, Toronto, Ontario, Canada

Steven K. Hoge, M.D., M.B.A.
New York University School of Medicine; Law and Psychiatry Program; Division of Forensic Psychiatry, Bellevue Hospital Center, New York, New York

Bruce R. Korf, M.D., Ph.D.
Department of Genetics, University of Alabama at Birmingham, Birmingham, Alabama

Alexia Koukopoulos, M.D.
Massachusetts General Hospital, Boston, Massachusetts

Stephanie Kurzenhäuser, Ph.D., Dipl.Psych.
Department of Psychology, University of Basel, Switzerland

Matthew B. McQueen, Sc.D.
Institute for Behavioral Genetics, University of Colorado, Boulder, Colorado

Ruta Nonacs, M.D.
Massachusetts General Hospital, Boston, Massachusetts

David L. Pauls, Ph.D.
Psychiatric and Neurodevelopmental Genetics Unit, Center for Human Genetic Research, Massachusetts General Hospital, Boston, Massachusetts

Holly L. Peay, M.S., C.G.C.
National Human Genome Research Institute, Social and Behavioral Research Branch, Bethesda, Maryland

Laura F. Petrillo, M.D.
Massachusetts General Hospital, Boston, Massachusetts

Beth Rosen Sheidley, M.S., C.G.C.

Genetic Counseling Program, Department of Biology, Brandeis University, Waltham, Massachusetts; Division of Genetics and Metabolism, Tufts–New England Medical Center, Floating Hospital for Children, Boston, Massachusetts

Jordan W. Smoller, M.D., Sc.D.

Harvard Medical School; Department of Epidemiology, Harvard School of Public Health; Department of Psychiatry, Massachusetts General Hospital; Psychiatric Genetics Program in Mood and Anxiety Disorders, Department of Psychiatry and Center for Human Genetic Research, Boston, Massachusetts

S. Evelyn Stewart, M.D.

Psychiatric and Neurodevelopmental Genetics Unit, Center for Human Genetic Research; Pediatric OCD Clinic; Adult OCD and Related Disorders Clinic, Massachusetts General Hospital, Boston, Massachusetts

Ming T. Tsuang, M.D., Ph.D., D.Sc.

Center for Behavioral Genomics, Department of Psychiatry, University of California, San Diego, La Jolla, California; Harvard Institute of Psychiatric Epidemiology and Genetics, Harvard Departments of Epidemiology and Psychiatry, Boston, Massachusetts; Veterans Affairs San Diego Healthcare System, San Diego, California

Adele C. Viguera, M.D.

Massachusetts General Hospital, Boston, Massachusetts; Cleveland Clinic, Neurological Institute, Cleveland, Ohio

Disclosure of Competing Interests

The following authors have competing interests to declare:

Lee S. Cohen, M.D.—*Grant support:* AstraZeneca, Berlex Laboratories, Eli Lilly, Forest, GlaxoSmithKline, Janssen, National Institute of Mental Health, Sepracor, Stanley Medical Research Institute, Wyeth-Ayerst; *Consultant:* Eli Lilly, GlaxoSmithKline, Janssen, Novartis, Ortho-McNeil, Wyeth-Ayerst; *Speaker's bureau:* AstraZeneca, Berlex Pharmaceuticals, Eli Lilly, Forest, GlaxoSmithKline, Janssen, Pfizer, Wyeth-Ayerst.

Stephen V. Faraone, Ph.D.—*Research support:* McNeil Pediatrics, National Institute of Child Health and Human Development, National Institute of Mental Health, National Institute of Neurological Disorders and Stroke,

Shire Laboratories; *Speaker's bureau:* McNeil Pediatrics; Shire Laboratories. *Dr. Faraone has had an advisory or consulting relationship with the following pharmaceutical companies:* Eli Lilly, McNeil Pediatrics, Novartis, Shire Laboratories.

Ruta Nonacs, M.D.— *Speaker's bureau:* GlaxoSmithKline.

Laura F. Petrillo, M.D.—*Salary support:* National Institute of Mental Health, Harvard Medical School Consolidated Departments of Psychiatry (through an Ethel Dupont Warren Award and a Livingston Award), Massachusetts General Hospital; *Grant support:* Janssen, Abbott Laboratories, AstraZeneca, Berlex Laboratories, Bristol-Myers Squibb, Eli Lilly, Forest Laboratories, GlaxoSmithKline, Sanofi-Synthélabo, Sepracor, the Stanley Foundation, Wyeth Pharmaceuticals.

Jordan W. Smoller, M.D., Sc.D.—*Honoraria:* Roche Pharmaceuticals Division; *Advisory board:* Roche Diagnostics Division.

Adele C. Viguera, M.D.— *Grant support:* AstraZeneca, Berlex Laboratories, Eli Lilly, Forest, GlaxoSmithKline, Harvard Medical School's Scholars in Medicine Fellowship (Claflin Award), Janssen, NARSAD: The Mental Health Research Association, National Institute of Mental Health, Pfizer, Sepracor, Stanley Medical Research Institute, Wyeth-Ayerst; *Speaker's bureau:* Eli Lilly, GlaxoSmithKline; *Honoraria:* Novartis, Wyeth-Ayerst; *Advisory board:* GlaxoSmithKline, Novartis.

The following authors have no competing interests to report:
Paul S. Appelbaum, M.D.
Anne S. Bassett, M.D., F.R.C.P.C.
Deborah Blacker, M.D., Sc.D.
Eva W.C. Chow, M.D., M.P.H., F.R.C.P.C.
Anja Dieckmann, Ph.D., Dipl.Psych.
Christine T. Finn, M.D.
Stephen J. Glatt, Ph.D.
Kathleen A. Hodgkinson, M.Sc.
Steven K. Hoge, M.D., M.B.A.
Bruce R. Korf, M.D., Ph.D.
Alexia Koukopoulos, M.D.
Stephanie Kurzenhäuser, Ph.D., Dipl.Psych.
Matthew B. McQueen, Sc.D.
David L. Pauls. Ph.D.
Holly L. Peay, M.S., C.G.C.
Beth Rosen Sheidley, M.S., C.G.C.
S. Evelyn Stewart, M.D.
Ming T. Tsuang, M.D., Ph.D., D.Sc.

Preface

The pace of research in genetics and genomics has been accelerating since the mid-1990s. Yet it is clear that we are only beginning to decipher the text that emerged from the sequencing of the human genome completed in 2003. We know the number and sequence of our genes but little about how most genes function in health and disease. Nevertheless, a combination of hope, hype, and genuine scientific discovery has created the expectation that genetic research will reveal fundamental insights into the etiology and pathophysiology of a broad range of medical illnesses, including psychiatric disorders. As of this writing, however, few specific genes have been established as contributing to the development of neuropsychiatric disorders.

What justification can there be, then, for a book addressing clinical aspects of psychiatric genetics? If specific genes and genetic tests have yet to emerge for common forms of psychiatric disorder, what relevance does psychiatric genetics have for clinicians? These are sensible questions, and they provide a context for us to describe our aims in compiling this volume. This book is intended to address several issues that have received little attention elsewhere and that we believe are of importance to clinicians.

First, the bewildering array of reported findings in genetics as a field and psychiatric genetics in particular can be difficult even for researchers in the field to keep up with. A search on Medline reveals that in the 5 years from 2002 through 2006, more than 5,400 English-language research articles were published about the genetics of major psychiatric disorders. Interpreting and evaluating the growing literature on psychiatric genetics is often difficult and requires familiarity with the vocabulary and methods involved in genetic research. In order to respond effectively when patients come to the office with questions about the latest media report that "the gene for" schizophrenia has been found, clinicians must understand the meaning and limitations of genetic discoveries. In Chapter 1, Glatt, Faraone, and Tsuang present a framework for understanding and critically evaluating the research literature in psychiatric genetics.

Second, even without identified susceptibility genes, the importance of familial and genetic factors in psychiatric illness has been established by family, twin, and adoption studies. Indeed, family history is the best-validated risk factor for disorders as varied as autism, attention-deficit/hyperactivity disorder, schizophrenia, bipolar disorder, recurrent major depression, and panic disorder. In our experience, an increasing number of patients and families are seeking information about familial risks of psychiatric illness, and this interest is likely to increase in the coming years as gene-identification studies further raise the profile of genetic research in psychiatry.

In a survey of practicing psychiatrists by Finn et al. (2005), more than 80% reported that they felt it is their role to discuss familial and genetic aspects of mental illness with patients and families, but fewer than 20% felt prepared or competent to do so. Moreover, survey respondents reported that they rarely refer such questions to genetics professionals (genetic counselors and medical geneticists). Thus, clinicians are addressing these issues in their practices despite feeling ill-prepared to inform or counsel patients and families. Another aim addressed in this book, then, is to provide a resource for clinicians who would like more information about the role and content of genetic counseling in psychiatry. In Chapter 2, Peay and Rosen Sheidley present an introduction to the principles and practice of genetic counseling that we hope will enhance clinicians' preparedness to approach issues of familial and genetic risk with patients and families. In Chapter 3, Kurzenhäuser and Dieckmann build on this introduction by discussing the psychological and quantitative aspects of risk estimation and communication in the context of genetic counseling. These crucial but often underappreciated issues have direct relevance to the impact and effectiveness of genetic counseling. The manner in which risks are estimated and discussed can have a profound effect on patients' understanding and psychological reactions to genetic information.

Third, we believe it is valuable for clinicians to be aware of the body of knowledge about the familial risk and genetic basis of psychiatric disorders. After the discussion of the tools for interpreting and communicating genetic information in Part 1, the five chapters in Part 2 provide substantive information about the genetics of mental illnesses, including clinical and epidemiological features, genetic epidemiology, molecular genetics, and implications for genetic counseling. In Chapters 4 through 7, the authors summarize aspects of major psychiatric disorders from childhood-onset disorders through dementia. Next, in Chapter 8, Finn provides a concise overview of neuropsychiatric manifestations of classic genetic disorders. Although many of these disorders are substantially less common than are primary psychiatric disorders, an awareness of their neuropsychiatric presentations can sometimes be crucial for differential diagnosis, risk estimation, and appropriate referral.

In Chapter 9 (Part 3), Koukopoulos and colleagues address a different aspect of reproductive risk about which patients and families often seek information and counseling: the course and treatment of psychiatric illness during pregnancy. The risk-benefit considerations related to medication use during pregnancy are complex and often misunderstood.

Finally, it is essential that researchers and clinicians interested in psychiatric genetics consider the ethical, legal, and social implications of genetic research and genetic counseling. This awareness is particularly important in the realm of psychiatric and behavioral genetics, whose early history included misguided and unethical practices based on pseudoscientific ideas. In Chapter 10, Hoge and Appelbaum review the cautionary tales that have emerged from this history and discuss the modern-day dilemmas that clinicians, families, and society may face as advances in genetic research move forward. In Chapter 11, the concluding chapter, Smoller and Korf discuss scientific progress in psychiatric genetics and the implications for clinical practice that may emerge in the coming years, including the prospects for genetic testing and personalized medicine.

To our knowledge, this book is the first of its kind: a volume devoted to psychiatric genetics that is written to be a resource primarily for clinicians who may or may not have extensive experience with genetic research or genetic medicine. We hope that the resulting volume is accessible, useful, and informative.

Jordan W. Smoller, M.D., Sc.D.

Beth Rosen Sheidley, M.S., C.G.C.

Ming T. Tsuang, M.D., Ph.D., D.Sc.

Reference

Finn CT, Wilcox MA, Korf BR, et al: Psychiatric genetics: a survey of psychiatrists' knowledge, opinions, and practice patterns. J Clin Psychiatry 66:821–830, 2005

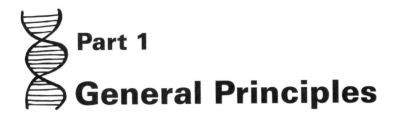

Part 1

General Principles

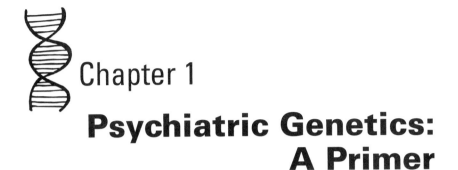

Chapter 1

Psychiatric Genetics: A Primer

Stephen J. Glatt, Ph.D.
Stephen V. Faraone, Ph.D.
Ming T. Tsuang, M.D., Ph.D., D.Sc.

Our goal in this text is to provide a practical resource that will help mental health clinicians 1) interpret the exponentially growing amount of information about genetics; 2) respond to patients' requests for genetic counseling, risk prediction, and counseling about reproductive and pregnancy-related issues; and 3) enhance their sophistication about the nature and implications of genetics for their practice. This first chapter serves to orient clinicians to the field of psychiatric genetics and the types of clinically relevant information yielded by psychiatric genetic research. The chapter begins with a brief overview of the theoretical underpinnings of the field. In the subsequent section, we provide a detailed description of the most popular methods employed in the field, including the interpretation of data obtained with each method. The chapter concludes with summary guidelines and caveats for reading and interpreting the scientific literature in psychiatric genetics and for generalizing the results of research studies to clinical practice.

Overview

Psychiatric genetics is an area of research in which human behavior and mental phenomena are studied in relation to inherited factors, or **genes**.[1] However, the term *psychiatric genetics* is actually shorthand for *psychiatric genetic* *epidemiology,* which more accurately reflects the discipline's alignment with the larger field of genetic epidemiology. **Genetic epidemiology** has been defined as "a science that deals with etiology, distribution, and control of disease in groups of relatives and with inherited causes of disease in populations" (Morton 1982). Genetic epidemiologists examine the distribution of illness within families with the goal of finding genetic *and* environmental causes of illness. Thus, in psychiatric genetic epidemiology, or psychiatric genetics, both environmental factors and genetic factors—and their interactions—are considered to be on an equal footing and to have an equal likelihood of influencing a given behavior, until subsequent research shows otherwise. These assumptions are then tested empirically, and the relative environmental and genetic contributions to a behavior can be determined.

It is crucial to recognize the importance that researchers in psychiatric genetics place on examining both genetic and environmental factors. Genetic epidemiologists have sometimes been accused (incorrectly) of ignoring the role of the environment in influencing human behavior. Of course, much of the literature in psychiatric genetics focuses exclusively on genetics. For instance, studies are conducted to demonstrate familiality, estimate **heritability**, and find genes for a particular trait. However, in many of these studies, a role for the environment is implicit, even if not mentioned directly. Thus, although a primary goal in psychiatric genetics is to clarify how genes influence psychiatric illness, most researchers agree that the pathway from **genotype** to **phenotype** cannot be understood without reference to environmental agents that trigger illness in susceptible individuals. Indeed, even the most heritable psychiatric disorders, such as schizophrenia and bipolar disorder, for which up to 85% of the liability is inherited, have considerable environmental components to their etiology.

Psychiatric genetic research on a particular disorder (or any relevant phenotype, including subthreshold psychopathology and biological traits) tends to follow a series of questions in a logical progression (Table 1–1). This sequence, which we have referred to as "the chain of psychiatric genetic research" (Faraone et al. 1999), proceeds as follows: First, we ask, Is the phenotype familial? or, in other words, Does it run in families? Second, What are the relative contributions of the genes and environment to the phenotype? Third, If genes mediate this transmission, where are they located? Fourth, What are the specific genes that influence risk for the phenotype? These questions are difficult to answer for any trait but are particularly so for phenotypes as complex as human behavior and psychiatric disorders. For-

---

[1]Terms in boldface type are defined in the glossary at the end of this book.

tunately, a wide variety of methods is available to help psychiatric genetic researchers resolve these issues. The list in Table 1–1 represents a sampling of some of the most popular and powerful methods available for answering the fundamental questions in the chain of psychiatric genetic research. We describe these methods in more detail in the next section.

Methods in Psychiatric Genetics

Psychiatric genetics is a multidisciplinary field with roots in human genetics, psychiatry, statistics, and epidemiology that date back about 100 years. The earliest work in the field involved clinical and behavioral genetic methods, such as family, twin, and adoption studies, which are effective for establishing whether and to what degree genetic factors influence a trait (Questions 1 and 2 in Table 1–1). Subsequently, the field branched out to include molecular genetic methods that could enable the isolation of regions on **chromosomes** and identification of specific genes mediating familial transmission of a trait through **linkage** and **association** analyses (Questions 3 and 4).

Thus, many of the tools for completing the chain of psychiatric genetic research are already available and have been for some time, while others have only recently reached maturity. It is clear, however, that even as molecular and computational technologies improve, clinical and behavioral genetic methods still have a very important role to play. For example, familial transmission has yet to be determined for many of the rarer, less severe, or otherwise understudied psychiatric disorders, such as some personality disorders. As a consequence, risk estimates are not available for family members of individuals affected with these disorders. Conversely, some heavily studied disorders, such as schizophrenia and bipolar disorder, have been the subject of sufficient numbers of family, twin, and adoption studies to justify subsequent molecular genetic analyses. This overview, therefore, necessarily presents a "moving target" of available methods in psychiatric genetics, and we acknowledge that some methods may no longer be commonly employed for certain disorders, others may not be ready for application to a given disorder pending completion of prior steps in the chain, and still others that are currently in development may ultimately supplant some of those described here.

Question 1: Is the Phenotype Familial?

The first question that must be asked and answered when attempting to delineate the genetic and environmental components of a disorder is, Does the phenotype run in families? or Is this phenotype familial?

TABLE 1–1.   The chain of psychiatric genetic research

Questions	Appropriate methods
1) Is the phenotype familial?	Family study
2) What are the relative contributions of genes and environment?	Twin study, adoption study
3) Where are the genes located?	Linkage analysis
4) What are the responsible genes?	Association analysis

Appropriate Method

This question can be answered through the use of a family study. The basic design of the family study begins with the ascertainment of a group of subjects who are affected with the disorder of interest (cases) and a comparable group of control subjects who do not have the disorder. Next, the biological relatives of these index subjects, or **probands,** are ascertained and evaluated for the presence of the disorder. The rate of the disorder among family members of affected probands is then compared with the rate of the disorder among family members of control probands to determine the familial risk or relative risk.

Rationale.   If a disorder has a genetic etiology, then biological relatives of case subjects should have a higher likelihood, compared with relatives of control subjects, of carrying the gene or genes that influenced illness in their relative, and thus they should be at greater risk for the illness themselves. In addition, the risk to relatives of cases should be correlated with their degree of relationship to the proband, or the proportion of genes they share in common. First-degree relatives such as parents, siblings, and children, share 50% of their genes, on average, with the proband. Thus, first-degree relatives of case subjects should be at greater risk for the disorder than second-degree relatives (grandparents, uncles, aunts, nephews, nieces, and half-siblings), because second-degree relatives share only 25% of their genes with the proband.

Possible outcomes and interpretation.   If the results of the family study indicate that the phenotype is not familial, then there is little reason or need to research the issue further with genetic methods, as absence of familiality argues strongly against a genetic component in the etiology of a disorder. If the phenotype is found to be familial, then there is some basis to suspect that it may also be heritable and, thus, that a gene or genes underlie this transmission. However, it is critical to understand (and convey to clients) that familiality does not establish heritability. For example, religion and language are familial traits, as often all members of the same family practice the same religion and speak the same language. These facts are due not to the transmission of "religion genes" or "language genes" through the family, but rather to the common environment and upbringing that those family members share.

Design considerations and limitations.   Several design features of a family study can influence the strength of the inferences that can be drawn regarding the degree of familiality of the disorder. (Many of these principles also apply to the other methods discussed in this chapter.) Ideally, a family study should use the blind case-control paradigm, wherein the individual assessing subjects for the presence or absence of the disorder has no information regarding the relationships between subjects. If this feature is not adopted, rater bias may be introduced, and risk estimates can be artificially deflated or, more likely, inflated by the rater's unconscious judgments of greater similarity among relatives.

The environment from which probands are selected for study can also influence the generalizability of results from family studies. For example, in order to increase the chances of ascertaining an adequate number of "true" cases, case probands are often selected from a source that is "enriched" with the diagnosis of interest (e.g., a clinic), because individuals who seek treatment and are given a clinical diagnosis are more likely to have experienced the level of distress and disability that the diagnostic nosology requires for psychiatric illness. The limitation of this strategy is that the ascertained sample may not be representative of affected patients in the larger population who do not attend that clinic.

The selection of control subjects should satisfy the comparability principles required for meaningful inferences in case-control epidemiological studies (Repsilber et al. 2005; Wacholder et al. 1992a, 1992b, 1992c). As with cases, multistage screening of control subjects decreases the probability of misclassifying as a control subject someone who has the disorder. Of course, since screened control subjects are selected for absence of the disorder of interest, they cannot be considered representative of the general population. An additional degree of comparability can be introduced if each case can be matched to a control subject on relevant variables. One problem here is defining what is and is not a "relevant" variable. Age, sex, and socioeconomic status are usually considered, but other variables may also be appropriate. However, matching should be used cautiously, to avoid the "matching fallacy" (Meehl 1970) and "overmatching" (Greenland and Morgenstern 1990). As discussed by Meehl (1970), matching based on specific variables often results in mismatches on other variables. In addition to creating unusual samples, this strategy may also lead to reduced statistical efficiency and biased estimates (Wacholder et al. 1992a). These problems are most severe when the matching variable is strongly associated with the disorder under study. These classic principles are still relevant, as even the latest genetic epidemiological tools, such as gene expression microarrays (Repsilber et al. 2005), rely on the comparability of cases and control subjects for derivation of valid inferences.

The presence and severity of these various biases must be considered when evaluating the results of family studies. They must also be considered when attempting to generalize the findings of family studies to the clinical setting, where familial risk estimates may influence decisions made by clients who seek genetic counsel.

Question 2: What Are the Relative Contributions of Genes and Environment?

Once a psychiatric disorder has been established to run in families, it becomes necessary to determine if that pattern is attributable to the inheritance of genes or to shared familial and other environmental factors. If a genetic contribution to the disorder is detected, it is also important to quantify that contribution relative to that made by environmental factors, because these findings may encourage or discourage future molecular genetic studies and also influence the decisions made by individuals seeking genetic counseling. These questions can be answered both by twin studies and by adoption studies. Both designs have several variations, each of which is useful for revealing a slightly different aspect of the nature and magnitude of genetic and environmental effects on the liability toward a given disorder. First, we consider the appropriate twin-study designs. Appropriate adoption-study designs are described in the next section.

Appropriate Method 1

In the twin study designs, identical (monozygotic [MZ]) and fraternal (dizygotic [DZ]) twin-pairs are ascertained if at least one member of the pair is affected with the disorder of interest. Twin-pairs are deemed **concordant** if both members of the pair have the disorder and are deemed **discordant** if only one member of the pair is affected. The ratio of concordant to discordant MZ twin-pairs is then compared with the ratio of concordant to discordant DZ twin-pairs.

Rationale.   Monozygotic twins are derived from the same zygote and thus share 100% of their genetic material. In contrast, DZ twins result from separate fertilizations and thus share, on average, 50% of their genes—no more or less than any other pair of siblings. Thus, a typical MZ twin-pair will have 50% more genes in common than a typical DZ twin-pair. The degree of similarity in environmental exposures between members of a MZ twin-pair should be no different than that between members of a DZ twin-pair, however. Thus, any difference in concordance for a disorder between the two types of twin-pairs can be attributed to the effects of the additional gene-sharing in the MZ twins. In other words, sharing 50% more genes in common can be attributed to be the sole factor responsible for any increased phenotypic similarity among MZ twin-pairs relative to DZ twin-pairs.

Possible outcomes and interpretation.   Concordance rates among twin-pairs can be calculated pairwise or probandwise, depending on the method of sampling employed. The *pairwise concordance rate* is defined as the proportion of twin-pairs in which both twins are affected with the disorder. We use this method of computing concordance when the probability of sampling any specific affected individual is so low that two affected co-twins are never independently sampled as probands. However, when the sampling probability is higher, the *probandwise concordance rate* is the method of choice. Probandwise concordance is the proportion of proband twins who have an affected co-twin.

Both types of concordance rates can be interpreted similarly, as long as the same method for determining concordance is used for both MZ and DZ twin-pairs in a sample. If the concordance for a disorder is higher among MZ twin-pairs than among DZ twin-pairs, the likelihood is high that there is a genetic contribution to that disorder; if MZ and DZ twin-pairs have approximately equal concordance rates, environmental factors are more strongly implicated.

Frequently, concordance rates among twin-pairs are used to estimate the heritability of a disorder. **Heritability** is a measure of the degree to which genetic factors influence variability in the manifestation of the phenotype. Phenotypic variability (V_p) is presumed to arise from two independent factors: genetic variability (V_g) and environmental variability (V_e). Heritability in the broad sense (h^2) is the ratio of genetic to phenotypic variances (i.e., $h^2 = V_g/V_p$), or the proportion of variance in the phenotype that is accounted for by variability in genetic factors. A heritability of 1.0 indicates that all variability in the phenotype is due to genetic factors alone. In contrast, a heritability of zero attributes all phenotypic variation to environmental factors.

Design considerations and limitations.   A major assumption, often cited as a challenge to the results of twin studies, is the so-called equal-environments assumption. A basic tenet underlying the partitioning of genetic and environmental variance is the assumption that MZ twin-pairs reared together have the same degree of exposure to similar environmental factors that reared-to-gether DZ twin-pairs have. However, common knowledge suggests that this is not a safe assumption, since many more MZ twin-pairs than DZ twin-pairs are treated identically and exposed to the same events. For example, MZ twin-pairs are far more likely to be dressed alike and engaged in the same activities than are DZ twin-pairs. Serious violation of the equal-environments assumption could result in increased phenotypic similarity among MZ twin-pairs relative to DZ twin-pairs that is due to environmental—not genetic—similarities between MZ twin-pairs. Thus, a portion of the variance in a phenotype that should be attributed to environmental factors is inadvertently ascribed to genetic factors, and heritability estimates are artificially inflated.

The equal-environments assumption can be entirely circumvented by introducing a twist in the basic design of the twin study. In one modification, only MZ twin-pairs who were reared separately (i.e., in different homes by different families) are included in the study. Because MZ twin-pairs reared apart do not share a common environment, any phenotypic similarity must be due to genetic factors. However, MZ twins with psychiatric illness are rare, and cases of such twins reared apart are even rarer; thus, this design cannot be routinely used. In another twist on the classic twin-study design, the children of discordant MZ twin-pairs are ascertained and included in a study. If a disorder is caused by a combination of genetic and environmental factors (as most psychiatric disorders are presumed to be), then the unaffected member of a discordant MZ twin-pair should still carry the genetic risk factor but have not been exposed to the relevant environmental factor. In this gene-by-environment interaction model, the children of the unaffected twin should have the same risk for the disorder as the children of the affected twin.

Appropriate Method 2

An alternative to the twin method for parsing the genetic and environmental contributions to a disorder is the adoption study. In an adoption study, ascertainment is targeted at individuals affected with a given disorder who were involved in an adoption, either as an adoptee or as an adoptive parent. Next, the biological and adoptive relatives of these probands are ascertained and evaluated for the presence of the disorder. The rate of the disorder among the biological relatives of probands is then compared with the rate of the disorder among adoptive relatives of the probands.

Rationale.   Children adopted at an early age have a genetic relationship to their biological parents and an environmental relationship to their adopted parents. Thus, adoption studies can be used to determine if biological or adoptive (environmental) relationships account for the familial transmission of disorders. If genes are important, then the familial transmission of illness should occur in the biological family but not in the adoptive family. In contrast, if culture, social learning, or other sources of environmental transmission cause a disorder, familial transmission should occur in the adoptive family but not in the biological family.

Possible outcomes and interpretation. The possible outcomes of an adoption study depend largely on study design, which can vary considerably; however, the primary outcome measure of each design is usually a ratio of the rate of disorder among the biological and adoptive relatives of probands. In the parent-as-proband design, rates of illness are determined in the adopted offspring of parents with and without the disorder. If genetic factors mediate the development of the disorder, then rates of illness should be greater in the adopted-away children of affected parents than in the adopted children of unaffected parents.

In the adoptee-as-proband design, researchers start by ascertaining affected and unaffected adoptees, and they then examine rates of the disorder among the biological and adoptive relatives of each group of probands. If the biological relatives of affected adoptees have higher rates of illness than the adoptive relatives of affected adoptees, then a genetic hypothesis is supported. In contrast, if the adoptive relatives show higher rates of illness, then an environmental hypothesis gains support.

The third design is the cross-fostering design, which compares rates of disorder among two groups of adoptees: 1) probands who were raised by affected adoptive parents but whose biological parents were unaffected and 2) probands who were raised by unaffected adoptive parents but whose biological parents were affected with the disorder. Higher rates of illness in the latter group of adoptees, compared with the former group, would support a genetic contribution to the development of the disorder; the opposite result would support a stronger environmental influence.

Design considerations and limitations. Despite their power to disentangle genetic and environmental factors, adoption studies must be viewed with some caution given the potential methodological problems that cloud their unambiguous interpretation. First, adoptees and their families are not representative of the general population, which may limit the generalizability of results. Furthermore, adoptees are at greater risk for psychiatric disorders, compared with nonadopted children (Hjern et al. 2002; Kotsopoulos et al. 1988; Tieman et al. 2005). The reasons for this difference are not clear. However, because of the increased risk for psychiatric disorders among adoptees, researchers are required to use an adoptee control group. For example, in the adoptee-as-proband design, the relatives of ill adoptees are compared with the relatives of well adoptees.

Another potential problem is the difficulty of finding a sample of adoptees who were separated from their parents at birth. If the child has lived with a parent for even a short period of time prior to adoption, the biological relationship will have been "contaminated" by environmental factors. Some might even argue that the child's contact with the mother immediately after birth or even in utero creates a residue of environmental influence that could affect subsequent psychopathology.

Question 3: Where Are the Genes Located?

Some disorders, including brain diseases such as Huntington's disease and some forms of Parkinson's disease (Jain et al. 2005), are transmitted according to traditional principles of Mendelian genetics. In contrast, most if not all psychiatric disorders are thought to have multifactorial polygenic etiologies in which numerous environmental and genetic factors have some role, while no individual factor is either necessary or sufficient for expression of the illness. Because single-gene variants of psychiatric disorders are considered the exception rather than the rule, most molecular genetic studies are designed so that they are suitable for detecting multiple genes with small effects on risk, none of which may be either necessary or sufficient to elicit illness on its own. Because of their partial effects on the development of illness, we refer to such genes as "risk genes" rather than "disease genes" per se. The two most common methods for locating chromosomal regions that may harbor risk genes for psychiatric disorders have been genetic linkage analysis and cytogenetic techniques.

Appropriate Method

The methods of cytogenetics have been in use in clinical genetics for many decades, and the pursuit of gross chromosomal abnormalities in psychiatric disorders predates the use of genetic linkage analysis using DNA markers. Cytogenetic methods (broadly involving staining and visualization of the chromosomes) are useful for identifying a multitude of irregularities in the physical structure of DNA, including insertions or deletions of DNA into the **genome,** duplications, inversions (where the DNA segment is reversed), and translocations (where parts of two chromosomes swap DNA segments). Some of the major successes of these methods in psychiatry include the mapping of a risk gene for schizophrenia (*DISC1*) to a translocation breakpoint on chromosome 1 (Millar et al. 2000), as well as the isolation of a deletion site on chromosome 22q that produces velocardiofacial syndrome/DiGeorge syndrome, which is characterized by a higher prevalence of psychotic disorders (Williams and Owen 2004).

Linkage analysis is another highly appropriate strategy for identifying regions of chromosomes that have a high likelihood of harboring risk genes for a disorder. Families are ascertained for linkage analysis through a proband affected with the disorder of interest. Pedigrees suitable for linkage analysis may range in size from as small as two family members (if both are affected with the disorder) to potentially any size, including extended pedigrees spanning several generations. Each individual is genotyped at a series of **DNA markers** (not necessarily in genes) spaced evenly throughout the genome, and the co-segregation of these DNA markers with the disorder of interest is tracked in each pedigree (Figure 1–1). Evidence for co-segregation at each marker **locus** is summed across pedigrees to derive an index of the likelihood of the obtained patterns of marker-phenotype co-segregation, given the sampled pedigree structures.

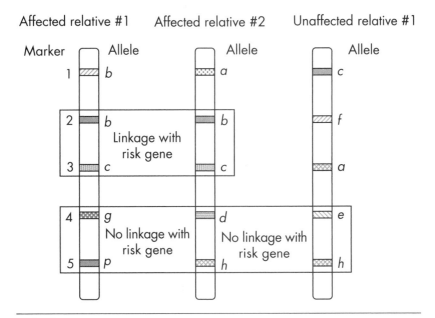

FIGURE 1–1.   Linkage analysis.

In linkage analysis, the co-occurence of a disorder with particular alleles of DNA markers is examined. In this example, two affected relatives from the same family have two alleles in common: one at marker locus 2 and one at marker locus 3. The co-inheritance of these marker alleles with the disease through this family suggests the presence of some unobserved risk-conferrring gene near these loci. In contrast, none of the relatives have any allele in common at marker loci 1 and 4, and at marker locus 5 the unaffected relative has the same allele as affected relative #2. Both of these scenarios argue against the presence of a risk-conferring gene in the proximity of these markers.

Rationale.   Linkage analysis is made possible by the **crossing over** that takes place between two homologous chromosomes during meiosis, the process whereby gametes are created. Genetic transmission occurs because we inherit one member of each pair of chromosomes from our mother and one from our father. However, these inherited chromosomes are not identical to any of the original parental chromosomes. During meiosis, the original chromosomes in a pair cross over each other and exchange portions of their DNA. After multiple crossovers, the resulting two chromosomes each consist of a new and unique combination of genes.

The probability that two genes on the same chromosome will recombine during meiosis is a function of their physical distance from one another. We say that two loci on the same chromosome are *linked* when they are so close to one another that crossing over rarely or never occurs between them. Closely linked genes usually remain together on the same chromosome after meiosis is complete. The greater the distance between loci on the same chromosome, the more likely it is that they will recombine.

The DNA markers used for linkage analysis are not presumed to be actual risk genes for the disorder; rather, they usually consist of DNA **polymorphisms** that lie between genes at approximately evenly spaced intervals, acting more like signposts or "mile markers" along the genome. Thus, when a DNA marker is observed to be linked to a disorder, we can only infer the presence of a nearby (but unobserved) risk gene, based on the co-inheritance of the marker with the phenotype that is influenced by that risk gene. In this design, the disorder serves as a proxy for the risk gene; thus DNA markers that co-segregate commonly with the disorder are presumed to co-segregate commonly with its underlying risk gene. Because the probability of co-segregation of two pieces of DNA is inversely proportional to the distance between them, the regularity of the co-segregation of the DNA marker and the phenotype gives an indirect indication of the genetic distance between the DNA marker and the unobserved risk gene.

Possible outcomes and interpretation.   The possible outcomes of a linkage analysis will vary depending on the structure of families ascertained for analysis. For example, linkage analysis can be performed with affected sibling-pairs, other affected relative-pairs, small nuclear families, or large extended pedigrees. Regardless of which family structure is the principal unit of analysis, the common output across methods is some index of the degree of phenotypic similarity of family members and the degree of genotypic similarity between those individuals at each DNA marker. The indices are summed across families to determine the overall evidence for linkage at a given locus in the full sample. If a given DNA marker co-segregates with the disorder through families more often than would be expected by chance, the marker is linked (i.e., is in relatively close physical proximity) to a risk gene that influences expression of the disorder. This evidence can then be used to direct dense DNA marker placement and more intensive linkage analysis across the linked chromosomal region in order to narrow the candidate region further and, ultimately, identify the responsible genetic variant by association analysis (discussed in the next section, in the context of Question 4).

Design considerations and limitations. Many methods exist for conducting genetic linkage analysis, and the possible outcomes of a linkage analysis will vary depending on the structure of families ascertained for analysis. The common output across methods is an index that is typically is expressed as a logarithm of the odds (or **lod score**) of obtaining the observed pattern of genetic and phenotypic marker similarity, given a certain pedigree structure. The results are summed across families in the sample to determine the overall evidence for linkage at a given locus, and generally accepted criteria exist for evaluating whether this evidence may be taken as "suggestive" or "significant" for linkage (Lander and Kruglyak 1995). It is important to recognize that linkage analysis merely identifies a chromosomal region likely to contain a risk gene. Typically, linked regions may contain many genes (sometimes hundreds) so the task of identifying the specific susceptibility locus underlying a linked locus requires other methods, including association analysis, discussed in the next section.

Question 4: What Are the Responsible Genes?

Once regions of certain chromosomes have been implicated from linkage analysis or cytogenetic studies as harboring a risk gene for a disorder, the next step is to identify the specific gene that is segregating through families to give rise to that linkage signal. Genes within a linked region are candidates for involvement in the phenotype based on their chromosomal location or position (i.e., they are "positional candidate genes"). Within a linked region or even in the absence of linkage evidence, a gene may also be a candidate if a compelling reason exists to suspect that the gene influences risk for a given disorder (i.e., is a "functional candidate gene").

Appropriate Method

In contrast to linkage analysis, which uses random DNA markers as proxies for nearby risk genes, genetic association analysis is the appropriate method for determining if a particular gene variant has a direct effect on risk for a particular disorder or is very tightly linked to such a gene. Association of candidate genes can be evaluated in an independent sample of cases with the disorder and matched control subjects (i.e., in a case-control study) or in small family units, where the transmission of variant and normal forms of the gene from parents to offspring can be monitored (i.e., in a family-based study).

Rationale. If a gene influences risk for a disorder, the association should be detectable as an increased frequency of the risk **allele** of the gene (or a tightly linked marker allele in a nearby gene) in case subjects relative to control subjects. Within the context of the family, the association would be detectable as an increased likelihood that an affected individual received the risk allele of the gene from his parent, when both the risk and normal forms of the gene were present in the parent and could have been transmitted with equal frequency and likelihood.

Possible outcomes and interpretation. In a case-control association study, we simply count the number of each type of allele of a gene that is found in case subjects and compare these counts with the allele distribution seen in the control group (Figure 1–2). This process can also be performed for genotypes. A simple statistical test (e.g., chi-square test) is then used to determine if the distribution of alleles observed in the group of cases is different from that seen in the control group. A difference in distribution of alleles is evidence for a genetic association with the disorder, where the allele that is overrepresented in the group of cases is considered the risk allele.

The degree of overrepresentation of the risk allele in case subjects relative to control subjects can be used to derive an **odds ratio**, which gives a numerical indication of the probability that an affected individual possesses the allele, in comparison to the probability that an unaffected individual possesses the allele. Association studies of this type can be performed for alleles or genotypes. In addition, a disorder can be tested for association with a **haplotype**, which is a pattern of alleles across several **syntenic** markers, or markers on the same chromosome. (For a description of the International HapMap Project, which is dedicated to cataloging the haplotype structure of the entire human genome, see International HapMap Consortium 2003.) If **linkage disequilibrium**, or unusually tight linkage, occurs between the markers in a haplotype, the markers will typically be inherited together, as no recombination will occur between them. This concept is particularly useful for family-based association studies. In family-based studies, we can use analogous statistics to determine if a difference from the expected equal inheritance of risk and normal alleles of a gene (or haplotypes within or across several genes) is detected in affected probands who could have received either allele from a parent (Figure 1–3). In a family-based study, the odds ratio estimates the **haplotype relative risk**, which

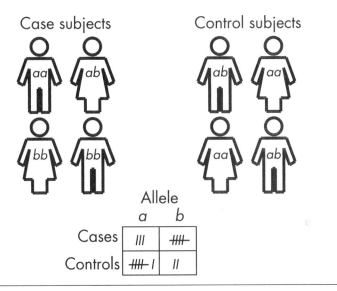

FIGURE 1–2. Case–control association study.

In a case-control association study, the numbers of each type of allele of a gene that is found in case subjects are counted, and those counts are compared with the allele distribution seen in the control group. A simple statistical test is then used to determine if the distribution of alleles observed in the group of case subjects is different from that seen in the control group. A difference in the distribution is considered evidence for a genetic association with the disorder, where the allele that is overrepresented in the group of cases (in this case, the *b* allele) is considered the risk allele.

represents the increase in the probability that the affected offspring received the risk allele (which is presumed to be on the same haplotype as the marker allele) rather than the normal allele.

If the odds ratio, relative risk, or other effect size attributed to a polymorphism is large enough to attain statistical significance, there are four possible explanations: 1) there is a true association with a causative risk allele, 2) the associated polymorphism is in **linkage disequilibrium** (i.e., is in close proximity and usually co-inherited) with the causal variant, 3) there is a confounding factor that introduces a systematic bias (e.g., **population stratification**, or background genetic differences between the case and control groups), or 4) the result is due to chance or random error.

Design considerations and limitations.   A major disadvantage of association studies is that the DNA marker must either be in the disease gene itself or at least be very tightly linked to it. This characteristic is in contrast with the linkage method, in which linkage can be detected over relatively large

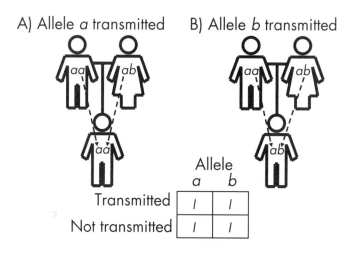

FIGURE 1–3.   Family-based studies.

Family-based studies follow the inheritance of particular alleles through families
that are affected with a particular disorder. (**A**) We know that the father has donated allele *a* to his affected son, because the father only has alleles of type *a* to donate.
The mother, however, can donate either allele *a* or allele *b* and, in this instance, has
donated allele *a*. Thus, allele *a* was transmitted, whereas allele *b* could have been
transmitted but was not. (**B**) In another parent-child trio, the father again donates
allele *a* to the child, but the child receives allele *b* from his mother. Thus, allele *b* was
transmitted, and allele *a* was not. If neither allele *a* nor allele *b* increases risk for the
disorder, then an equal number of alleles *a* and *b* would be inherited by affected
offspring from the parent that had two different alleles to give. A simple statistical
test is used to determine if any difference from the expected equal inheritance of
these alleles is found in the sample of multiple parent-child trios.

distances. Thus, with linkage analysis, it is possible to "scan the genome,"
which is a shorthand way of saying that if we use many markers, we can test
for linkage to all chromosomal loci. In contrast, for a traditional candidate
gene association study to succeed, we must know where to look for the
gene, based either on positional grounds arising from a linkage signal or on
functional grounds arising from the known or presumed pathology of the
disorder.

Neither basis for selecting a candidate gene is without limitations. For a
gene to become a positional candidate gene, it must map to a chromosomal
region that has been observed to show linkage to the disorder. However,
genes with a small but reliable effect on risk may not necessarily generate
a notable linkage signal and thus may never come under study. On the
other hand, selecting genes for association analysis based on their potential

involvement in the disease process is risky as well. Because our understanding of the biological basis of most psychiatric disorders is far from comprehensive, the pursuit of candidate genes typically progresses incrementally through genes that are expressed within systems widely implicated in the disorder. This process clearly is not optimal, as the probability of selecting the right candidate gene (from approximately 25,000 human genes) and the right polymorphism (from more than 10,000,000 in the human genome) for analysis is remote. This approach is essential for clarifying the nature of dysfunction within recognized candidate pathways; however, it is far from optimal for identifying additional novel risk genes outside of these systems. The recent advancement of laboratory and statistical methods for genomewide association analysis should allow for a more unbiased examination of association patterns throughout the genome and may help resolve this dilemma in coming years (Thomas et al. 2005).

Another limitation of association studies is that they are notoriously difficult to replicate, perhaps owing to their propensity toward false-positive results (Ioannidis et al. 2001). The problem of false-positive results is exacerbated by the fact that close linkage is not the only cause of disease-marker associations. For example, the frequencies of DNA marker alleles may vary among ethnic groups, cohorts of different ages, or other isolated segments of a population. Thus, if case and control groups are not drawn from the same populations and carefully matched on all potentially relevant factors, spurious differences in allele frequencies between groups will emerge because of the population admixture alone (Freedman et al. 2004).

Family-based association methods help to overcome some of the problems posed by ethnicity and population admixture. In these methods, the parents or siblings of patients are included as control subjects. Because each parent transmits only one allele to a child, the allele that is not transmitted to the child is used as the control allele. The statistical test involves comparisons of the transmitted versus the nontransmitted allele. Because both alleles come from the same parent, there are no differences in ethnicity between the case and control alleles.

Guidelines and Caveats

We conclude this brief overview of psychiatric genetics with a summary of guidelines and caveats regarding the translation of psychiatric genetic research into clinically relevant applications.

Family Studies

By demonstrating that a disorder "runs in the family," family studies can provide the initial impetus for seeking specific genetic factors underlying transmission of that disorder. The results of a well-controlled family study can provide important risk estimates to family members of affected individuals. Familial risk estimates are available for many psychiatric disorders (see Table 1–2). Although these estimates can be informative for individuals in evaluating their own risk, the use of these estimates to influence reproductive decisions is not straightforward and must be done with due caution. In either case, it is imperative that clients in genetic counseling settings are informed about the difference between familial and genetic transmission.

The results of family studies can show that a disorder aggregates in families, but they cannot establish that such aggregation is a direct action of genes segregating through those families. Thus, the increased risk posed to these individuals should not necessarily be "blamed" on "faulty genes"; rather, clients should be assisted in understanding that genes as well as other shared familial experiences can influence the familial resemblance for the disorder.

Generalizing the results of family studies to clinical settings is further complicated by the heterogeneity of most psychiatric disorders. Although familial risk estimates are derived from carefully controlled research studies that ascertained particular types of patients and families, a much wider variety of affected individuals and families exists in the real world. Thus, the results of a particular family study or series of family studies may not be directly applicable to all at-risk individuals.

From a clinical perspective, the lack (or low level) of familiality of a psychiatric disorder would also be important information to convey in a genetic counseling setting. For example, an individual who has a relative affected with a nonfamilial psychiatric disorder could be reassured that his or her risk for developing the same illness is no greater than the average risk in the population. Real-world examples of such a scenario are scarce, as most, if not all, psychiatric disorders studied to date have shown evidence for some degree of familiality.

Twin and Adoption Studies

Twin and adoption studies (especially the much more common twin studies) are the premier methods for determining if the familial transmission of a psychiatric disorder is due to genetic or common environmental factors. To date, all DSM-IV-TR (American Psychiatric Association 2000) psychiatric disorders that have been the subject of a twin study have been shown to have some degree of heritability (Table 1–2). (The lone exception is dysthymia, which was found to be influenced solely by environmental factors.) Estimates of heritability derived from concordance rates in twin studies define the upper limit of the percentage of the variance in liability toward a disorder that is attributable to genes; however, heritability is an aggregate measure of genetic influences that does not tell us how many genes may be involved, how strong the effects of individual genes are, or how important genes are in a given family. For example, the heritability of major depressive disorder has been estimated to be between 29% and 42% (Kendler et al. 2006), but the illness seems to be transmitted in some families in a manner that suggests a much stronger genetic influence conveyed by a single major locus (Maher et al. 2002).

Relative risk estimates derived from a family study can illustrate what an individual's risk for a disorder is, given the degree of the biological relationship to an affected individual. In conjunction with relative risk estimates, heritability estimates can sometimes be usefully presented in genetic counseling sessions to illustrate the percentage of increased risk that is due to genetic or environmental factors. Yet, because a heritability estimate does not indicate how much of an individual's illness is genetic, this information can also be misleading in genetic counseling

Other important caveats about interpreting heritability must also be noted. In this chapter, we have tried to define the types of information that can and cannot be inferred by a heritability estimate. Thus, a heritability of 80% would suggest that 80% of the variability in whether an individual becomes affected with the illness is inherited and that 20% is not inherited. A heritability of 80% does not mean that genes account for 80% of the factors that caused a given individual to develop an illness. As with the results of family studies, the results of twin studies are subject to limitations on their interpretability that stem from their design and sampled populations. Thus, the genetic heterogeneity of an illness cannot be conveyed by a single heritability estimate derived from one sample of twins. For example, while most forms of bipolar disorder are considered to be multifactorial in origin (i.e., the result of both genetic and environmental factors), some pedigrees have been identified in which the disorder seems to segregate in a dominant fashion as the result of a single major gene effect (Craddock et al. 1994). In such families, the heritability and familial risk of the illness would be expected to be much higher than in "typical" families, who are affected by the illness in a less straightforward and reliable manner.

Genetic Linkage and Association Analyses

In psychiatric genetics, linkage signals are seen not as diagnostic indices but as intermediaries between the phenotype of interest and the polymorphisms that are actually responsible for increasing risk for the disorder. Thus, linkage analysis has little or no real utility in clinical genetic counseling environments. On the other hand, mutation screening of polymorphisms that were initially identified by association analysis is becoming a popular

TABLE 1–2. Results of family and twin studies of psychiatric disorders

Psychiatric disorder	RR (λ_s)	Heritability (h^2)
Autism	22	93
Tourette's syndrome	12	90
Schizoaffective disorder	11	85
Bipolar disorder	8	84
Schizophrenia	12	84
Narcissistic personality disorder	–	79
OCPD	–	78
Cannabis abuse	6	76
ADHD	4	75
Conduct disorder	–	74
Anorexia nervosa	11	71
Stuttering	5	70
Antisocial personality disorder	–	69
Borderline personality disorder	–	69
Obsessive-compulsive disorder	4	68
Histrionic personality disorder	–	67
Stimulant abuse	–	66
Hallucinogen abuse	–	65
Gender identity disorder	–	62
Oppositional defiant disorder	–	61
Nicotine dependence	–	60
Sleepwalking	–	60
Sedative abuse	–	59
Alzheimer's disease	2	58
Dependent personality disorder	–	57
Bulimia nervosa	4	55
Dyslexia	–	53
Dissociative identity disorder	–	48
Pathological gambling	4	46

TABLE 1–2. Results of family and twin studies of psychiatric disorders *(continued)*

Psychiatric disorder	RR (λ_s)	Heritability (h^2)	
Panic disorder	5	43	
Suicide	10	43	
Nightmare disorder	–	41	
Agoraphobia	4	38	
Opiate abuse	10	38	
Postpartum psychosis	11	38	
PTSD	–	38	
Major depression	4	37	
Narcolepsy	–	37	
Alcohol abuse	2	36	
Cocaine abuse	4	32	
Generalized anxiety disorder	6	32	
Insomnia	–	32	
Schizoid personality disorder	4	29	
Seasonal affective disorder	–	29	
Simple phobia	4	29	
Avoidant personality disorder	4	28	
Paranoid personality disorder	4	28	
Schizotypal personality disorder	5	28	
Social phobia	4	25	
Enuresis	–	24	
Dysthymia	–	0	

Note. ADHD=attention-deficit/hyperactivity disorder; OCPD=obsessive-compulsive personality disorder; PTSD=posttraumatic stress disorder; RR = relative risk.

diagnostic and predictive tool in clinical settings and genetic counseling situations, as more genes are found to either cause or influence risk for a disorder (http://www.genetests.org). For example, commercial testing is available for *BRCA1* and *BRCA2* mutations that increase risk for breast and ovarian cancer and for *APC* mutations that elevate risk for colon cancer. These tests are available only for rare forms of these disorders that are known to be caused by mutations in a single gene. However, the majority of cases of breast, colon, and other cancers, as well as of psychiatric disorders, have multifactorial etiologies in which numerous genetic and environmental contributors each make a small contribution to risk and no single gene is either necessary or sufficient to produce illness on its own. As such, information about these risk genes is much less useful in clinical settings, because it includes only the probability of becoming affected, given possession of the gene. Thus, even if an individual possesses the copy of a gene that increases risk for a disorder in the population, he or she is far from destined to develop the illness.

Extreme caution is required when attempting to generalize the results of genetic association studies to clinical and genetic counseling settings, due to the probabilistic nature of risk associated with susceptibility genes in complex disorders. In this context, the uncertainty and fear caused by knowing one's status regarding a sole risk gene may be unwarranted and may outweigh any potential benefits gained by knowing the resultant risk estimate associated with that gene. If, in the future, a panel of risk genes for a disorder becomes available, and these genes can collectively predict risk for a disorder with a high degree of certainty, genetic testing might have sufficient clinical utility to be feasible. The recent emergence of easy-to-use chip-based genotyping platforms may ultimately provide the means for assembling a panel of known risk genes for a disorder on one glass slide, drawing a client's blood in the clinic, and determining a risk profile. Eventually, the risk for a disorder that could be estimated from the presence of specific risk alleles of many risk genes could replace traditional risk estimates derived from family studies. Much work remains to be done before this vision can be realized, especially in psychiatry, where no single risk gene has yet been unequivocally associated with a particular disorder.

Conclusions

Psychiatric genetic researchers have a powerful toolbox of methods at their disposal for determining the genetic and environmental causes of mental illnesses. These methods span a wide spectrum, from clinical and behavioral genetic methods to molecular biological assays, and reflect the present status of psychiatric genetics as a truly multidisciplinary field. In addition, new methods such as transcriptomics (i.e., the analysis of gene transcription rates through mRNA quantification) and proteomics (i.e., the analysis of gene translation rates by protein quantification) are pushing the boundaries of psychiatric genetics. In a strict sense, these new methods are not genetic techniques and thus may fall under the larger rubric of molecular psychiatry, or even biological psychiatry. However, these techniques examine gene products whose expression is influenced by both genetic and environmental factors, and, in this sense, examining such molecules is entirely consistent with the approach of genetic epidemiology, which is to identify both genetic and environmental causes of disease.

Despite this progress, major contributions of psychiatric genetic research to the diagnosis, treatment, prediction, and prevention of psychiatric disorders have yet to be realized. Several limitations of genetic research and its effect on clinical practice must be acknowledged and overcome. Most important, the etiological heterogeneity of psychiatric disorders must be embraced as the rule rather than the exception. Identifying phenotypic factors that differentiate genetic subtypes will allow the future derivation of reasonable and reliable estimates of familial risk and heritability that are based on the particular features of the affected family and its members. It is nevertheless exciting to visualize the potential contributions to clinical psychiatry and genetic counseling, including reduced uncertainty in formulating primary and differential diagnoses; individually tailored pharmacotherapy and disease management; early identification and intervention, leading to better prognosis; and ultimately, effective prevention programs. As technologies improve, experimental capacity increases, and computational methods become more efficient, it is expected that the rate of discovery of risk genes for psychiatric disorders will also accelerate. The identification of specific genetic risk factors for psychiatric disorders will then facilitate the identification and quantification of environmental risk factors that interact with these genes to produce illness. A thorough understanding of these determinants of mental illness will allow the considerable promise of psychiatric genetics to be fulfilled.

References

American Psychiatric Association: Diagnostic and Statistical Manual of Mental Disorders, 4th Edition, Text Revision. Washington, DC, American Psychiatric Association, 2000

Craddock N, Owen M, Burge S, et al: Familial cosegregation of major affective disorder and Darier's disease (keratosis follicularis). Br J Psychiatry 164:355–358, 1994

Faraone SV, Tsuang D, Tsuang MT: Genetics of Mental Disorders: A Guide for Students, Clinicians, and Researchers. New York, Guilford, 1999

Freedman ML, Reich D, Penney KL, et al: Assessing the impact of population stratification on genetic association studies. Nat Genet 36:388–393, 2004

Greenland S, Morgenstern H: Matching and efficiency in cohort studies. Am J Epidemiol 131:151–159, 1990

Hjern A, Lindblad F, Vinnerljung B: Suicide, psychiatric illness, and social maladjustment in intercountry adoptees in Sweden: a cohort study. Lancet 360:443–448, 2002

International HapMap Consortium: The International HapMap Project. Nature 426:789–796, 2003

Ioannidis JP, Ntzani EE, Trikalinos TA, et al: Replication validity of genetic association studies. Nat Genet 29:306–309, 2001

Jain S, Wood NW, Healy DG: Molecular genetic pathways in Parkinson's disease: a review. Clin Sci (London) 109:355–364, 2005

Kendler KS, Gatz M, Gardner CO, et al: A Swedish national twin study of lifetime major depression. Am J Psychiatry 163:109–114, 2006

Kotsopoulos S, Côté A, Joseph L, et al: Psychiatric disorders in adopted children: a controlled study. Am J Orthopsychiatry 58:608–612, 1988

Lander E, Kruglyak L: Genetic dissection of complex traits: guidelines for interpreting and reporting linkage results. Nat Genet 11:241–247, 1995

Maher BS, Marazita ML, Zubenko WN, et al: Genetic segregation analysis of recurrent, early onset major depression: evidence for single major locus transmission. Am J Med Genet (Neuropsychiatr Genet) 114:214–221, 2002

Meehl PE: Nuisance variables and the ex post facto design, in Minnesota Studies in the Philosophy of Science. Edited by Radner M, Winokur S. Minneapolis, University of Minnesota Press, 1970, pp 373–402

Millar JK, Wilson-Annan JC, Anderson S, et al: Disruption of two novel genes by a translocation co-segregating with schizophrenia. Hum Mol Genet 9:1415–1423, 2000

Morton NE: Outline of Genetic Epidemiology. Basel, Switzerland, Karger, 1982

Repsilber D, Fink L, Jacobsen M, et al: Sample selection for microarray gene expression studies. Methods Inf Med 44:461–467, 2005

Thomas DC, Haile RW, Duggan D: Recent developments in genomewide association scans: a workshop summary and review. Am J Hum Genet 77:337–345, 2005

Tieman W, van der Ende J, Verhulst FC: Psychiatric disorders in young adult intercountry adoptees: an epidemiological study. Am J Psychiatry 162:592–598, 2005

Wacholder S, McLaughlin JK, Silverman DT, et al: Selection of controls in case-control studies. I. Principles. Am J Epidemiol 135:1019–1028, 1992a

Wacholder S, Silverman DT, McLaughlin JK, et al: Selection of controls in case-control studies. II. Types of controls. Am J Epidemiol 135:1029–1041, 1992b

Wacholder S, Silverman DT, McLaughlin JK, et al: Selection of controls in case-control studies. III. Design options. Am J Epidemiol 135:1042–1050, 1992c

Williams NM, Owen MJ: Genetic abnormalities of chromosome 22 and the development of psychosis. Curr Psychiatry Rep 6:176–182, 2004

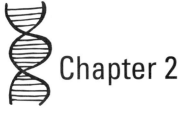

Chapter 2

Principles of Genetic Counseling

Holly L. Peay, M.S., C.G.C.
Beth Rosen Sheidley, M.S., C.G.C.

There is no doubt that psychiatric illness can be devastating to affected individuals and their family members. In addition to dealing with symptoms and treatment plans, many families struggle with guilt and blame regarding causation of the illness, fears of disorder recurrence in at-risk family members, and difficult reproductive choices. Yet, some health care professionals find it difficult to imagine the benefits of genetic counseling for mental illness, given that currently no genetic testing is available. When a client asks about whether there will be another occurrence of a psychiatric illness in the family, the only honest answer is that we simply cannot predict with certainty. Many providers are tempted to end the discussion at that point, but in most cases this conclusion is deeply dissatisfying to both the client and the provider. Even in the absence of highly predictive testing, our knowledge about the etiology of psychiatric disorders allows us to provide additional information, including education about the causes and natural history of psychiatric disorders, risk assessment based on an evaluation of the fam-

We thank Barbara Bowles Biesecker for thoughtful comments. This work was supported in part by the Intramural Research Program of the National Human Genome Research Institute, National Institutes of Health.

ily history and empiric risks, psychological support, and assistance with life planning.

The often-stated goals of research in psychiatric genetics are to use genetic findings to develop more effective treatments and to identify patients who may respond better to specific drug therapies based on their genotype. In addition, such research may lead to presymptomatic genetic testing and a better understanding of environmental risk factors that could be modified to reduce individual risk. As we learn more about specific genetic and environmental risk factors, gather more accurate empiric risks, and begin to use genetic factors to guide diagnosis or treatment, the demand for genetic counseling is likely to increase. The results of several studies (see Table 2-1) have shown that patients with mental illness and their families are interested in genetics services and that consumer interest will increase if genetic testing for psychiatric disorders becomes available. Experience suggests, however, that theoretical interest in genetic testing exceeds actual uptake of testing (Evers-Kiebooms and Decruyenaere 1998).

The great majority of the genes that researchers identify will be genes of small effect that confer an increased risk the magnitude of which will likely be low or uncertain. As we have learned from experience with apolipoprotein E (*APOE*) alleles and risk assessment for Alzheimer's disease, determining whether and how to incorporate genetic susceptibility information into risk assessment and counseling will be challenging (American College of Medical Genetics/American Society of Human Genetics Working Group on ApoE and Alzheimer Disease 1995; Green 2002; Roberts et al. 2005). Specific challenges include understanding test validity and utility, disorder pathophysiology, and client responses to uncertain risk information. As is the case in *APOE* testing, genetic susceptibility testing for psychiatric illness, should it become available, will not allow us to definitively predict the future mental health of any individual. Because of the predictive limitations, genetic counseling for common, complex disorders involves, and will continue to involve, empowering the client by providing understandable information about etiology, a carefully tailored risk assessment, and assistance in managing uncertainty.

Patients and their families will bring questions about inheritance to mental health care providers. Ideally, such providers would possess the core competencies in genetics set forth by the National Coalition for Health Professional Education in Genetics (NCHPEG) (http://www.nchpeg.org/core/corecomps-3rd_ed_aug07.pdf) and would be able to fully participate in the world of "genomic medicine" (Guttmacher et al. 2001; Collins and Guttmacher 2001). At a minimum, providers should be able to appreciate the limitations of their genetics expertise, understand the social and psychological implications of genetics services, and know how and when to make a referral to a genetics professional (NCHPEG core competencies). Our goals in this chapter are to help mental health providers identify patients who may need genetic counseling; to introduce basic concepts related to genetic education, risk assessment, and psychosocial support; and to offer recommendations for when a referral to a genetics professional may be appropriate.

What Is Genetic Counseling?

Many health care providers discuss family history with their patients, consider issues of heredity when developing a treatment plan, and/or order genetic tests (Acheson et al. 2000, 2005). All are elements of the genetic counseling process. Currently, however, most genetic counseling is provided to patients by genetic counselors, medical geneticists, nurse geneticists, and other health care professionals with expertise in genetics. The term *genetic counselor* has in recent years become synonymous with master's-level professionals trained specifically for the purpose of providing genetic counseling. The first class of 10 genetic counseling students graduated from Sarah Lawrence College in 1971. There are now more than 2,000 genetic counselors worldwide, with approximately 150 new graduates in North America each year from a total of 32 master's-level training programs (approximately 70 training program exist worldwide). Traditionally genetic counselors have worked in prenatal or pediatric settings within academic medical centers. Increasingly they are moving into primary care, public health, and specialty areas such as oncology, neurology, infertility, and psychiatry. The definition of genetic counseling, adopted in 2005 by the National Society of Genetic Counselors (http://www.nsgc.org/consumer/definition.cfm), underscores the dynamic nature of the counseling process:

> Genetic counseling is the process of helping people understand and adapt to the medical, psychological, and familial implications of genetic contributions to disease. This process integrates
>
> - Collection and interpretation of family and medical histories to assess the chance of disease occurrence or recurrence
> - Education about inheritance, testing, management, prevention, resources, and research
> - Counseling to promote informed choices and adaptation to the risk or condition.

Common indications for genetic counseling are listed in Table 2–2.

Although the field of genetic counseling is relatively young, it is rapidly expanding and evolving. The intense effort into genetic research for common, complex disorders, including cardiovascular disease, cancer, asthma,

TABLE 2–1. Studies evaluating interest in psychiatric genetics services among affected individuals and family members

Study	Design and population	Selected findings
DeLisi and Bertisch 2006	Survey with 48 members of multiplex schizophrenia families	83% would want genetic testing for gene of small effect; 56% would want prenatal testing; 71% would see a genetic counselor
Jones et al. 2002	Survey of 147 individuals with bipolar disorder	87% agreed/strongly agreed that predictive testing should be available; 78% agreed/strongly agreed that testing for minors should be available; 25% agreed/strongly agreed that prenatal testing with the option of termination should be available
Lyus 2007	Survey of 68 individuals with schizophrenia and 145 relatives	74% of relatives and 72% of affected individuals thought genetic counseling would be useful to them; 94% had not been offered genetic counseling
Meiser et al. 2005	Qualitative interviews with 15 individuals with bipolar disorder from multiplex families and 7 unaffected relatives	Majority were interested in genetic testing with definitive answer or 70% lifetime risk; approximately 50% were interested in presymptomatic genetic testing of adolescents; limited interest in prenatal testing
Milner et al. 1999	Survey of 65 members of the Alliance for the Mentally Ill	Approximately 77% endorsed prenatal testing for bipolar disorder, 8.5% for schizophrenia and autism, 70% for depression, 65% for attention-deficit/hyperactivity disorder, and 55% for panic disorder

TABLE 2–1. Studies evaluating interest in psychiatric genetics services among affected individuals and family members *(continued)*

Study	Design and population	Selected findings
Schulz et al. 1982	Survey of 12 individuals with schizophrenia and 32 of their family members	58% of patients, 75% of parents, and 63% of siblings felt that genetic counseling with empiric risk assessment was helpful; 25% of patients, 58% of parents, and 38% of siblings felt it was necessary
Smith et al. 1996	Survey of 48 members of a bipolar disorder support group (affected individuals, partners, family members, and friends)	83% would seek susceptibility testing for children if there were prophylactic treatment available; 68% would test in the absence of such treatment
Trippitelli et al. 1998	Survey of 45 patients with bipolar disorder and their spouses	85.4% of affected individuals definitely and 14.6% probably would be tested for "gene for bipolar disorder"; 77% of affected individuals indicated that minors should definitely or probably be tested; 46.3% of spouses definitely and 34.1% probably would be tested; 43.9% of affected individuals and spouses would definitely or probably test a fetus

Note. We report data only for affected individuals and family members. Some studies included other research populations as well.

TABLE 2–2. **Common indications for genetic counseling**

Preconception/Prenatal

>   Mother will be 35 years old or older at delivery

>   Abnormal results from a maternal serum screen or fetal ultrasound

>   Personal or family history of a known or suspected genetic disorder, birth defect, or chromosomal abnormality

>   Potential or known exposure to a known or suspected teratogen, including psychotropic medications

>   Mother has a medical condition known or suspected to affect fetal development

>   Recurrent pregnancy losses

>   Consanguinity of parents

>   Ethnic predisposition to certain genetic disorders

>   History of infertility (male or female)

Pediatric

>   Abnormal newborn screening results

>   One or more major malformations in any organ system

>   Abnormalities in growth

>   Mental retardation or developmental delay

>   Autism and autistic-like behaviors

>   Blindness or deafness

>   Presence of a known or suspected genetic disorder or chromosomal abnormality

>   Family history of a known or suspected genetic disorder, birth defect, or chromosomal abnormality

Adolescent/Adult

>   Suspicion of a genetic disorder/syndrome

>   Family history indicating increased risk for common, chronic disease

>>   Cardiovascular disease

>>   Cancer

>>   Metabolic syndrome

>>   Dementia

>>   Psychiatric disorders

>   Risk assessment for pregnancy planning

Source.   Modified from Gene Tests: Medical Genetics Information Resource (online database). Educational Materials: About Genetic Services. Copyright, University of Washington, Seattle. 1993–2007. Available at: http://www.genetests.org. Accessed March 7, 2007. Used with permission.

and psychiatric disorders, is enhancing our understanding of disease etiology, improving our ability to predict familial recurrence, and in some cases leading to genetic susceptibility tests. These advances are fueling professional interest in common disorders and leading to an increased public demand for genetics services; for example, there has been strong public interest in genetic counseling for cancer (Bennett et al. 2003). The successful incorporation of genetics into the care of common, chronic disorders will require nongenetics health care professionals to take a more active role in genetic education and counseling. To that end, a wide array of genetics education materials have been developed (for additional information visit the NCHPEG website [http://www.nchpeg.org]).

Bennett et al. (2003) described the goals of genetic counseling to include reducing the client's anxiety, enhancing the client's sense of control and mastery over life circumstances, increasing the client's understanding of the disease and options for testing and disease management, and providing the individual and family with the tools required to adjust to potential outcomes. Ultimately, genetic counseling seeks to help patients personalize what is often threatening information in order to clarify their values and strengthen their coping mechanisms (Bennett et al. 2003). Given these goals, the potential benefits of psychiatric genetic counseling are evident. Mental health professionals can appreciate the significant anxiety that many affected individuals and their relatives bring to conversations about disease causation and the possibility of recurrence. Skilled genetic counseling, especially when followed by long-term psychological support, can help clients personalize and cope with genetic risk for what often are considered to be highly burdensome disorders with limited aspects of control.

Historically, genetic counseling was rooted in a nondirective ethos that advocated the importance of facilitated decision making instead of advice giving. Genetic counseling for common disorders challenges that paradigm because there often are no immediate decisions to be made, and at times clear prevention and management strategies are warranted. The newer public health–oriented model of genetic counseling focuses on understanding disorder etiology, internalization and management of risk and uncertainty, anticipatory guidance and facilitated life planning, and (in some cases) education about prevention and management. Genetic counseling for psychiatric disorders includes another layer of complexity in that the known environmental risk factors are largely outside of one's control, minimizing clients' ability to significantly reduce the risk of disorder onset. This aspect of psychiatric disorders requires thorough and thoughtful discussion with patients.

We encourage providers to continue the practice of noncoercive counseling in prenatal or preconception situations. For example, if a patient asks whether she should have children, we do not directly answer her question based on our own judgments. Having never "walked in her shoes," we do not have the necessary knowledge to answer. Instead, we help her weigh the pros and cons of having children (who would have an increased chance to later become affected) and assist her in making a decision that is consistent with her desires, values, and beliefs.

In addition to emphasizing the principle of nondirectiveness, the profession of genetic counseling espouses several goals, including voluntary utilization of services, equal access, client education, complete disclosure of information, attention to psychosocial and affective dimensions in counseling, confidentiality, and protection of privacy (Baker et al. 1998). These goals are familiar in any medical setting, but they are made more challenging in the context of genetic counseling because of the complex nature of genetic information. For example, because genetic information generally applies to more than one individual in the family, the familial implications of genetic risk assessment must be considered and clients must be informed about the importance of family disclosure. In addition, the focus on common disorders of adolescent or adult onset raises several areas of concern. First, should genetic susceptibility tests become available for psychiatric disorders, we undoubtedly will have to consider the wisdom of testing minors. Second, our growing ability to predict who is at increased risk for disorders with adolescent or adult onset challenges the distinction between mental illness and mental wellness—for example, how should we interpret mild depressive symptoms in an at-risk adolescent? How should the at-risk individual perceive his or her own mental health? This blurring of the line between sick and well may lead to stigmatization and negative psychological consequences in at-risk individuals. Conversely, however, the ability to predict who is at increased risk may result in reduced anxiety and facilitated life planning for those found to be at lower risk. For those at higher risk, it would allow education and counseling, assisted psychological adjustment and life planning, early treatment, and perhaps risk reduction strategies.

Who Seeks Psychiatric Genetic Counseling?

Patients and/or their family members may seek genetic counseling for a wide variety of reasons. In our experience, most clients who seek genetic counseling are quite concerned about risks for recurrence and consider psychiatric illness to be burdensome. Although some clients make reproductive choices partly based on genetic risk assessment, many plan to or already have children and are concerned about the chances that offspring will develop symptomatic illness. Frequently families look for guidance about what constitutes normal versus abnormal behaviors in children, adolescents, and young adults. These families benefit from discussions about early symptoms, the importance of prompt treatment, and exploration of what constitutes a reasonable level of vigilance.

Although the population of persons who seek genetic counseling is largely self-referred and may not be representative of the general psychiatric population, studies have revealed a high perception of illness burden in spouses and relatives (Chakrabarti et al. 1992; Perlick et al. 1999; Schulz et al. 1982; Smith et al. 1996; Targum et al. 1981). There is mixed support for the idea that affected individuals and family members are making, or would have made, reproductive decisions based on genetic information (Meiser et al. 2005; Targum et al. 1981; Trippitelli et al. 1998). Individuals with extensive family histories of illness or with relatives who have had a severe course of illness may be more motivated to seek counseling (Tsuang 1978), which is appropriate, because those families likely are at the highest genetic risk.

Consider the following scenarios commonly encountered in psychiatric genetic counseling, which may also arise during appointments with primary care and mental health care providers:

- A 28-year-old woman with bipolar disorder asks what the chances are that she'll have a child with a mood disorder and is concerned about the potential teratogenic risk of her medication.
- A 78-year-old man with obsessive-compulsive disorder raises concerns that his granddaughter may be exhibiting obsessions and compulsions.
- The 37-year-old brother of a man with schizophrenia wants to know how likely it is that his young children may become ill.
- A couple who are in the process of adopting a baby have just found out that there is a significant family history of mental illness, and they seek guidance about whether to proceed with the adoption.
- An individual who has experienced a depressive episode and has a family history of bipolar disorder asks what the chances are that he will go on to develop bipolar disorder.

Each instance is unique, and yet ultimately the central questions are the same: Why did the disorder happen? and Will it happen again in the family? In that sense, psychiatric genetic counseling is no different from genetic counseling for any indication. However, it is important to remember that with mental illness, more so than with many other medical conditions, there is the possibility for discrimination and stigmatization based on affected and at-risk status. This possibility may have a significant impact on family relationships, disclosure of information to the counselor, and ultimately the outcome of the counseling session.

Components of a Typical Genetic Counseling Session

The elements of a genetic counseling interaction include assessing family and environmental history to determine disease risk, offering genetic testing if indicated, assisting in diagnosis and disease prevention and management, and offering psychosocial and ethical guidance to help patients make informed, autonomous health care and reproductive decisions (Ciarleglio et al. 2003). When performing psychiatric genetic counseling, we focus on education about etiology, risk assessment and risk communication, psychological support, anticipatory guidance, and facilitation of life planning.

Although caution is warranted when describing any interaction with a client as "typical," we present the following case study to illustrate the components that commonly structure a genetic counseling session. In doing so, we hope to demonstrate the most important concepts and goals of each element of the counseling interaction. Keep in mind that the order in which the components are presented, the relative importance of each component, and the amount and complexity of the information provided vary considerably from client to client. We often begin with education about the etiology of the disease, because we find that clients are more likely to understand risk assessment if they first have an appreciation for the genetics of complex disorders. In addition, many individuals and families have their own "stories" about the cause of a particular illness. By thoughtfully discussing what is known about etiology and helping the client integrate that knowledge into his or her belief about causation, the clinician has an opportunity to dispel erroneous beliefs and address issues of guilt and shame. Doing so early in the genetic counseling process may be enormously helpful.

Case Study

A 28-year-old woman with bipolar disorder, Ms. C, asks you what the chances are that she will have children with a mood disorder. She is engaged, and she and her fiancé have discussed her becoming pregnant in the next few years.

Education About Etiology

Ms. C reports that she attributes much of her illness to an upbringing marred by neglect. She is conflicted about her perception of risk for her children. On the one hand, she expects the risk to any children she might have to be rather low, as she would never put her children in such a negative environment. On the other hand, Ms. C is concerned that she will not be able to provide the "perfect environment" and that, despite her best efforts, she could inadvertently cause a mood disorder in her children. She reports that she also thinks that some people, based on their genes, are more easily harmed by a poor environment, and she wonders if this may be the case in her family.

Complex disorders are indeed complex. Research findings suggest that in the majority of families, psychiatric disorders are caused by multiple susceptibility genes of relatively small effect acting in concert with one or more environmental triggers. (In genetics terms, "environment" is a catch-all phrase meaning anything outside of the genome that can affect the expression of a gene, including in utero environment during development, shared and nonshared family environment, exposures to harmful substances, and medical history.)

How can the provider best convey the complicated information to his or her clients? To help Ms. C understand what is known about the cause of bipolar disorder, the provider should use language that is understandable to her and should define any medical terms. We find it useful to begin by discussing the idea of susceptibility, where risk is caused by several genes of small effect together with environmental risk factors. The provider should explain the suspected environmental risk factors and reiterate the small role that shared environmental factors, including much of the parenting style in the family, seem to play in disorder causation (McGuffin et al. 2003). The provider should anticipate that this discussion may bring up contradictory feelings in the client. Most of the suspected environmental risk factors, as well as which genes are passed down to future generations, are outside of the control of family members; this lack of control may contribute to feelings of helplessness. On the other hand, families may benefit from knowing that even "perfect parenting" is unlikely to prevent the onset of a psychiatric illness; this awareness may reduce feelings of guilt. One of the primary counseling goals is to help clients manage the vulnerability and uncertainty that results from increased genetic risk for psychiatric disorders. In Ms. C's case, the provider should be aware that her endorsement of neglect as a contributing factor may provide her a sense of control over recurrence. The discussion of etiology may make her feel more vulnerable, and this possibility should be explored.

Although educating clients about the etiology of psychiatric disorders may seem difficult, our clinical experience and some research findings suggest that many clients may be primed for such education because they already endorse a multifactorial cause of neuropsychiatric illnesses, including both genetic/biological and lifestyle/environmental causes (Bassett et al. 2004; Gamm et al. 2004; Meiser et al. 2005; Schulz et al. 1982; Targum et al. 1981). By helping clients understand the idea of complex genetics, the provider helps prevent clients' endorsement of genetic determinism, the idea that having a genetic risk equals having the disorder in question.

Family History

> Ms. C initially reports that no one else in her family has bipolar disorder. When asked specific questions, however, she states that her mother and one of her sisters have serious, recurrent depression and that her maternal grandfather was hospitalized several times for violent, suicidal behavior. When asked about her fiancé's family history, Ms. C indicates that it does not include any individuals known to have psychiatric disorders.

Ms. C's case is not unusual in that she initially denied a family history of bipolar disorder, but once the provider probed the history, it became clear that other family members had disorders that may be etiologically related to bipolar disorder. Providers often must be systematic and persistent in order to obtain information that is as accurate and complete as possible. Of course, accuracy of the family history is affected by the evolution of diagnostic criteria, provider variations in applying diagnoses, symptoms that overlap between diagnoses, and the progressive nature of psychiatric illness within an individual. Whenever possible, the provider should obtain medical records and/or evaluate affected individuals in the family. It is important to keep in mind that the stigma related to psychiatric illness might make an individual reluctant or unwilling to share a personal or family history, that the client may not be aware of affected individuals in the family, and that in some cases clients who are affected might have trouble providing family history information because of their symptoms or alienation from their family.

The provider should (at minimum) complete a three-generation pedigree, including the following information:

- Any history of psychiatric symptoms, treatments, or diagnoses of any type, including the history of seemingly well family members
    - For individuals with psychiatric symptoms or diagnoses, age at symptom onset and, if applicable, age at diagnosis should be determined.
    - Special vigilance is needed in asking about disorders known to cluster in families, e.g., major depression and dysthymia in families that include persons with bipolar disorder.
- Information about both sides of the family
    - Given the high rate of assortative mating (i.e., individuals with a personal or family history more frequently having children with others who have a personal or family history) in psychiatric disorders and the high prevalence of these disorders in the general population, it is critical to evaluate both sides of the family.

- Birth defects, unusual illnesses, or learning problems, which could signify an increased possibility of a genetic syndrome
- The age and sex of at-risk consultands, which may play a role in risk assessment.

Risk Assessment and Risk Communication

> The provider and Ms. C discuss the different psychiatric diagnoses and symptoms found in her family. The provider explains that the disorders may be causally related, reviews empiric risks, and discusses the limitations of empiric risks for any individual or family. The risk to any children that Ms. C might have may be greater than the empiric risks because there are several symptomatic people in her family contributing to the risk. The provider and Ms. C discuss the spectrum of disorders for which close family members are at increased risk, including bipolar disorder and major depression. The provider ensures that Ms. C has a reasonably accurate understanding of the information provided and then asks how she perceives the estimated risk for her children. Does the risk sound higher than she expected, about equal to what she expected, or lower than she expected? How is her perception of the risk likely to affect her choice to have children or to affect how vigilant she will feel the need to be during their lives?

Risk assessment for common disorders often is challenging, and in most cases genetic testing is not available to inform risk status. Therefore, risk assessment is based on the family history and environmental history, coupled with empiric risks. By definition empiric risks do not apply to any one individual or family, and the population-based figures should be used with full awareness of their limitations.

In any consideration of psychiatric disorders, several additional issues complicate genetic risk assessment.

- Heterogeneity within diagnostic groups and the frequent occurrence of comorbidity make it more difficult to evaluate whether disorders may be etiologically related in a family. The high prevalence of psychiatric disorders confounds the issue, because some illnesses may be unrelated to other illnesses in the family.
- It may be difficult to evaluate *for what disorder* family members are at risk. Family studies have indicated that on a research population level, no psychiatric diagnosis occurs in a vacuum. That is, if a relative has one psychiatric illness, family members are at empirically increased risk for a range of other disorders as well.
- The typical teenage/young-adult onset of major psychiatric disorders could confound pedigree assessment, because it is possible that individ-

uals who are genetically susceptible and will become symptomatic have not yet experienced onset of illness.

- While research suggests that the vast majority of psychiatric illness is complex in etiology, at this time we cannot rule out any mode of inheritance in any particular family.

It is important to keep in mind that, as with all common disorders, some families are at low risk and some are at high risk. Higher-risk families tend to include several affected individuals (with the same or etiologically related disorders) who may have early onset and/or more severe illness. For example, some research suggests that an earlier age at symptom onset in persons with schizophrenia and related disorders is associated with higher risk to their relatives (Asarnow et al. 2001; Husted et al. 2006; Nicolson et al. 2003). Explanations for high-risk families may include a gene of major effect, an unusual clustering of genes of small effect, or unusually significant environmental risk factors. It often is impossible to determine which factor is most likely in a high-risk family, but the risk to relatives may be considerably higher than the average risk indicated by empiric risks.

A client's perception of risk is influenced by many factors, including the perceived burden of the disorder (Walter and Emery 2005), emotional closeness with the affected relative and experience of the relative's illness (Walter et al. 2004), preconceived notions about the level of risk prior to genetic counseling (Shiloh and Sagi 1989), level of uncertainty in the risk estimates and disease outcome (Lippman-Hand and Fraser 1979), motivation to have children (Lippman-Hand and Fraser 1979; Schulz et al. 1982), and perceived control over illness onset (Walter et al. 2004). The individual providing genetic counseling should explore these issues with clients and help them integrate genetic risk information into their perceptions of risk and burden. Clients frequently internalize risk information by modifying it into qualitative or binary forms (Lippman-Hand and Fraser 1979), and thus providers should be wary of using exact risk recollection as a proxy for the success of genetic counseling.

In many cases clients overestimate the risk for recurrence of psychiatric disorders, and in these instances genetic counseling can be reassuring. Even when clients have a realistic preconceived idea of recurrence risks, genetic counseling can empower clients by validating their concerns about close relatives. Often clients express that the confirmation itself is therapeutic. The provider can help clients anticipate what may happen if they (or their children) began to exhibit symptoms. For example, when counseling families where children or adolescents are at increased risk, the provider can recommend a low threshold of symptoms for seeking psychiatric care and can discuss how early symptoms of the relevant disorder(s) may exhibit.

Clients should leave the session with a basic understanding of the limits of current abilities to predict risk. The provider should convey the limitations of empiric risks and of risk assessment based on family history. Patients should be made aware that empiric risks are drawn from research cohorts and that the risks may or may not accurately reflect the level of risk in their family. Rather, the information gives an estimate of the likely magnitude of risk, *after* taking into account the complete family history. In addition, the individual providing genetic counseling should explore the client's reaction to the uncertain information and provide tools to help manage that uncertainty.

The number of available susceptibility tests for common disorders will increase in the coming years, and those tests may be used to help inform risk assessment. However, in many cases, risk assessment becomes *more* complicated when susceptibility tests are available. For example, in complex disorders, genetic heterogeneity is a key aspect of the difficulty of risk assessment, even with the assistance of susceptibility tests (Liu et al. 2004). The predictive value of genetic tests for Mendelian disorders is much greater than the predictive value of susceptibility tests for common disorders. The family history is likely to remain important in the interpretation of test results for common disorders, because it may help determine the likelihood of expression of the phenotype.

Psychological Support, Anticipatory Guidance, and Facilitation of Life Planning

Ms. C clearly has thought about what it would mean to have a child with a mood disorder, and she welcomes a discussion about how she would react if she had a child who became ill. She is interested to hear about early signs of a mood disorder, many of which she can recognize from her own childhood and early adolescence, and feels empowered by a discussion of early identification of and treatment for mood symptoms. The provider reminds Ms. C that, should she have children who are affected with a mood disorder, more effective treatments are likely to be available by the time they exhibit symptoms. She also is interested to learn that she is at increased risk to experience symptoms during the postpartum period and is pleased to know that the provider will help her anticipate how to maximize her health during that time. She states that she still strongly desires children. She and her fiancé will continue, however, to consider their choice in light of an increased risk for mood disorders in their offspring.

When providing genetic education, it is vital that providers also offer psychological support to help clients and families interpret the information in meaningful ways. Part of this process includes anticipatory guidance: exploring what would it be like if different outcomes came to pass, for example, if one's child were to be affected with bipolar disorder. This approach leads to empowerment of the client and the ability to use the information provided to make life plans, including decisions about whether to have children, the level of vigilance regarding possible psychiatric symptoms in children the client already has, and whether the client feels that he or she has all of the relevant information. Although psychological support, anticipatory guidance, and facilitation of life planning are the least systematically taught elements of genetic counseling, research suggests that these factors are important elements of the benefit that patients derive from the genetic counseling process (Bernhardt et al. 2000; D. Roter, personal communication, February 2006).

Integrating Genetic Counseling Into Clinical Care

All health care providers will be affected by the rapid advances in genetic medicine (Burke 2004). Providers of mental health care are uniquely positioned to recognize and address hereditary issues for their patients, given the ongoing patient contact and long-term provider-patient relationship. We encourage mental health care providers to obtain detailed family history information. This task is best done in person, whether by starting fresh or *building on* (not simply relying on) family history forms that patients complete on their own. There is no substitute for a frank, in-depth, one-on-one discussion about the family history.

For mental health professionals, the goals of the family history are to assess recurrence risk and to determine when consultation and referral may be indicated. In some instances, the focus of counseling may need to shift away from complex inheritance to a more specific etiology and in some instances may include genetic testing. Clues that indicate increased family risk and thus are an indication for consultation with or referral to a genetic counselor include

- A history of birth defects, mental retardation or developmental delay, dementia of early onset, psychiatric symptoms with ataxia, unexplained medical crises, and/or metabolic disease, which are suggestive of a possible Mendelian syndrome or chromosomal etiology
- Occurrence of a psychiatric illness in several family members in multiple generations, which is suggestive of a possible gene of major effect or the clustering of genes of small effect in a family
- Occurrence of psychiatric illness on both sides of an at-risk individual's family, especially in cases where both parents are affected, which can lead to risks of recurrence of more than 50%.

Other common issues leading to referrals from mental health care providers to genetic counselors include

- Teratogen concerns in an affected woman who is pregnant or considering pregnancy
- Autism or autistic features in a child (an underlying genetic cause is identified in 10%–15% of cases)

Ideally, the team providing psychiatric genetic counseling will include a mental health care provider and a genetics professional, both of whom can benefit from the other's expertise. Because the mental health care provider has an established relationship with the patient, he or she might choose to consult with the genetics professional as needed and address the patient's questions directly. In the event of a complicated history suggesting increased genetic risk, the provider should consider referral. (To identify a genetic counselor in a local geographic area, contact the National Society of Genetic Counselors [http://www.nsgc.org].) The identification of a high-risk family, and more significantly a family with a genetic syndrome, may significantly alter the assessment of recurrence risk for family members, have implications for psychiatric and nonpsychiatric medical care, and also may provide the opportunity for presymptomatic or prenatal testing.

Future Issues

It is not difficult to imagine a time in the not-so-distant future when diagnoses and treatment choices will be made with the assistance of genetic information. In fact, pharmacogenetic studies are now being used to aid psychopharmacology. It would be naive to think that patients and their family members will not ask about the familial implications of genetic test results, even if the purpose of the test is to tailor the treatment plan. The increasing sophistication of genetic studies will result in data that allow more accurate risk assessment, which likely will increase the demand for psychiatric genetic counseling. If it is possible to identify individuals at increased risk, especially in high-risk families, then requests for predictive genetic testing (probably involving very young adults or minors) may become common.

The need for health care providers to be educated in genetics will increase as we learn more about the causes of common disorders; conversely, the need for genetics professionals to be educated about psychiatry also will increase as we learn more about the causes of psychiatric illness. Efforts are under way to improve these gaps in knowledge, but at least in the short term the most effective solution involves a team that includes genetics and mental health professionals. It is the authors' hope that the true revolution in knowledge about psychiatric genetics stemming from research into the etiology of psychiatric disorders will lead to strong and lasting collaborations between genetics and mental health professionals.

References

Acheson LS, Wiesner GL, Zyzanski SJ, et al: Family history-taking in community family practice: implications for genetic screening. Genet Med 2:180–185, 2000

Acheson LS, Stange KC, Zyzanski S: Clinical genetics issues encountered by family physicians. Genet Med 7:501–508, 2005

American College of Medical Genetics/American Society of Human Genetics, Working Group on ApoE and Alzheimer Disease: Statement on use of apolipoprotein E testing for Alzheimer disease. JAMA 274:1627–1629, 1995

Asarnow RF, Nuechterlein KH, Fogelson D, et al: Schizophrenia and schizophrenia-spectrum personality disorders in the first-degree relatives of children with schizophrenia: the UCLA family study. Arch Gen Psychiatry 58:581–588, 2001

Baker DL, Schuette JL, Uhlmann WR: A Guide to Genetic Counseling. New York, Wiley-Liss, 1998

Bassett SS, Havstad SL, Chase GA: The role of test accuracy in predicting acceptance of genetic susceptibility testing for Alzheimer's disease. Genet Test 8:120–126, 2004

Bennett RL, Hampel HL, Mandell JB, et al: Genetic counselors: translating genomic science into clinical practice. J Clin Invest 112:1274–1279, 2003

Bernhardt BA, Biesecker BB, Mastromarino CL: Goals, benefits, and outcomes of genetic counseling: client and genetic counselor assessment. Am J Med Genet 94:189–197, 2000

Burke W: Genetic testing in primary care. Annu Rev Genomics Hum Genet 5:1–14, 2004

Chakrabarti S, Kulhara P, Verma SK: Extent and determinants of burden among families of patients with affective disorders. Acta Psychiatr Scand 86:247–252, 1992

Ciarleglio LJ, Bennett RL, Williamson J, et al: Genetic counseling throughout the life cycle. J Clin Invest 112:1280–1286, 2003

Collins FS, Guttmacher AE: Genetics moves into the medical mainstream. JAMA 286:2322–2324, 2001

DeLisi LE, Bertisch H: A preliminary comparison of the hopes of researchers, clinicians, and families for the future ethical use of genetic findings on schizophrenia. Am J Med Genet B Neuropsychiatr Genet 141:110–115, 2006

Evers-Kiebooms G, Decruyenaere M: Predictive testing for Huntington's disease: a challenge for persons at risk and for professionals. Patient Educ Couns 35:15–26, 1998

Frank E, Targum SD, Gershon ES, et al: A comparison of nonpatient and bipolar patient-well spouse couples. Am J Psychiatry 138:764–768, 1981

Gamm JL, Nussbaum RL, Biesecker BB: Genetics and alcoholism among at-risk relatives. I: Perceptions of cause, risk, and control. Am J Med Genet A 128:144–150, 2004

Green RC: Risk assessment for Alzheimer's disease with genetic susceptibility testing: has the moment arrived? Alzheimer's Care Quarterly 3:208–214, 2002

Guttmacher AE, Jenkins J, Uhlmann WR: Genomic medicine: who will practice it? A call to open arms. Am J Med Genet 106:216–222, 2001

Husted J, Greenwood CM, Bassett AS: Heritability of schizophrenia and major affective disorder as a function of age, in the presence of strong cohort effects. Eur Arch Psychiatry Clin Neurosci 256:222–229, 2006

Jones I, Scourfield J, McCandless F, et al: Attitudes towards future testing for bipolar disorder susceptibility genes: a preliminary investigation. J Affect Disord 71:189–193, 2002

Lippman-Hand A, Fraser FC: Genetic counseling: provision and reception of information. Am J Med Genet 3:113–127, 1979

Liu W, Icitovic N, Shaffer ML, et al: The impact of population heterogeneity on risk estimation in genetic counseling. BMC Med Genet 5:18, 2004

Lyus VL: The importance of genetic counseling for individuals with schizophrenia and their relatives: potential clients' opinions and experiences. Am J Med Genet B Neuropsychiatr Genet May 24, 2007 (epub ahead of print)

McGuffin P, Rijsdijk F, Andrew M, et al: The heritability of bipolar affective disorder and the genetic relationship to unipolar depression. Arch Gen Psychiatry 60:497–502, 2003

Meiser B, Mitchell PB, McGirr H, et al: Implications of genetic risk information in families with a high density of bipolar disorder: an exploratory study. Soc Sci Med 60:109–118, 2005

Milner KK, Han T, Petty EM: Support for the availability of prenatal testing for neurological and psychiatric conditions in the psychiatric community. Genet Test 3:279–286, 1999

Nicolson R, Brookner FB, Lenane M, et al: Parental schizophrenia spectrum disorders in childhood-onset and adult-onset schizophrenia. Am J Psychiatry 160:490–495, 2003

Perlick D, Clarkin JF, Sirey J, et al: Burden experienced by care-givers of persons with bipolar affective disorder. Br J Psychiatry 175:56–62, 1999

Roberts JS, Cupples LA, Relkin NR, et al: Genetic risk assessment for adult children of people with Alzheimer's disease: the Risk Evaluation and Education for Alzheimer's Disease (REVEAL) study. J Geriatr Psychiatry Neurol 18:250–255, 2005

Schulz PM, Schulz SC, Dibble E, et al: Patient and family attitudes about schizophrenia: implications for genetic counseling. Schizophr Bull 8:504–513, 1982

Shiloh S, Sagi M: Effect of framing on the perception of genetic recurrence risks. Am J Med Genet 33:130–135, 1989

Smith LB, Sapers B, Reus VI, et al: Attitudes towards bipolar disorder and predictive genetic testing among patients and providers. J Med Genet 33:544–549, 1996

Targum SD, Dibble ED, Davenport YB, et al: The Family Attitudes Questionnaire: patients' and spouses' views of bipolar illness. Arch Gen Psychiatry 38:562–568, 1981

Trippitelli CL, Jamison KR, Folstein MF, et al: Pilot study on patients' and spouses' attitudes toward potential genetic testing for bipolar disorder. Am J Psychiatry 155:899–904, 1998

Tsuang MT: Genetic counseling for psychiatric patients and their families. Am J Psychiatry 135:1465–1475, 1978

Walter FM, Emery J: "Coming down the line"–patients' understanding of their family history of common chronic disease. Ann Fam Med 3:405–414, 2005

Walter FM, Emery J, Braithwaite D, et al: Lay understanding of familial risk of common chronic diseases: a systematic review and synthesis of qualitative research. Ann Fam Med 2:583–594, 2004

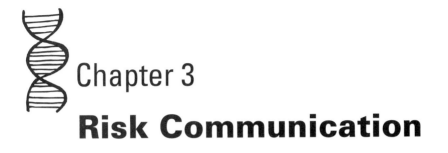

Chapter 3

Risk Communication

Simple Tools to Foster Understanding

Stephanie Kurzenhäuser, Ph.D., Dipl.Psych.
Anja Dieckmann, Ph.D., Dipl.Psych.

Hardly a month passes without a new entry in the already impressive list of inherited disorders and risk factors that can be detected through genetic testing. It is widely believed that genetic testing will soon be part of everyday medical care and will be key in detecting vulnerability to disease and determining drug response in healthy individuals (Henneman et al. 2004). For psychiatric disorders, which have a complex, multifactorial etiology that includes genetic elements (Maier 2003), the benefits of genetic testing are currently limited. However, the increasing availability of molecular tests for syndromic subtypes of major illnesses has wider implications. It has already brought about a change in counseling practice (Bassett 2001), because such subtypes have specific recurrence risk that counselors must consider. From the perspective of a client with a family history of a particular disorder, the desire for certainty is the main reason for seeking genetic counseling (Helm-

We thank Matthias Elstner for feedback on an earlier version of this chapter, Laura Wiles for editing the manuscript, and the Jacobs Foundation for their financial support to the first author (grant to Hertwig & Wänke).

chen 2000; Meincke et al. 2003). This hope for certainty may have been boosted by the availability of new genetic technologies.

Many people seem to project the illusion of certainty onto this new technology. More than other screening methods for health risks, the new genetic technologies may prompt this illusion because of their association with the typical image of genetic endowment as a blueprint or program with fixed and unavoidable consequences (Davison et al. 1994). Consequently, the results of genetic screening might be taken as if they represented immutable fate. Indeed, the public seems to overestimate the accuracy and predictive power of genetic testing (Davison et al. 1994). However, many of these diagnostic technologies (e.g., DNA fingerprinting, HIV tests, and gene scans), while excellent, do not offer certainty; they merely quantify in statistical terms the chance with which an event has occurred or will occur. Therefore, to understand the value and limitations of these technologies, people must come to terms with the statistical information associated with the test results (Kurzenhäuser and Hertwig 2006).

How can people become competent consumers of the crucial information rendered available by genetic technologies? Despite the public's interest in the topic of genetic technologies, most people see themselves as only moderately genetically literate (Henneman et al. 2004). Moreover, counseling quality may suffer because of the widespread problem of inadequate understanding of numbers, known as *innumeracy* (Gigerenzer 2002; Paulos 1988). Counselors should be aware that people may be ignorant of the multitude of risks and uncertainties involved in genetic testing[1] and, when provided with statistical information, may be confused by the numbers.

Only for a very few diseases, let alone psychiatric diseases, do the laws of *Mendelian inheritance* apply. One example is Huntington's disease, an autosomal dominant neurodegenerative condition caused by a single gene mutation on chromosome 4. An individual with a parent affected by Huntington's disease has a 50% chance of inheriting the gene mutation that leads to the disease. On the surface this relationship appears straightforward. However, age at onset, severity of symptoms, and duration of illness may vary from person to person even within a family. These differences are known as *variable expressivity.* Another genetic phenomenon that may complicate

---

[1]Commonly, the term *risk* is used for outcomes with known probabilities, while the term *uncertainty* applies when one lacks empiric data to assign numbers to the possible alternative outcomes (Bottorff et al. 1998; Gigerenzer 2002). Following this distinction, we focus on risks in this chapter, but one should be aware that the line between risks and uncertainties is not clear-cut. In the case of uncommon family constellations, for instance, there might not be enough reliable data to quantify the uncertainty.

the interpretation of a family history or genetic testing for single gene mutations is *reduced penetrance*, which refers to instances in which an individual does not express the expected phenotype despite having a specific genotype. Reduced penetrance and variable expressivity introduce additional levels of uncertainty and complicate clients' ability to understand what is meant by the presence of a certain genotype. Risk assessment is further complicated by the fact that for many disorders there is *genetic heterogeneity*. That is, different genotypes can cause the same phenotype, and each genotype can be associated with a very different risk. Moreover, in the case of *multifactorial etiology*, genes interact with other factors in ways that are not yet well understood and thus are very difficult to quantify.

In addition, for disorders for which diagnostic tests are available, there is *diagnostic uncertainty*: people without a certain genetic aberration are sometimes falsely identified as carriers (false-positive test result), and carriers are sometimes not recognized (false-negative test result). Such errors are very rare, but they do happen. False negatives may be due to genetic heterogeneity and mutations that have not yet been identified as being associated with a particular disease, and false positives may result from human error in the laboratory, for example, confusing blood samples or entering erroneous data into the computer.

For major psychiatric disorders, such as mood disorders, schizophrenia, and dementia, assessment of risk is even more complicated. Psychiatric disorders are in most instances not due to single gene mutations. Simple rules of inheritance do not apply, and psychiatric disorders, although familial, result from a complex but poorly understood interaction between genetic and environmental factors. In addition, most of the causal factors have yet to be identified, and consequently little or no genetic testing is available.

In face of these multiple sources of uncertainty associated with interpreting genetic risk information, it is not surprising that genetic counselors have difficulty conveying risk information in a way that reliably promotes recipients' understanding and ability to use the information appropriately (Bottorff et al. 1998; Marteau and Dormandy 2001). For instance, many recipients of genetic counseling appear to feel the need to convert statistical information (e.g., a 20% chance) into categorical, definite terms (e.g., high vs. low risk), thus removing the probabilistic aspect of the statement (Bottorff et al. 1998). Nevertheless, advising clients on the probability of developing or transmitting a disorder is a crucial part of the genetic counseling process, as defined by Harper (1993, p. 3):

> Genetic counseling is the process by which patients or relatives at risk of a disorder that may be hereditary are advised of the consequences of this disorder, the probability of developing or transmitting it, and of the ways in which this may be prevented, avoided or ameliorated.

An understanding of recurrence risk was an essential component of the American Society of Human Genetics' definition of genetic counseling as long ago as 1975. Strong consensus currently exists that health professionals are ethically obliged to provide this type of statistical information, thus enabling patients to make informed decisions (Marteau and Dormandy 2001). Indeed, some go so far as to call information about the recurrence rate "the sine qua non of counseling" (Lippman-Hand and Fraser 1979, p. 117). Ideally, genetic counselors should have tools at hand to overcome their clients' and, possibly, their own innumeracy.

Statistical innumeracy, we emphasize, is not simply a problem within the individual mind or a problem of lack of knowledge. The problem lies in the failure to communicate risk in ways that are understandable and that allow a person to draw conclusions from the risk (e.g., the predictive value of a genetic test result). To address this problem, cognitive psychologists have identified tools for communicating risk in a way that fosters insight and that can help both laypeople and experts improve their comprehension of statistical information.

In what follows, we present different representations of statistical information that invite misunderstandings and hamper the ability to draw appropriate conclusions from the information. Specifically, we focus on three numerical formats that have been repeatedly demonstrated to cloud people's minds: single-event probabilities, conditional probabilities, and relative risks. For each of these formats, we propose alternative ways of representing statistical information that facilitate people's understanding. Thus, our contribution goes beyond redescribing the mistakes people make and their various over- and underestimations of genetic risks in terms of heuristics they might apply and biases to which they might fall prey (Shiloh 1994). Rather, for concrete pieces of numerical information that must be conveyed in the counseling session, we describe methods of helping people overcome mistakes and misperceptions. We also provide a brief overview of related findings on the visual representation of numerical risks.

Before we focus on different numerical formats, we critically review another suggestion that has been raised in response to people's repeated demonstration of problems in understanding numerical information: namely, providing verbal rather than numerical information.

Verbal or Numerical Risk Information?

Understanding risks is a challenging task for many people. The types of numerical information that are most often used to convey risk information—fractions and proportions—prove especially demanding for the average person (Lipkus et al. 2001). Even experts and educated people have problems performing mental operations with probabilities (Kahneman and Tversky 1974; Lipkus et al. 2001). In view of these problems, it has been suggested that numerical information should be replaced with simple verbal categorizations of risk (i.e., "high," "moderate," or "low" risk) (Heilbrun et al. 1999).

Enabling people to thoroughly understand numerical expressions of risk is not a trivial task (Weinstein 1999), and representations intended to foster understanding will not invariably succeed. However, numbers appear to be better suited than words for communicating risk. First, verbal quantifiers such as "high" or "moderate" are less precise than numbers, thus inviting more varied interpretations and resulting in an even less accurate understanding (Burkell 2004; Marteau et al. 2000; but see Marteau et al. 2001 for an exception). For example, what seems a "moderate" risk from the counselor's perspective might well seem a "high" risk from the patient's viewpoint (Burkell 2004). Second, even though most people like to *provide* information in categorical terms, they prefer to *receive* information numerically if they must use the information as the basis of a decision (Wallsten et al. 1993). For instance, in genetic counseling for breast and ovarian cancer, 73% of the counselees expressed a preference for the risk to be described in quantitative formats (Hallowell et al. 1997). In addition, a numerical statement of risk can increase trust in and comfort with the risk information, compared with a purely verbal statement (Gurmankin et al. 2004).

To conclude, even though people often translate numerical into categorical risk information during their decision-making process (Bottorff et al. 1998), they expect numbers to begin with, and they appear to benefit more from numbers–if represented in the right way–than from words.

Numerical Risk Information

Single-Event Probabilities

To communicate risk in the form of a single-event probability means to make a statement of this type: "The probability that an event will happen is x%." Such a statement can be confusing, because a single-event probability leaves open the class of events to which the probability refers. The following example illustrates this ambiguity (Gigerenzer 2002):

> A psychiatrist prescribed fluoxetine to his mildly depressed patients. He would inform them that they had a "30% to 50% chance of developing a sexual problem" such as impotence or loss of sexual interest. Hearing this, patients were concerned and anxious, but they did not usually ask further questions. After learning about the ambiguity of single-event probabilities,

the psychiatrist changed his way of communicating risks and chose an alternative, mathematically equivalent format. He told patients that of every 10 people for whom he prescribes fluoxetine, 3–5 will experience a sexual problem. Psychologically, this way of communicating the risk of side effects made a difference. It seemed to put patients more at ease, and they asked questions such as what to do if they were among the three to five people. The psychiatrist realized that he had never checked how his patients understood what "a 30% to 50% chance of developing a sexual problem" meant. It turned out that many had thought that something would go wrong in 30% to 50% of their sexual encounters.

The important insight from this doctor-patient interaction is that the psychiatrist's initial approach to risk communication left the reference class unclear. A *reference class* is the answer to the question "Percentage of what?" Did the percentage refer to a class of people (patients who take fluoxetine), to a class of events (a given person's sexual encounters), or to some other class? Whereas the psychiatrist's reference class was the total number of his patients taking fluoxetine, his patients' reference class was their own sexual encounters. Only by chance did the psychiatrist choose a different way of communicating the risk of side effects and subsequently realize his patients' previously unobserved misunderstandings.

When risks are solely communicated in terms of single-event probabilities, people have little choice but to fill in a class spontaneously. This tendency was demonstrated in a recent study that asked pedestrians in one American city (New York) and four major European cities about their understanding of a probabilistic weather forecast ("30% chance of rain tomorrow") (Gigerenzer et al. 2005). Only in New York did a majority of participants supply the standard meteorological interpretation, namely, that when the weather conditions are like today, in 3 of 10 cases there will be (at least a trace of) rain the next day. In each of the European cities, this interpretation was judged as the *least* appropriate. The preferred interpretation in Europe was that it will rain tomorrow "30% of the time," followed by "in 30% of the area." In other words, numerical probabilities can be interpreted by members of the public in multiple, possibly even mutually contradictory ways.

The ambiguity of a single-event probability and the resulting misunderstandings are not limited to the risks of side effects and precipitation. Single-event probabilities can also have far-reaching consequences when they are, for instance, used by expert witnesses to explain DNA evidence in court (Koehler 1996b), used by clinical psychologists and psychiatrists to predict the possibility that a mentally ill patient will commit violent acts (Slovic et al. 2000), and used by medical organizations to communicate the benefits and risks of treatments (Gigerenzer 2002).

A straightforward way to reduce confusion about the meaning of single-event probabilities is always to communicate the reference class to which the single-event probabilities pertain. For instance, "30% probability of rain tomorrow" does not refer to how long, in what area, or how much it will rain. It means that in 3 of 10 times when meteorologists make this prediction, there will be at least a trace of rain the next day. Alternatively, one may avoid confusion by replacing ambiguous single-event statements with frequency statements. For instance, the psychiatrist in the previous example may simply explain to patients that "three of every ten patients have a side effect when taking this drug" (Gigerenzer and Edwards 2003).

This finding is relevant for genetic counseling, especially for counseling involving relatively rare genetic conditions. For example, the 22q deletion syndrome, also known as DiGeorge syndrome or velocardiofacial syndrome, involves a microdeletion on chromosome 22q. Its highly variable phenotype includes learning disabilities, palatal anomalies, cardiac defects, typical facial features, and psychiatric illnesses. Schizophrenia is the most common psychiatric illness associated with this syndrome (Hodgkinson et al. 2001). Newborns are not systematically screened for 22q deletion syndrome, and its true prevalence can therefore only be estimated. Regardless of the uncertainty concerning the actual prevalence of the syndrome, however, rather than stating the estimated prevalence as approximately 0.024%, one should use the more graphic expression that the syndrome occurs in approximately one of 4,000 live births (duMontcel et al. 1996).

At the same time, incidence rates expressed as frequencies are perceived as riskier than incidence rates expressed as probabilities (Siegrist 1997; Slovic et al. 2000). A suggested explanation for this perception is that frequencies evoke stronger affective reactions because they lead to imagination of concrete cases, while such images are rarely evoked in response to probabilities (Slovic et al. 2000). People's imagination seems to focus on the numerator, such that a condition that occurs in 20 of 100 cases is perceived as riskier than one that occurs in 2 of 10 cases (Slovic et al. 2000). Counselors should be aware of these effects and can reduce fears by using the smallest possible numerator, for example, 1 of 5 cases.

Finally, cognitive psychologists have investigated how different ways of *framing* numerical information affect judgment and decision making (for reviews, see Edwards et al. 2001 and Wilson et al. 1988). Framing is the expression of logically equivalent information (whether numerical or verbal) in different ways (Gigerenzer and Edwards 2003). One type of framing that is especially relevant for communicating clinical risk is gain versus loss framing, because it concerns the implications of accepting or declining tests. *Loss framing* considers information about the potential losses or risks of not undertaking an action (e.g.,"failing to detect disease X early can cost you your life"); *gain framing* emphasizes the benefits of undertaking the action (e.g., "detecting disease X early can save your life"). Evidence suggests that loss framing is more effective than gain framing in promoting detection behaviors such as undertaking screening and other diagnostic tests (Banks et al. 1995; Rothman and Salovey 1997). An explanation for this finding is that people perceive detection behaviors as being risky in the short term (even though beneficial in the long term) because they can reveal a negative or even threatening health status, and it is an established fact that risk-seeking behavior can be induced by using loss frames (Rothman and Salovey 1997). Prevention behaviors (e.g., using sunscreen to avoid skin cancer) on the other hand are not seen as risky and are therefore promoted more effectively with gain-framed messages (Detweiler et al. 1999). The finding that different presentations of risk information can influence patients' behavior and decisions in different ways is a challenge to the ideal of informed consent (Edwards et al. 2001; Gigerenzer and Edwards 2003), and health professionals should be aware of the risk for manipulation and over-directiveness. Health professionals such as genetic counselors should consistently use transparent representations that foster understanding and should balance the use of frames, for example by using both gain and loss frames (Edwards et al. 2001).

Conditional Probabilities

Even with prior experience of diagnostic testing, patients often have little knowledge about the accuracy of such tests (Hamm and Smith 1998). Limited knowledge, in turn, is often tantamount to the belief that diagnostic tests are more accurate and more predictive than they actually are (Black et al. 1995). Genetic testing in particular is perceived to be extremely predictive, perhaps even infallible (Davison et al. 1994; Koehler 1996b). Thus, for many people, it comes as a surprise that the results of diagnostic tests do not predict outcomes with certainty. For instance, in a recent survey in the Netherlands, 32% of respondents thought that if the results of prenatal tests such as chorionic villus sampling and amniocentesis were negative, the child would definitely be healthy (Henneman et al. 2004). Believing that a negative test result means having zero risk is a misunderstanding that abets an illusory sense of certainty.

Similarly, positive test results can also be wrong. At a conference on AIDS in 1987, it was reported that of 22 blood donors in Florida who were notified of having tested HIV-positive with the enzyme-linked immunosorbent assay (ELISA) test, 7 committed suicide (Stine 1996; see Gigerenzer 2002). For them, the positive test result was tantamount to a death sentence. How would they have reacted had they known, for example, that even with the combined ELISA and Western blot tests–now the standard procedure in HIV testing–the predictive value of a positive test in German men who do not belong to a risk group is only 50%? That is, even with the combined tests, one of two positive test results is wrong (Gigerenzer 2002). Such misunderstandings stem in part from the way that the test results are presented (Marteau et al. 2000). When attempting to comprehend the results of genetic tests, people should be made aware that these tests are not fail-safe and can result in incorrect as well as correct identifications. The chance of each outcome is typically expressed in terms of conditional probability, illustrated in the following statement about the sensitivity of a test: "If a child has a genetic disease, the probability of a positive result of prenatal test X is 90%." Such conditional probabilities are easily misunderstood. Specifically, the conditional probability of a positive test result given a genetic disease (a test's sensitivity) is confused with the inverse probability of genetic disease given a positive test result (a test's predictive value).

Experts are not immune to this confusion. In one study, experienced doctors read the following information about a screening test for colorectal cancer (Hoffrage and Gigerenzer 1998):

> The probability of colorectal cancer in a certain population is 0.3% [base rate]. If a person has colorectal cancer, the probability that the hemoccult test is positive is 50% [sensitivity]. If a person does not have colorectal cancer, the probability that she or he still tests positive is 3% [false-positive rate].

The doctors were then asked to estimate the probability that someone who tests positive actually has colorectal cancer. The formula needed to solve this diagnostic inference problem is Bayes's rule (see Figure 3–1, left side), and the correct estimate for the test's positive predictive value is 5%. Yet, answers ranged from 1% to 99%, and every second doctor estimated the probability as 50% (the sensitivity) or 47% (the sensitivity minus false-positive rate).

As this example shows, information about the performance of diagnostic tests that is given in terms of conditional probabilities often leads to an overestimation of the predictive value of a positive test result. People tend to assume that the predictive value lies in the order of magnitude of the test's sensitivity, ignoring the usually low prevalence of the disease that is tested. This tendency might also contribute to the belief that diagnostic tests are more predictive than they actually are (Davison et al. 1994; Hamm and Smith 1998).

The difficulties that people have in reasoning with conditional probabilities are often presented as if they were natural consequences of flawed mental software (Bar-Hillel 1980). This view, however, overlooks the fun-

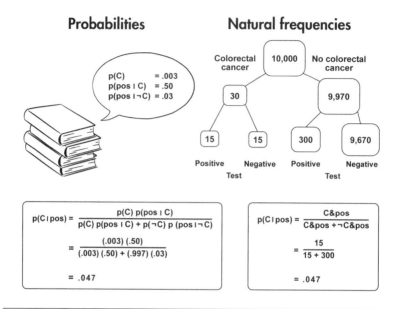

FIGURE 3–1.   Calculation of the probability (p) of colorectal cancer (C) given a positive test result (pos).

Natural frequencies facilitate the computation of p(C1pos). Computation using Bayes's rule for probabilities (left side) involves more calculations than computation using natural frequencies (right side).

¬C=no colorectal cancer.

Source.   Right side from Hoffrage et al. 2005.

damental fact that the human mind processes information through external representations and that the choice of representations can improve or impair our understanding of statistical information. Consider the following alternative representation of the information just presented:

> Of every 10,000 people, 30 have colorectal cancer. Of these 30, 15 will have a positive hemoccult test. Of the remaining 9,970 people without colorectal cancer, 300 will still test positive. How many of those who test positive actually have colorectal cancer?

As before, the correct answer is 5%, that is, 15 of 315. In responding to this *natural frequency representation,* 16 of 24 physicians gave the correct answer. In contrast, only 1 of 24 physicians could give the correct answer when the statistical information was expressed as probabilities (Hoffrage and Gigerenzer 1998).

Representation matters because the statistical reasoning that is required, for instance, to calculate the positive predictive value of a test (Bayesian reasoning) is relatively simple with natural frequencies but becomes cumbersome when conditional probabilities are introduced (see Figure 3–1). The results of previous studies have shown that physicians (Berwick et al. 1981) and laypeople (Koehler 1996a) have great difficulty understanding the predictive value of test results typically presented in terms of probabilities and percentages. One reason is that the conditional probabilities given in our example refer to groups of people that differ widely in number. The 50% (the sensitivity) refers to the (small) group of people with colorectal cancer, but the 3% (the false-positive rate) refers to a different (much larger) group of people without colorectal cancer. This switch of reference class can confuse the minds of physicians and patients alike. Natural frequencies, in contrast, all refer to the same class of observations and therefore carry implicit information about base rates. This characteristic reduces the number of computations required to determine the positive predictive value of a test (Hoffrage and Gigerenzer 1998). Natural frequencies also correspond to the way in which humans have experienced statistical information over most of their history (for a discussion of this explanation and alternative explanations, see Hoffrage et al. 2002).

Note that an isolated number, such as 15, is not by itself a natural frequency; it becomes a natural frequency only because of its relation to other numbers in a natural frequency tree (such as the tree shown in Figure 3–1) (Hoffrage et al. 2002). Natural frequencies are a distinct class of frequencies, different from other kinds of frequencies. Consider the following version of the earlier example:

> Of every 1,000 people, 30 have colorectal cancer. Of every 1,000 people who have colorectal cancer, 500 will have a positive hemoccult test. Of every 1,000 people who do not have colorectal cancer, 30 will still test positive. How many of those who test positive actually have colorectal cancer?

In this example, frequency information has been normalized, that is, every piece of information refers to a reference class of the same size, here 1,000 people. The benefit of normalization is that the numbers can be easily compared with each other. However, normalization does have a cost. Because normalized frequencies do not stem from the sequential partitioning of one population, they cannot be displayed in a natural frequency tree as in Figure 3–1, and the calculation of the positive predictive value becomes more difficult—that is, subject to the same difficulties encountered when trying to derive predictive value from other normalized information such as percentages and probabilities.

Representing risk in terms of natural frequencies fosters statistical reasoning. This finding is robust for laypeople and experts (Brase 2002; Hertwig and Hoffrage 2002; Kurzenhäuser and Lücking 2004). Although the beneficial effect of natural frequencies occurs without providing more knowledge through training or instruction—just by changing the representation of information—people can be explicitly encouraged to translate conditional probabilities into natural frequencies. Teaching people to change representations turns out to be much more effective in improving diagnostic inferences than training them to apply mathematical formulas such as Bayes's rule (Kurzenhäuser and Hoffrage 2002; Sedlmeier and Gigerenzer 2001).

Relative Risks

In addition to single-event probabilities and conditional probabilities, another source of misunderstandings in communicating risk is *relative risk*, illustrated in the following example. Women who ask what the effect of mammography screening is on the risk of dying from breast cancer often hear the following answer: By undergoing mammography screening, women over age 40 years reduce their risk of dying from breast cancer by 25%. This number is a *relative risk reduction*, which is the relative decrease in the number of breast cancer deaths among women who participate in mammography screening, compared with the number of deaths among women who do not participate. This number is mute on the underlying raw frequencies. The frequencies for these data are derived from four Swedish randomized trials for women between age 40 and 74 years (Nyström et al. 1996; see Table 3–1): Of 1,000 women who did not participate in mammography screening, 4 died of breast cancer. Of 1,000 women who did participate in mammography screening, 3 died of breast cancer. Screening thus saved the life of 1 of 4 women who would otherwise have died from breast cancer, which is a reduction of 25%.

Relative risk reduction is not the only way to represent the benefit of mammography. Alternatively, its benefits can be framed in terms of *absolute risk reduction*, namely, the proportion of women who die from breast cancer without undergoing mammography screening minus those who die despite being screened. Screening reduces the number of people who die from 4 to 3 in 1,000. That is, the absolute risk reduction is 1 in 1,000, which is 0.1%. Still another representation of the same information is the *number needed to treat*, which is the number of people who must participate in the screening to save one life. This number can be derived from the absolute risk reduction. The number of people who need to be screened to save one life is 1,000, because the screening prevents 1 in 1,000 deaths.

TABLE 3–1. Overview of the benefits of mammography screening

Participation in mammography screening?	Breast cancer deaths in 10 years per 1,000 women over age 40 years
Yes	3
No	4

Source.   Data from Nyström et al. 1996.

The relative risk reduction looks more impressive than the absolute risk reduction. Health organizations inform patients about the benefits of mammography screening almost exclusively in terms of the relative risk reduction, and it is not surprising that people are more likely to prefer an intervention if it is advertised in terms of relative risk reduction than in terms of absolute risk reduction (Gigerenzer 2002; Sarfati et al. 1998). It has been suggested that people draw incorrect conclusions from reports of relative risk reduction. Again, misunderstandings may be caused by confusion about the reference class. In the example, although relative risk reduction refers to women dying of breast cancer, absolute risk reduction and number needed to treat refer to all women in the relevant age group who participate in screening. Indeed, the fact that people frequently overestimate the benefits of screening programs (Black et al. 1995) is consistent with the possibility that they assume that the relative risk reduction (e.g., 25%) applies to those who participate in screenings when in fact it refers to the people who die without having been screened.

Similarly, a relative risk increase sounds more impressive and might thus excessively stoke fears. In the mid-1990s, an official statement concerning side effects of oral contraceptives was publicized in Great Britain, warning that "combined oral contraceptives containing desogestrel and gestodene are associated with around a two-fold increase in the risk of thromboembolism" (Jain et al. 1998). The warning caused great concern among British women and their physicians. Many women stopped taking birth control pills, resulting in an increase in unwanted pregnancies and abortions (Jain et al. 1998). If the same information about thromboembolism had been expressed in absolute terms, it would have been clear how frequent this dangerous side effect actually was. The study had shown that of every 14,000 women who do not take the pill, one has thromboembolism, whereas among every 14,000 women who take the pill, this number is two. In terms of absolute risk, the chance of thromboembolism increases from one to two in 14,000 women, which is less than 0.01% (cf. Gigerenzer 2002).

In the psychiatric genetics literature, the risk of developing a disease given a certain genotype is also often expressed relative to the risk in the general population. We have already mentioned that the 22q microdeletion is associated with an increased risk of developing schizophrenia. This risk can be expressed in relative terms as a 25 times increased risk, compared with the general population (Hodgkinson et al. 2001; Murphy et al. 1999; Pulver et al. 1994). To give counselees the opportunity to judge the absolute numbers that underlie this 25-fold increase, we recommend conveying the information in absolute terms: In the general population, one in 100 people will develop schizophrenia in their lifetime; among people with 22q deletion syndrome, 25 in 100 people will develop schizophrenia in their lifetime.

Both absolute and relative representations of the raw frequencies are mathematically correct. Yet, they suggest different amounts of benefit or harm and thus are likely to elicit different expectations. We propose that risks can be communicated more effectively in absolute rather than relative terms, to give the client a chance to realistically assess the absolute order of magnitude. At a minimum, both pieces of information should be provided (Gigerenzer and Edwards 2003).

Visual Representation of Risk

Visual representations may substantially improve comprehension of risk (Edwards et al. 2002). First, they attract people's attention because information is displayed in concrete, visual terms, and second, they can reveal data patterns that may be undetected otherwise (e.g., line graphs can convey trends in data [Lipkus and Hollands 1999]). Risks can be communicated visually in many ways. For example, the risk of developing a specific disease can be displayed in bar charts, pie charts, grids, or so-called risk ladders.[2] Sedlmeier and Gigerenzer (2001) tested Bayesian reasoning tutorials that taught people to translate probabilities into natural frequencies and represent them either in the form of a natural frequency tree or a frequency grid (see Figure 3–2 for an example of both representations). Both tutorials were associated with a pronounced and stable increase in performance and were superior to more traditional rule training for teaching Bayes's formula.

---

[2]Here, the probability of several risks are indicated on one common scale to allow for risk comparisons, such as depicting the number of cancer deaths expected from different levels of radon exposure in comparison to the number of deaths expected from smoking different numbers of cigarettes per day (Lipkus and Hollands 1999).

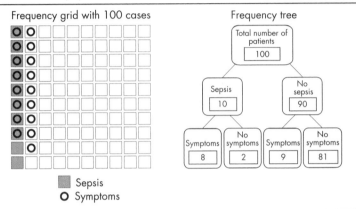

Task: You are working in an outpatient clinic where the record shows that during the past year, 10% of the walk-in patients had sepsis. A patient walks in with high fever and chills, and you also note that he has skin lesions. According to the record:
- If a patient has sepsis, there is an 80% chance that he or she will have these symptoms.
- If a patient does not have sepsis, there is still a 10% chance that he or she will show these symptoms.

Frequency grid with 100 cases

Frequency tree

Total number of patients
100

Sepsis
10

No sepsis
90

Symptoms
8

No symptoms
2

Symptoms
9

No symptoms
81

■ Sepsis
O Symptoms

FIGURE 3–2.   Representation of a typical Bayesian reasoning task using a frequency grid and a frequency tree.

In a tutorial for teaching Bayesian reasoning, the participants in one group were trained to translate the given probabilities into cases in a frequency grid (left side), participants in another group were trained to translate the probabilities into a frequency tree (right side), and participants in a third group were trained to use Bayes's formula (not shown).

Source.   Adapted from Sedlmeier and Gigerenzer 2001.

No single graphic format will perform optimally in all situations, because the effectiveness of a display will be affected by several factors such as data complexity, the involvement of the recipient, and the type of material (Lipkus and Hollands 1999). Simpler displays are more appropriate for a take-home information brochure than for material a counselor will guide a client through in a face-to-face session. It is therefore not surprising that the evidence for the efficiency of visual representations in fostering comprehension of risks has been mixed (Lipkus and Hollands 1999; Wright 1999). The same is true for the use of videos and more interactive media (Marteau and Dormandy 2001). More systematic and theoretical research is needed to explore the types of graphics and visual materials that are best matched to particular risk communication tasks. Nevertheless, some tentative guidelines for maximizing the effectiveness of graphic displays can already be extrapolated from the existing literature. For instance, the reader's task (e.g., reading one exact value or comparing two risks) should be taken into account when choosing the type of display, and the number of mental operations should be minimized (see Lipkus and Hollands 1999 for a comprehensive review of the existing literature).

Conclusions

Genetic counselors face a dilemma: clients prefer numerical formats (Hallowell et al. 1997), but numbers have been shown to be often misunderstood. We suggest that this dilemma can be resolved by replacing numerical formats that regularly cause confusion with formats that are more easily understood, such as frequency formats.

Misunderstandings associated with three formats commonly used to convey statistical information—single-event probabilities, conditional probabilities, and relative risks—may arise from confusion about the reference class. We have shown how to lift the mental fog by clarifying the reference class and using transparent representations such as natural frequencies.

More specifically, natural frequencies have three main advantages. First, they specify the reference class, thus avoiding misconceptions caused by single-event probabilities and relative risk statements. Second, as a replacement for conditional probabilities in Bayesian reasoning tasks, natural frequencies refer to the same reference class and thus avoid typical errors resulting from the difficult integration of probabilities that refer to different base rates. Finally, natural frequencies simplify the necessary computations involved in Bayesian reasoning, because they are integers and require fewer calculation steps.

Visual displays can boost understanding, although more research is needed to find out which visual formats are best suited to presenting different types of information. Where conclusive advice from the literature is lacking, counselors should feel encouraged to experiment with different representations and report their experiences with these formats. For instance, Shiloh (1994) suggested that educational aids such as tossing coins or making bets may highlight the uncertainties inherent in genetics and may be used to foster statistical reasoning.

There is, of course, more to the counseling process than good statistical reasoning on the part of the counselor and the client (Marteau and Dormandy 2001), but without statistical reasoning, the results of the best diagnostic technology will be of little value in clarifying risk.

References

Banks SM, Salovey P, Greener S, et al: The effects of message framing on mammography utilization. Health Psychol 14:178–184, 1995

Bar-Hillel M: The base-rate fallacy in probability judgments. Acta Psychol 44:211–233, 1980

Bassett AS: Psychiatric genetics in the 21st century. Can J Psychiatry 46:121–122, 2001

Berwick DM, Fineberg HV, Weinstein MC: When doctors meet numbers. Am J Med 71:991–998, 1981

Black WC, Nease RF Jr, Tosteson AN: Perceptions of breast cancer risk and screening effectiveness in women younger than 50 years of age. J Natl Cancer Inst 87:720–731, 1995

Bottorff JL, Ratner PA, Johnson JL, et al: Communicating cancer risk information: the challenges of uncertainty. Patient Educ Couns 33:67–81, 1998

Brase G: Which statistical formats facilitate what decisions? The perception and influence of different statistical information formats. J Behav Decis Making 15:381–401, 2002

Burkell J: What are the chances? Evaluating risk and benefit information in consumer health materials. J Med Libr Assoc 92:200–208, 2004

Davison C, Macintyre S, Smith GD: The potential social impact of predictive genetic testing for susceptibility to common chronic diseases: a review and proposed research agenda. Sociol Health Illn 16:340–371, 1994

Detweiler JB, Bedell BT, Salovey P, et al: Message framing and sunscreen use: gain-framed messages motivate beach-goers. Health Psychol 18:189–196, 1999

DuMontcel ST, Mendizabal H, Ayme S, et al: Prevalence of 22q11 microdeletion. J Med Genet 33:719, 1996

Edwards A, Elwyn G, Covey J, et al: Presenting risk information—a review of the effects of "framing" and other manipulations on patient outcomes. J Health Commun 6:61–82, 2001

Edwards A, Elwyn G, Mulley A: Explaining risks: turning numerical data into meaningful pictures. BMJ 324:827–830, 2002

Gigerenzer G: Reckoning with Risk: Learning to Live With Uncertainty. London, Penguin Books, 2002

Gigerenzer G, Edwards A: Simple tools for understanding risks: from innumeracy to insight. BMJ 327:741–744, 2003

Gigerenzer G, Hertwig R, van den Broek E, et al: "A 30% chance of rain tomorrow": how does the public understand probabilistic weather forecasts? Risk Anal 25:623–629, 2005

Gurmankin AD, Baron J, Armstrong K: The effect of numerical statements of risk on trust and comfort with hypothetical physician risk communication. Med Decis Making 24:265–271, 2004

Hallowell N, Statham H, Murton F, et al: "Talking about chance": the presentation of risk information during genetic counseling for breast and ovarian cancer. J Genet Couns 6:269–286, 1997

Hamm RM, Smith SL: The accuracy of patients' judgments of disease probability and test sensitivity and specificity. J Fam Pract 47:44–52, 1998

Harper P: Practical Genetic Counselling. London, Butterworth, 1993

Heilbrun K, Philipson J, Berman L, et al: Risk communication: clinicians' reported approaches and perceived values. J Am Acad Psychiatry Law 27:397–406, 1999

Helmchen H: Ethische Implikationen der Neurowissenschaften in der Klinik [Ethical aspects of clinical neuroscience]. Nervenarzt 71:700–708, 2000 (German)

Henneman L, Timmermans DRM, van der Wal G: Public experiences, knowledge and expectations about genetics and the use of genetic information. Community Genet 7:33–743, 2004

Hertwig R, Hoffrage U: Technology needs psychology: how natural frequencies foster insight in medical and legal experts, in Etc: Frequency Processing and Cognition. Edited by Sedlmeier P, Betsch T. New York, Oxford University Press, 2002, pp 285–302

Hodgkinson K, Murphy J, O'Neill S, et al: Genetic counselling for schizophrenia in the era of molecular genetics. Can J Psychiatry 46:123–130, 2001

Hoffrage U, Gigerenzer G: Using natural frequencies to improve diagnostic inferences. Acad Med 73:538–540, 1998

Hoffrage U, Gigerenzer G, Krauss S, et al: Representation facilitates reasoning: what natural frequencies are and what they are not. Cognition 84:343–352, 2002

Hoffrage U, Kurzenhäuser K, Gigerenzer G: Understanding the results of medical tests: why the representation of statistical information matters, in Science and Medicine in Dialogue: Thinking Through Particulars and Universals. Edited by Bibace R, Laird JD, Noeller KL, et al. Westport, CT, Praeger, 2005, pp 89–98

Jain BP, McQuay H, Moore A: Number needed to treat and relative risk reduction. Ann Intern Med 128:72–73, 1998

Kahneman D, Tversky A: Judgment under uncertainty: heuristics and biases. Science 185:1124–1131, 1974

Koehler JJ: The base rate fallacy reconsidered: descriptive, normative, and methodological challenges. Behav Brain Sci 19:1–53, 1996a

Koehler JJ: On conveying the probative value of DNA evidence: frequencies, likelihood ratios, and error rates. University of Colorado Law Review 67:859–886, 1996b

Kurzenhäuser S, Hertwig R: How to foster citizens' statistical reasoning: implications for genetic counseling. Community Genet 9:197–203, 2006

Kurzenhäuser S, Hoffrage U: Teaching Bayesian reasoning: an evaluation of a classroom tutorial for medical students. Med Teach 24:516–521, 2002

Kurzenhäuser S, Lücking A: Statistical formats in Bayesian inference, in Cognitive Illusions: Fallacies and Biases in Thinking, Judgment, and Memory. Edited by Pohl R. Hove, England, Psychology Press, 2004, pp 61–77

Lipkus IM, Hollands JG: The visual communication of risk. J Natl Cancer Inst Monogr 25:149–163, 1999

Lipkus IM, Samsa G, Rimer BK: General performance on a numeracy scale among highly educated samples. Med Decis Making 21:37–44, 2001

Lippman-Hand A, Fraser FC: Genetic counseling: provision and reception of information. Am J Med Genet 3:113–127, 1979

Maier W: Psychiatric genetics: overview on achievements, problems, perspectives, in Psychiatric Genetics: Methods and Reviews. Edited by Leboyer M, Bellivier F. Totowa, NJ, Humana Press, 2003, pp 3–20

Marteau TM, Dormandy E: Facilitating informed choice in prenatal testing: how well are we doing? Am J Med Genet 106:185–190, 2001

Marteau TM, Saidi G, Goodburn S, et al: Numbers or words? A randomized controlled trial of presenting screen negative results to pregnant women. Prenat Diagn 20:714–718, 2000

Marteau TM, Senior V, Sasieni P: Women's understanding of a "normal smear test result": experimental questionnaire based study. BMJ 322:526–528, 2001

Meincke U, Kosinski CH, Zerres K, et al: Psychiatrische und ethische Aspekte genetischer Diagnostik am Beispiel der Chorea Huntington [Psychiatric and ethical aspects of genetic diagnosis exemplified by Huntingdon's chorea]. Nervenarzt 74:413–419, 2003 (German)

Murphy KC, Jones LA, Owen MJ: High prevalence of schizophrenia in adults with velo-cardio-facial syndrome. Arch Gen Psychiatry 56:940–945, 1999

Nyström L, Larsson LG, Wall S, et al: An overview of the Swedish randomised mammography trials: total mortality pattern and the representivity of the study cohorts. J Med Screen 3:85–87, 1996

Paulos JA: Innumeracy: Mathematical Illiteracy and Its Consequences. New York, Vintage Books, 1988

Pulver AE, Nestadt G, Goldberg R, et al: Psychotic illness in patients diagnosed with velo-cardio-facial syndrome and their relatives. J Nerv Ment Dis 182:476–478, 1994

Rothman AJ, Salovey P: Shaping perceptions to motivate healthy behavior: the role of message framing. Psychol Bull 121:3–19, 1997

Sarfati D, Howden-Chapman P, Woodward A, Salmond C: Does the frame affect the picture? A study into how attitudes to screening for cancer are affected by the way benefits are expressed. J Med Screen 5:137–140, 1998

Sedlmeier P, Gigerenzer G: Teaching Bayesian reasoning in less than two hours. J Exp Psychol Gen 130:380–400, 2001

Shiloh S: Heuristics and biases in health decision making: their expression in genetic counseling, in Applications of Heuristics and Biases to Social Issues. Edited by Heath L, Tindale RS, Edwards J, et al. New York, Plenum, 1994, pp 13–30

Siegrist M: Communicating low risk magnitudes: incidence rates expressed as frequency versus rates expressed as probability. Risk Anal 17:507–510, 1997

Slovic P, Monahan J, MacGregor DG: Violence risk assessment and risk communication: the effects of using actual cases, providing instruction, and employing probability versus frequency formats. Law Hum Behav 24:271–296, 2000

Stine GJ: Acquired Immune Deficiency Syndrome: Biological, Medical, Social, and Legal Issues, 2nd Edition. Englewood Cliffs, NJ, Prentice Hall, 1996

Wallsten TS, Budescu DV, Zwick R, et al: Preference and reasons for communicating probabilistic information in numerical or verbal terms. Bull Psychon Soc 31:135–138, 1993

Weinstein ND: What does it mean to understand a risk? Evaluating risk comprehension. J Natl Cancer Inst Monogr 25:15–20, 1999

Wilson DK, Purdon SE, Wallston KA: Compliance to health recommendations: a theoretical overview of message framing. Health Educ Res 3:161–171, 1988

Wright P: Designing healthcare advice for the public, in Handbook of Applied Cognition. Edited by Durso FT, Nickerson RS, Schvaneveldt RW, et al. New York, Wiley, 1999, pp 695–723

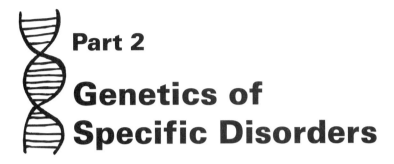

Part 2

Genetics of Specific Disorders

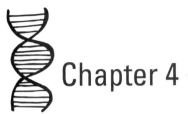

Chapter 4

Genetics of Childhood-Onset Psychiatric Disorders

S. Evelyn Stewart, M.D.
David L. Pauls, Ph.D.

Our aim in this chapter is to provide a clinically relevant resource to help clinicians interpret the exponential growth of information about genetics in childhood-onset psychiatric disorders. Since the late 1980s there have been major advances in our understanding of the phenomenology, prevalence, and development of childhood psychiatric disorders. In a recent epidemiology study, in which a representative sample of 1,420 children ages 9–13 years at baseline were evaluated annually until age 16 years, it was observed that the 3-month prevalence of any psychiatric disorder was on average 13.3% (Costello et al. 2003). However, during the study period, 36.7% of the participants were determined to have at least one diagnosable psychiatric disorder. The authors concluded that "the risk of having at least 1 psychiatric disorder by 16 years is much higher than point estimates would suggest." Clearly, childhood psychiatric disorders represent a major health concern. Considerable research has been focused on whether genetics plays a role in the manifestation of these conditions, and major advances have been reported for a significant number of childhood disorders.

It is beyond the scope of this chapter to discuss what is known about the genetics of each childhood-onset disorder; hence we focus on four of the more commonly studied illnesses: attention-deficit/hyperactivity disorder (ADHD), autistic disorder, obsessive-compulsive disorder (OCD), and Tourette's disorder. For each disorder, we describe the clinical phenotype and epidemiology. This description is followed by an overview of genetic epidemiology, including family studies, twin studies, and adoption studies. Subsequently, we summarize findings within molecular genetics, including findings of linkage studies, segregation analyses, and candidate gene studies. Finally, we discuss implications for genetic counseling, recurrence risk estimation, and communication of risks for each of these disorders.

Attention-Deficit/Hyperactivity Disorder

Clinical Phenotype and Epidemiology

Attention-deficit/hyperactivity disorder is a common neuropsychiatric and behavioral disorder of childhood onset. The prevalence of ADHD is 8%–12% worldwide (Faraone et al. 2003); it is among the most frequently observed neurobehavioral problems in the pediatric age group. Males are affected approximately four times as often as females (Staller and Faraone 2006). Although a variety of etiologies have been identified for some cases (Faraone 2004), in the majority of individuals no single etiological factor is evident. Subtypes of ADHD are defined in DSM-IV-TR (American Psychiatric Association 2000) by the presence of at least six symptoms of inattention, hyperactivity/impulsivity, or both. At least some of these symptoms must be present by age 7 years, and these symptoms must have a duration of at least 6 months. Furthermore, they must be present in more than one setting.

Genetic Epidemiology

Cumulative results from several lines of study suggest that genetic factors play an important etiological role in ADHD. This research includes twin and adoption studies, genomewide scans, and candidate gene studies. However, progress in this field has been limited by the presence of multiple genes of small effect rather than genes of major effect, by clinical heterogeneity of the disorder, and by the interaction between genes and the environment (Buitelaar 2005).

Family Studies

Family history studies provide support for the hypothesis that hyperactivity is familial (Faraone 2004). Early studies reported increased hyperactivity in relatives of hyperactive children versus relatives of control subjects, demonstrating that ADHD is vertically transmitted within families. In the first study in which relatives were directly assessed with structured interviews (Biederman et al. 1986), an increased rate of ADHD was found in relatives of ADHD males (31.5%), compared with relatives of control subjects (5.7%). Risk for ADHD among parents of ADHD-affected children was increased between two- and eightfold (Faraone and Biederman 2000). Two double-blind, case-control studies confirmed the familiality of ADHD while controlling for gender, socioeconomic status, and family intactness (Biederman et al. 1990, 1992; Faraone and Biederman 2000; Faraone et al. 1992). Increased risk for ADHD has also been associated with parental substance use disorders and low birth weight (Knopik et al. 2005; Wilens et al. 2002). Unfortunately, family studies cannot disentangle genetic and environmental causes of ADHD. Thus, twin and adoption studies can be used to determine whether genes account for familial transmission.

Twin Studies

Approximately 20 ADHD twin studies have been conducted to date in the United States, Europe, and Australia (Faraone 2004). The mean heritability estimate from these studies was calculated to be 76% (Faraone 2004). In a large study (102 monozygotic [MZ] and 111 same-sex dizygotic [DZ] twin-pairs), Goodman and Stevenson (1989) found higher concordance on inattentiveness and hyperactivity in same-sex MZ twins, compared with same-sex DZ twins. They concluded that heritability accounted for 30% to 50%, and common environment effects accounted for less than 30% of the variance in inattention and hyperactivity. Stevenson (1992) reported on a multiple regression analysis of data from 91 MZ and 105 same-sex DZ twins; the results demonstrated a significant genetic contribution to activity and attention levels. In more recent longitudinal twin studies, stability of ADHD symptoms over 5 years was found to be due to genetic influences (Larsson et al. 2004; Rietveld et al. 2004).

Adoption Studies

Adoption studies also suggest a genetic component in ADHD. Two such studies found lower levels of familial hyperactivity in adoptive versus control parents of different hyperactive children (Cantwell 1975; Morrison and Stewart 1973). Both of these studies are biased by the inability to compare family ADHD rates of the biological and adoptive parents of the same hyperactive children. However, in a study by Sprich et al. (2000) examining 25 adopted children and 50 control subjects, 6% of adoptive parents, 18% of biological parents, and 3% of control parents had ADHD. This research demonstrated that ADHD-affected children resemble families of their biological parents more than those of their adoptive parents or of control parents, supporting the role of genetics in this disorder.

Molecular Genetics

Segregation Analysis

In a segregation analysis of a quantitative ADHD trait, which involved 495 families ascertained for substance abuse in the father, a sex-dependent Mendelian co-dominant model was best fitting (Maher et al. 1999).

Linkage Scans

Several genomewide linkage scans and fine mapping studies of ADHD have been conducted to identify regions of chromosomes that contain causal ADHD genes. In 126 affected sib-pairs, four regions showed evidence of linkage (LOD>1.5): 5p12, 10q26, 12q23, and 16p13 (Fisher et al. 2002). Analyses of affected sib-pairs found evidence of linkage on 16p13 (LOD= 4) (Smalley et al. 2002) and on 17p11 (LOD=2.98) (Ogdie et al. 2003). In a fine-mapping study, high likelihood regions for susceptibility genes included 5p13, 6q12, 16p13, and 17p11 (Ogdie et al. 2004). Another affected sib-pair study found a peak at 7p13 (LOD=3.0) and also a peak (previously noted in autistic disorder) at 15q15 (LOD=3.5) (Bakker et al. 2003). A further genomewide scan from a Colombian population isolate implicated 8q12, 11q23, 4q13, 17p11, 12q23, and 8p23 (Arcos-Burgos et al. 2004), and a study of sib-pairs with ADHD and reading disability identified a region at 14q32 (single-point LOD=3.9) (Gayan et al. 2005).

Candidate Gene Studies

In studies of candidate genes influencing dopaminergic, noradrenergic, serotonergic, and other neurochemical systems, statistical association has been used to determine whether they influence ADHD susceptibility. A representative summary of these studies follows. The dopamine transporter (DAT) gene (*SLC6A3*) is perhaps the most-studied candidate gene in ADHD, as stimulants proven to effectively treat ADHD block the dopamine transporter. Meta-analyses have failed to support this gene as a likely candidate (Curran et al. 2001; Maher et al. 2002; Purper-Ouakil et al. 2005; Wohl et al. 2005), although a pooled study analysis demonstrated some effect (Faraone 2004). Meta-analyses (Maher et al. 2002; Purper-Ouakil et al. 2005; Wohl et al. 2005) and a pooled analysis (Faraone 2004) have reported associations with genes coding for dopamine receptors D_4 (*DRD4*) and D_5 (*DRD5*) and for dopamine beta-hydroxylase enzyme (DBH) but not with the catechol-*O*-methyltransferase gene (*COMT*). *DRD1IP* (Laurin et al. 2005) has also been associated with ADHD.

In the multitude of noradrenergic system gene studies to date, no association was demonstrated with receptor genes *ADRA2A* (Roman et al. 2003) or *ADRA2C* after Bonferroni correction (De Luca et al. 2004), but inconsistent association was reported for the norepinephrine transporter (NET) gene (*SLC6A2*) (De Luca et al. 2004; Xu et al. 2005; Yang et al. 2004).

Numerous serotonergic system candidate genes have been studied. The serotonin transporter (5-HTT) gene (*SLC6A4*), possibly the best-studied gene in psychiatric genetics, was significantly associated with ADHD in a pooled analysis (Faraone 2004). In the same analysis, a pooled odds ratio for all serotonin 5-HT$_{2A}$ receptor gene (*HTR2A*) studies was nonsignificant, but significant association was found with the serotonin 5-HT$_{1B}$ receptor gene (*HTR1B*) (Faraone 2004). Few positive or negative studies of the gene coding for the enzyme tryptophan hydroxylase (TPH) have been conducted (Sheehan et al. 2005; Walitza et al. 2005).

Other genes that have been studied in ADHD include acetylcholine receptor genes (*CHRNA4* and *CHRNA7*) (Todd et al. 2003), a glutamate receptor gene (*GRIN2A*) (Adams et al. 2004; Turic et al. 2004), and genes coding for synapotosome-associated protein 25 kDa (SNAP-25) (Mill et al. 2004), brain-derived neurotrophic factor (BDNF) (Kent et al. 2005), interleukin-1 (IL-1) (Misener et al. 2004), and myelin oligodendrocyte glycoprotein (MOG) (Barr et al. 2001).

Genetic Counseling, Risk Estimation, Communication, and Genetic Testing

Given the lack of definitive molecular genetic findings, genetic counseling for ADHD must rely on empiric risk figures that have been obtained from family studies. Before providing any information about risk to prospective offspring, the genetic counselor should obtain a complete and comprehensive family history for the presence of ADHD in all relatives in the extended family. The accuracy of this history is critical, although it is often difficult and/or impossible for the counselee to provide reliable information about childhood behaviors for aunts and uncles, first cousins, and grandparents. It is optimal to obtain this kind of information from family members who are contemporaries of the relatives in question. Obviously direct interviews are the best way to obtain reliable information from all relatives, but those interviews are generally beyond the scope of the counseling session. In that case, it is probably most conservative to assume a positive family history and provide the empiric risk estimates for the recurrence of ADHD, explaining that the actual risk estimate is impossible to obtain for the specific individual.

For ADHD, the relative risk for the recurrence of the disorder is approximately two to three times greater than the risk in the general population. Relative risk is defined as the probability that an individual who has an affected relative will develop the disorder, compared with the prevalence of the condition in the general population. The population prevalence of ADHD has been estimated to be about 8%–12% in the United States population. Thus, the chance that an individual who has an affected relative with ADHD will develop ADHD is approximately 15%–30%. Unfortunately, more precise estimates cannot be given because there is no laboratory-based test that can identify individuals at risk on the basis of biological differences. As several Mendelian disorders, chromosome anomalies, and mitochondrial disorders may include ADHD as one manifestation (e.g., fragile X syndrome, Klinefelter's syndrome, neurofibromatosis, Prader-Willi syndrome, Smith-Magenis syndrome, Turner's syndrome, tuberous sclerosis, Williams syndrome, and X-linked adrenoleukodystrophy) (Bastain et al. 2002), it is imperative that the presence of such diagnoses be ruled out prior to communicating risk estimates based on empiric risk figures (see Table 4–1). In most instances a specific underlying genetic diagnosis would lead to a significantly different recurrence risk estimate and differing availability of preimplantation diagnosis and/or prenatal diagnosis.

Autistic Disorder

Clinical Phenotype and Epidemiology

Autistic disorder is a severe childhood developmental disorder characterized by unusual behaviors and difficulties in the areas of social interaction, cognition, and communicative abilities (Rutter et al. 1994; Volkmar et al. 1994). Most individuals with autistic disorder also exhibit mental retardation (Bull et al. 1998). Restricted patterns of interest, unusual responses to the environment, and adaptive deficits are common and are often severe to profound (Volkmar et al. 1993, 1994).

In early epidemiological studies autistic disorder rates of 10 cases per 10,000 children were reported (Bryson et al. 1988). The results of more recent studies have suggested that the prevalence is higher, with rates from 0.7 to 21.1 (median 4–5) per 10,000 in nearly 30 studies (Volkmar and Pauls 2003). Even higher rates have been noted more recently—as many as 60 per 10,000 children—along with the concern that autism is increasing in frequency. These different prevalence estimates may be due to methodological differences, growing public awareness, and, possibly most important of all, changes in DSM diagnostic criteria (Wing and Potter 2002). Currently, at least one in 1,000 children in the population will receive a diagnosis of autistic disorder (Fombonne 2003).

Autistic disorder is three to four times more common among males than among females. One possible explanation for this difference is that males have a lower threshold than females for brain dysfunction, suggesting that more severe brain dysfunction or higher genetic loading is required for a female to develop autistic disorder. The relevant hypotheses predict that to develop autistic disorder, females would probably have more severe cognitive impairment, and this pattern has been noted (Dawson et al. 1998).

Genetic Epidemiology

Family Studies

The evidence for a genetic contribution to autistic disorder comes from twin and family studies (Santangelo and Folstein 1999). Data from several epidemiological twin and family studies have been previously reviewed (Folstein and Rosen-Sheidley 2001; Lamb et al. 2002; Rutter 2000). Collectively, these studies provide substantial evidence that autism spectrum disorders are among the most heritable complex disorders. Family studies have consistently shown that the rate of autistic disorder among siblings of autistic probands is significantly higher than the population prevalence (Bolton et al. 1994; Jorde et al. 1991; Piven et al. 1990; Smalley et al. 1991; Szatmari et al. 1993). Although the actual recurrence risk of autistic disorder for siblings is low (2%–7%), the relative risk is 50–200 times higher than the population prevalence of autistic disorder (Bailey et al. 1996).

Twin Studies

All twin studies of autistic disorder (Bailey et al. 1995; Folstein and Rutter 1977; Steffenburg et al. 1989) have demonstrated that the concordance rates for MZ twins are significantly higher than those for DZ twins. With a concordance rate in MZ twins of 60%–90% (Bacchelli and Maestrini 2006), the heritability of autistic disorder is greater than 90% (Volkmar and Pauls 2003).

Molecular Genetics

Segregation Analyses

Although the genetic basis of autistic disorder is well established, the mode of genetic transmission is not yet known. Complex segregation analyses do not point to one unambiguous model (Gurling 1986; Jorde et al. 1991; Ritvo et al. 1985; Tsai et al. 1981). Jorde et al. (1991) analyzed data from 185 families ascertained in an epidemiological survey and found that the transmission pattern was inconsistent with single-gene inheritance. Subsequently, Pickles et al. (1995) used a latent-class approach to examine twin data (Bailey et al. 1995) and family history data (Bolton et al. 1994) and reported evidence of epistatic oligogenic inheritance.

TABLE 4–1. Summary of prominent genetic findings for childhood psychiatric disorders to date

Disorder	Population prevalence (%)	Family study recurrence risk (%)	Twin study heritability/ concordance rates (%)	Linkage study peak regions	Candidate genes with prior positive reports[a]	Genetic syndromes/ diagnoses with similar symptoms[b]
ADHD	8%–12%	32% (male proband) (OR=2–8)	76%	LOD>3: 5q15, 7p13, 16p13 LOD>2: 9q33	*DAT/SLC6A3, DRD4, DRD5, DBH, HTR1B, 5-HTT, SNAP-25*	Fragile X syndrome, neurofibromatosis, tuberous sclerosis, Klinefelter's syndrome, Turner's syndrome, Prader-Willi syndrome, Williams syndrome, Smith-Magenis syndrome, X-linked adrenoleuko-dystrophy
Autistic disorder	0.05%	2%–7% (RR=50–200)	>90%	LOD>3: 15q Nonparametric linkage>3: 1q, 2q, 7q, 21q	*RELN, SLC6A4, NLGN3, NLGN4X*	Fragile X syndrome, Rett syndrome, tuberous sclerosis, Down syndrome, Sanfilippo's syndrome, phenylketonuria, Smith-Magenis syndrome, Cohen syndrome, Angelman's syndrome, Smith-Lemli-Opitz syndrome, adenylsuccinate lyase deficiency

TABLE 4–1. Summary of prominent genetic findings for childhood psychiatric disorders to date (*continued*)

Disorder	Population prevalence (%)	Family study recurrence risk (%)	Twin study heritability/ concordance rates (%)	Linkage study peak regions	Candidate genes with prior positive reports[a]	Genetic syndromes/ diagnoses with similar symptoms[b]
OCD	1%–3%	8% (OR=4)	4.5%–6.5% (children) 27%–47% (adults)	LOD>2: 3q, 9p	*SLC1A1, 5-HTT, GRIN2B, DLGAP3*	Velocardiofacial syndrome, homocystinuria, Prader-Willi syndrome, Williams syndrome
Tourette's disorder	0.01%–1%	7%–18% (OR=5–10)	53%–56% MZ vs. 8% DZ	LOD>3: 11q LOD>2: 4q, 8p, 17q −log(P)>2: 3q, 4p, 6p −log(P) =4.42: 2p	*DRD2, DRD3, DRD4, DBH,* tryptophan oxidase	Chromosomal anomalies

Note.   ADHD=attention-deficit/hyperactivity disorder;   DZ=dyzygotic twin concordance;   MZ=monozygotic twin concordance; OCD=obsessive-compulsive disorder; OR=odds ratio; RR=relative risk.

[a]It is important to note that candidate gene studies often suffer from misleading false positive findings. Few, if any, candidate genes have been consistently replicated in childhood-onset psychiatric illnesses.

[b]Consider genetic testing only if symptoms or family history is suggestive.

Linkage Scans

Autistic disorder linkage studies have been limited to families of affected sib-pairs, given the complex inheritance and the small size of autism families. Since 1998, more than 10 genome scans for autistic disorder have been reported (Bacchelli and Maestrini 2006). Most have identified a region of interest on chromosome 7q (designated as AUTS1). However, the actual linkage peaks and significance of the findings vary considerably across studies. In a recent meta-analysis of six genome scans, the 7q22–q32 region reached genomewide significance (Trikalinos et al. 2006). Two other regions that have been implicated by more than one group are on chromosomes 2q and 17q.

Independent of the genome screens, there is evidence that the region on chromosome 15q11–13 contains an autistic disorder–related gene. Numerous cases with chromosomal duplications or deletions in this region have been reported in association with the autistic disorder phenotype (Baker et al. 1994; Bundey et al. 1994; Cook et al. 1998; Gillberg et al. 1991; Schroer et al. 1998). Linkage disequilibrium was also reported between autistic disorder and the region of *GABRB3*, the gamma-aminobutyric acid (GABA) receptor subunit gene (Cook et al. 1998; Martin et al. 2000; Nurmi et al. 2001; Shao et al. 2002). The plethora of potential susceptibility loci identified and the lack of success in narrowing the linkage intervals using molecular cytogenetic and/or linkage approaches have resulted in many investigative teams launching candidate gene studies.

Candidate Gene Studies

Over the last 10 years, more than 100 candidate genes for autistic disorder have been reported. Unfortunately, no gene has yet been irrefutably identified. A comprehensive evaluation of these studies is beyond the scope of this review. Bacchelli and Maestrini (2006) provided a partial review focusing on four examples: the reelin gene (*RELN*), the 5-HTT gene (*SLC6A4*), and two neuroligin genes (*NLGN3* and *NLGN4X*)–and summarized research examining these genes and the strengths and weaknesses of the studies. The authors noted that these genes have been examined by many research groups and represent important models for illustrating the potential problems of candidate gene studies. In this review, examples also highlight the difficulty of interpreting current candidate gene studies and the unfortunate irreproducibility of results in autistic disorder. The key problems with candidate gene studies include 1) differences in ascertainment and inclusion criteria of patients and families, 2) clinical heterogeneity, 3) etiological heterogeneity (both genetic and nongenetic factors probably contribute to the manifestation of autistic disorder), 4) low statistical power of most studies reported to date, and 5) the complexity of the underlying genetic and nongenetic mechanisms.

Genetic Counseling, Risk Estimation, Communication, and Genetic Testing

Given the lack of definitive molecular genetic findings, genetic counseling for autistic disorder must rely primarily on empiric risk figures that have been obtained from family studies. As noted for ADHD, before providing any information about risk to prospective offspring, the genetic counselor should obtain a complete and comprehensive family history for the presence of autistic disorder and related conditions in all relatives in the extended family. The accuracy of this history is critical, although it is often difficult and/or impossible for the counselee to provide reliable information about childhood behaviors for aunts, uncles, first cousins, and grandparents. It is optimal to obtain this kind of information from family members who are contemporaries of the relatives in question. Obviously direct interviews are the best way to obtain reliable information from all relatives, but such interviews are generally beyond the scope of the counseling session. In that case, it is probably most conservative to assume a positive family history and provide the empiric risk estimates for the recurrence of autistic disorder, explaining that the actual risk estimate is impossible to obtain for the specific individual. For autistic disorder, the relative risk for the recurrence of the disorder is approximately 40–50 times greater than the risk in the general population.

As with ADHD, a number of genetic diseases, including Mendelian disorders and cytogenetic abnormalities (translocations, insertions, and deletions), are associated with autistic-like features. Thus, it is critical to rule out these disorders as possible causes of the presenting behaviors. Autistic behaviors are included among the symptoms of fragile X syndrome, Rett syndrome, tuberous sclerosis, duplication of 15q11–q13, Down syndrome, Sanfilippo's syndrome, *MECP2*-related disorders, phenylketonuria, Smith-Magenis syndrome, 22q13 deletion, adenylosuccinate lyase deficiency, Cohen syndrome, Smith-Lemli-Opitz syndrome, and Angelman's syndrome (Cohen et al. 2005). Thus, genetic testing may be a necessary first step in the counseling process to rule out any cases that may be due to single gene disorders or cytogenetic abnormalities (see Table 4–1). If such an abnormality is present, empiric risk estimates would not apply and in such cases, preimplantation diagnosis and prenatal diagnosis would also become viable options.

Obsessive-Compulsive Disorder

Clinical Phenotype and Epidemiology

Obsessive-compulsive disorder is listed as an anxiety disorder in DSM-IV-TR. It is characterized by repetitive thoughts, images, impulses, or actions that are distressing or time-consuming or that affect functioning. Obsessions may be focused on aggressive, sexual, religious, symmetry, and contamination-related thoughts. Compulsions include washing, counting, checking, repeating, hoarding, ordering, and mental rituals. Patients with OCD frequently experience more than one symptom type at one time, and symptoms change over the course of the illness. Although OCD was previously thought to be rare in children and adolescents, research over the last two decades has identified this disorder as one of the most common of all psychiatric illnesses affecting youth. Lifetime prevalence in pediatric populations has been reported to be in the range of 1%–3% in epidemiological studies (Stewart et al. 2003, 2004).

Genetic Epidemiology

Family Studies

Evidence for the importance of genetic factors in OCD has come from twin and family aggregation studies (Pauls and Tourette Syndrome Association International Consortium on Genetics 2001; Pauls et al. 2002). Early family studies of obsessive-compulsive neurosis reported rates in relatives ranging between 4.5% and 19.8% (Brown 1942; Kringlen 1965; Lewis 1935). Several adult studies used a control group and found higher rates among relatives of cases (Nestadt et al. 2000b; Pauls et al. 1995). The findings of higher rates were confirmed in a meta-analysis of five OCD family studies involving 1,209 first-degree relatives (Hettema et al. 2001), in which a significantly increased risk of OCD was found among relatives of probands (8.2%) versus control subjects (2.0%) (odds ratio=4.0). In studies ascertained through children or adolescents, familial risk appears to be even higher (9.5%–17%) than that for later-onset OCD (Bellodi et al. 1992; Chabane et al. 2005; do Rosario-Campos et al. 2005; Lenane et al. 1990; Leonard et al. 1992; Reddy et al. 2001; Riddle et al. 1990). In studies by Nestadt, Pauls and others, approximately one-half of the OCD cases were familial (Cavallini et al. 1999; Eapen et al. 1993; Nicolini et al. 1993). These findings, together with results from twin studies, provide compelling evidence that genetic factors play an important role in the manifestation of some forms of OCD.

Twin Studies

Although twin studies can provide compelling evidence for the role of genetic factors in complex neuropsychiatric disorders, no large systematic twin studies have focused exclusively on OCD. In 1986, Rasmussen and Tsuang (1986) summarized the twin OCD literature and reported that 32 of 51 (63%) unconfirmed and 13 of 20 (65%) confirmed MZ twins included in previous studies were concordant for OCD. However, the extent to which genetic factors contributed was not possible to decipher, because no data for DZ twins were presented. Subsequent twin studies found rate differences as high as 40% between MZ and DZ concordance (Andrews et al. 1990). In a more recent review of OCD twin studies starting in 1929, the authors concluded that obsessive-compulsive symptoms are heritable, with genetic influences in children ranging from 45% to 65% (van Grootheest et al. 2005) and in adults ranging from 27% to 47% (van Grootheest et al. 2005). However, twin studies do not provide conclusive evidence that unique genes are important for the manifestation of OCD.

Molecular Genetics

Molecular genetic studies have begun to provide evidence that specific genes may play a role in the manifestation of OCD.

Segregation Analyses

Several segregation analyses have been conducted examining the familial patterns of OCD transmission. In several studies, a dominant model provided a better fit than the other Mendelian models (Cavallini et al. 1999; Hanna et al. 2005; Nestadt et al. 2000a). In the others, neither an autosomal dominant nor an autosomal recessive model could be ruled out (Nicolini et al. 1991), and only the model of no transmission could be rejected (Alsobrook et al. 1999). Results of these combined segregation analyses suggest that the transmission of OCD in families is difficult to model. However, the most parsimonious solution suggests that there are at least some genes of major effect. It is highly likely that OCD is an oligogenic disorder, with several genes important for the expression of the syndrome.

Linkage Scans

At the present time, four linkage studies for OCD or OCD symptoms have been published (Hanna et al. 2002; Shugart et al. 2006; Willour et al. 2004; Zhang et al. 2002). Hanna and colleagues (2002) completed a genomewide scan of 56 individuals in seven families and found suggestive evidence for linkage to markers on chromosomes 9p (LOD=2.25 before fine mapping and LOD=1.97 after fine mapping) and 19q (LOD=1.73). Willour et al.

(2004) replicated findings with signals that lie within 0.5 cM (<350 kb) of Hanna's original 9p24 linkage peak (heterogeneity LOD=2.26). In a study focusing on the hoarding component of OCD in sib-pairs affected with Tourette's disorder, Zhang et al. (2002) found linkages to three regions in three chromosomal regions (4q, 5q, and 17q). Most recently, a linkage scan was conducted on the Johns Hopkins sib-pair study sample, with findings suggestive for susceptibility loci on chromosomes 3q, 7p, 15q, 6q, and 1q (Shugart et al. 2006). The maximum LOD score was on 3q and was equal to 2.67, which is not at the level of genomewide significance.

Candidate Gene Studies and Animal Models

Several central neurotransmitters, including serotonin, dopamine, and glutamate, and their associated enzymes have been implicated in the pathophysiology of OCD, as have the opioidergic and neuropeptidergic systems. Related candidate gene research has been thoroughly reviewed elsewhere (Pauls and Stewart, in press), and representative studies are referenced in this section.

The efficacy of serotonin reuptake inhibitors in OCD has led to many serotonin-related candidate gene studies. Serotonin-related genes considered in OCD, including genes coding for 5-HTT (Hanna et al. 1998; Mundo et al. 2002) and receptors 5-HT_{2A} (Enoch et al. 2001), 5-HT_{2B} (Kim et al. 2000), 5-HT_{2C} (Cavallini et al. 1998), and 5-HT_{1B} (Mundo et al. 2002), have yielded some positive results, although predominantly negative results have been found. In a recent study meriting replication, a 5-HTT gain-of-function variant was associated with OCD (Hu et al. 2006). The gene for the serotonin enzyme TPH does not appear to be associated with OCD (Walitza et al. 2004).

Dopamine-related genes studied in OCD include the dopamine transporter (DAT1) gene (Billett et al. 1998; Rowe et al. 1998) and *DRD2, DRD3,* and *DRD4* (Cruz et al. 1997). Dopamine-enzyme-related genes, including those for COMT (Alsobrook et al. 2002), adjacent regions (Kinnear et al. 2001), and monoamine oxidase A (MAO A) have all been studied (Camarena et al. 2001). Monoamine oxidase A low-activity alleles were associated with OCD in females only (Camarena et al. 2001), and MAO A high-activity and COMT low-activity alleles were associated with OCD in males only (Karayiorgou et al. 1999).

Glutamate-related genes reportedly associated with OCD include *GRIK* (Delorme et al. 2004; Stewart et al. 2007b), *GRIN2B* (Arnold et al. 2004; Stewart et al. 2007b), and *SLC1A1* (Arnold et al. 2006; Dickel et al. 2006; Stewart et al. 2007a). Other genes that have been associated with OCD include the white matter–related genes *OLIG2* (Stewart et al. 2007c) and *MOG* (Zai et al. 2004).

Given the complexity of the OCD phenotype, it is unlikely that any of these candidate genes have a major effect on the disorder, and few if any genes have been consistently replicated in large samples. Because current therapeutic agents have major influence on the serotonergic and dopaminergic systems, and may influence glutamate, some of the genes associated with these systems may be important for effective treatment, but that does not necessarily imply that those same genes would be involved in the etiology of OCD.

Very recently, a potential mouse model for OCD was proposed. This model was created by "knocking out" the *SAPAP3* (or *DLGAP3*) gene, involved in glutamate signal transduction within the basal ganglia. When the gene was inactivated, OCD-like excessive grooming behavior and increased anxiety emerged; these changes were reversed with the addition of a selective serotonin reuptake inhibitor medication, frequently used in OCD (Welch et al. 2007). Reversal also occurred with selective expression of *SAPAP3* in the striatum.

Genetic Counseling, Risk Estimation, Communication, and Genetic Testing

As is the case for ADHD and autism, genetic counseling for OCD must rely on empiric risk figures that have been obtained from family studies. To date there have been no replicated findings implicating a specific causal mutation for OCD. Again, before providing any information about risk to prospective offspring, the genetic counselor should obtain a complete and comprehensive family history for the presence of OCD and related conditions in all relatives in the extended family. As indicated for ADHD, it is again critical to obtain accurate information about all members of the extended family, and this may prove even more difficult for OCD, because many affected individuals are secretive about their symptoms and hide them from family members. Again, direct interviews are the best way to obtain reliable information from all relatives, but interviews of that type are generally beyond the scope of the counseling session. In the absence of any family data for OCD, it is best to assume a positive family history and provide the empiric risk estimates for the recurrence of OCD, explaining that the actual risk estimate is impossible to obtain for the specific individual. For OCD, the relative risk for the recurrence of the disorder is approximately five to six times greater than the risk in the general population. The population prevalence of OCD has been estimated to be about 2% in the United States population. Thus, the chance that an individual who has an affected relative with OCD will develop OCD is approximately 10%–12%.

Unfortunately, more precise estimates cannot be given because we have no laboratory-based test that can identify individuals at risk on the basis of biological differences. There has been a report of OCD in velocardiofacial (22q11 deletion) syndrome, and if clinically suggested, this syndrome should be ruled out with laboratory investigation (Gothelf et al. 2004). Obsessive-compulsive disorder may also manifest in individuals with other underlying genetic disorders, such as homocystinuria, Prader-Willi syndrome, and Williams syndrome. As noted with ADHD and autistic disorder, such diagnoses should be ruled out before risk estimates based on empiric risk figures are communicated to families (see Table 4–1).

Gilles de la Tourette's Syndrome

Clinical Phenotype and Epidemiology

Gilles de la Tourette's syndrome, or Tourette's disorder as it is called in DSM-IV-TR, is a neuropsychiatric disorder emerging early in development. Tourette's disorder is characterized by the presence of both multiple motor and one or more vocal tics that 1) occur many times a day (usually in bouts) nearly every day or intermittently through a period of more than 1 year, 2) have onset before age 18 years, and 3) are not due to other neurological causes (American Psychiatric Association 2000). Most patients with Tourette's disorder have symptoms and severity that change over time, with a typical diminution of symptoms in adolescence (Leckman et al. 1998). For nearly a century after its original description in 1885, Tourette's disorder was considered to be a rare neuropsychiatric disorder. However, research over the last three decades has found that it is much more common than previously thought; it is now estimated to affect between 0.5% and 1% of the general population (Pauls 2003). It is also three times more common in males than in females (Stewart et al. 2003).

Genetic Epidemiology

Family studies of Tourette's disorder have demonstrated that it is a familial disorder (Hebebrand et al. 1997; Pauls et al. 1991b; Walkup et al. 1996), and twin studies have provided additional evidence that genetic factors are important in its expression (Hyde et al. 1992; Price et al. 1985).

Family Studies

In 10 family studies conducted since 1980, rates of Tourette's disorder in relatives ranged between 1.9% and 17.9% (Scharf and Pauls 2007). An approximate 5- to 10-fold increased risk exists in first-degree relatives of probands with Tourette's disorder, compared with the general population (7%–18% and 1%–2%, respectively). Patterns within Tourette's disorder and OCD families (Pauls and Leckman 1986; Pauls et al. 1986, 1991b) suggest that there is a genetic relationship between these illnesses (do Rosario-Campos et al. 2005; Pauls et al. 1995). There may also be a relationship with increased ADHD in relatives affected by Tourette's disorder (Stewart et al. 2006). Furthermore, when these diagnoses are considered as a spectrum, bilineal transmission is commonly observed in families of Tourette's disorder probands (McMahon et al. 1996; Walkup et al. 1996).

Twin Studies

Evidence from twin studies supports the belief that Tourette's disorder has a strong genetic component. As summarized by Scharf and Pauls (2007), concordance rates for Tourette's disorder in MZ and DZ twins were 53%–56% and 8%, respectively, in the two twin studies conducted to date (Hyde et al. 1992; Price et al. 1985). For combined TD and other tic disorders, these rates were 77%–94% and 23%, respectively. Both studies indicate that there must be nongenetic factors that either contribute directly to the Tourette's disorder phenotype or reduce the expressivity of Tourette's disorder susceptibility genes.

Adoption Studies

In the one adoption study conducted for Tourette's disorder to date, tic frequencies were compared in first-degree relatives of 22 adopted versus 641 nonadopted Tourette's disorder patients (Shapiro et al. 1988). Rates of Tourette's disorder or other tic disorders in relatives were 0% in the adoption families and 35% in the nonadoption families. In the two adoption families for whom data on biological relatives were available, both had a relative with tics. This finding suggests that the increased frequency of Tourette's disorder in twins and other family members of Tourette's disorder probands is due to shared inherited factors, rather than shared environmental factors.

Molecular Genetics

Segregation Analyses

Early segregation analyses of Tourette's disorder family study data consistently found autosomal dominant inheritance (Eapen et al. 1993; Pauls and Leckman 1986), but the results of subsequent studies (Hasstedt et al. 1995; Pauls et al. 1991a; Seuchter et al. 2000; Walkup et al. 1996) suggested that the mode of inheritance is more complex. Although the mode of inheritance of Tourette's disorder is not simple, it is clear that it has a significant genetic basis and that some individuals with Tourette's disorder, chronic tic disorder, and OCD manifest variant expressions of the same genetic factors. A number of investigators have documented a wide range of phenotypes that unfold throughout development. A more complete understanding of the genetic basis of Tourette's and related disorders and of the role of relevant genotypes will be vital for understanding this developmental process.

Linkage Scans

Several genome scans have been completed on small Tourette's disorder samples. The Tourette Syndrome Association International Consortium for Genetics ("A Complete Genome Scan in Sib Pairs Affected by Gilles de la Tourette Syndrome" 1999) reported suggestive evidence for three genomic regions on 4p, 4q, and 8p from analyses of 92 sib-pairs from 76 affected sib-pair families. In a South African Afrikaner sample, association was reported with markers on chromosomes 2p11, 8q22, and 11q23–24 (Simonic et al. 1998, 2001). A follow-up linkage study in one large French Canadian kindred yielded a lod score of 3.24 on 11q23 (Merette et al. 2000). In a multigenerational family study, promising results were found for two regions (19p13.3 and 5p13–q11.2) (Barr et al. 1999). A region on 17q containing genes *CD7* and *TBCD* has also shown positive linkage results in three multigenerational families (Paschou et al. 2004). The most recent linkage study, which included 304 affected sib-pair families and 18 large multigenerational families, yielded significant evidence for linkage to a region on chromosome 2p (Tourette Syndrome Association International Consortium for Genetics 2007). Work is currently under way to replicate this result.

Candidate Gene Studies

A number of candidate gene studies have also been completed for Tourette's disorder, including studies of genes related to dopamine, noradrenaline, serotonin, and GABA (Scharf and Pauls 2007). Because dopamine antagonists (e.g., haloperidol and pimozide) have been the mainstay of recent therapy for tic disorders, the majority of candidate genes studied involved neuronal dopaminergic function (e.g., receptors and/or transporters). Twenty different candidate genes have been evaluated by linkage analyses in large, multigenerational Tourette's disorder families from the United States, Canada, and Great Britain (Scharf and Pauls, submitted for publication). None of the genes were found to be linked to either Tourette's disorder or Tourette's disorder/chronic motor tics. In addition, 16 different candidate genes were analyzed in case-control or family-based association studies of Tourette's disorder patients. Seven genes were reported to have positive associations in at least one study (*DRD2, DRD3, DRD4, DAT1, DBH, MAOA,* and the tryptophan oxidase gene). However, no replicated association has been found for any of these genes other than *DAT1* (Tamok et al. 2007; Yoon et al. 2007).

Other approaches have been employed in the search for Tourette's disorder susceptibility loci. In a recent study, an association was found between the slit and Trk-like 1 gene (*SLITRK1*) and Tourette's disorder (Abelson et al. 2005). *SLITRK1* was examined because of its proximity to a de novo chromosomal inversion on chromosome 13q31.1 in a child with Tourette's disorder. A frameshift mutation and two independent occurrences of the identical variant in the binding site for microRNA hsa-miR-189 were identified among 174 unrelated probands. These variants were not observed in 3,600 control chromosomes. In addition, *SLITRK1* mRNA and hsa-miR-189 showed an overlapping expression pattern in brain regions previously implicated in Tourette's disorder. It has been suggested that this may be a rare variant associated with a small number of Tourette's disorder cases.

Genetic Counseling, Risk Estimation, Communication, and Genetic Testing

Again, as with ADHD, autistic disorder, and OCD, there is no definitive molecular genetic evidence for genes that cause Tourette's disorder. Thus, genetic counseling for Tourette's disorder must rely on empiric risk figures that have been obtained from family studies. Once again, in the absence of any family data, it is best to assume a positive family history and provide the empiric risk estimates for the recurrence of Tourette's disorder, explaining that the actual risk estimate is impossible to obtain for the specific individual. For Tourette's disorder, the relative risk for the recurrence of the disorder is approximately 10–20 times greater than the risk in the general population. The population prevalence of Tourette's disorder has been estimated to range between 1/1000 to 1/100 in the general population. Thus, the chance that an individual who has an affected relative with Tourette's disorder will develop the disorder is approximately 10%–15%, and between 25%–30% if chronic tics and OCD are assumed to be part of the inherited spectrum of Tourette's disorder in these families. Unfortunately, more precise estimates cannot be given because we have no laboratory-based test that can identify individuals at risk on the basis of biological differences. Since there are reports of chromosome anomalies in individuals with Tourette's disorder, karyotyping should be considered if clinically indicated.

Conclusions

Despite major advances in our understanding of childhood-onset psychiatric disorders in recent decades, the complex genetic basis of these disorders remains incompletely understood. This chapter focused on four of the more commonly studied childhood-onset psychiatric disorders: ADHD, autistic disorder, OCD, and Tourette's disorder. Implications for genetic counseling, recurrence risk estimation, and communication of risk were discussed for each of these disorders. Findings regarding population prevalence, recurrence estimates based on family studies, and heritability rates are summarized in Table 4–1. Linkage scan peak regions, candidate genes of interest, and similar presenting genetic syndromes to be considered for these disorders are also summarized in the table.

References

Abelson JF, Kwan KY, O'Roak BJ, et al: Sequence variants in SLITRK1 are associated with Tourette's syndrome. Science 310:317–320, 2005

Adams J, Crosbie J, Wigg K, et al: Glutamate receptor, ionotropic, N-methyl-D-aspartate 2A (GRIN2A) gene as a positional candidate for attention-deficit/hyperactivity disorder in the 16p13 region. Mol Psychiatry 9:494–499, 2004

Alsobrook JP II, Leckman JF, Goodman WK, et al: Segregation analysis of obsessive-compulsive disorder using symptom-based factor scores. Am J Med Genet 88:669–675, 1999

Alsobrook JP II, Zohar AH, Leboyer M, et al: Association between the COMT locus and obsessive-compulsive disorder in females but not males. Am J Med Genet B Neuropsychiatr Genet 114:116–120, 2002

American Psychiatric Association: Diagnostic and Statistical Manual of Mental Disorders, 4th Edition, Text Revision. Washington, DC, American Psychiatric Association, 2000

Andrews G, Stewart G, Allen R, et al: The genetics of six neurotic disorders: a twin study. J Affect Disord 19:23–29, 1990

Arcos-Burgos M, Castellanos FX, Konecki D, et al: Pedigree disequilibrium test (PDT) replicates association and linkage between DRD4 and ADHD in multigenerational and extended pedigrees from a genetic isolate. Mol Psychiatry 9:252–259, 2004

Arnold PD, Rosenberg DR, Mundo E, et al: Association of a glutamate (NMDA) subunit receptor gene (GRIN2B) with obsessive-compulsive disorder: a preliminary study. Psychopharmacology (Berl) 174:530–538, 2004

Arnold PD, Sicard T, Burroughs E, et al: Transported gene (SLC1A1) associated with obsessive-compulsive disorder. Arch Gen Psychiatry 63:769–776, 2006

Bacchelli E, Maestrini E: Autism spectrum disorders: molecular genetic advances. Am J Med Genet C Semin Med Genet 142:13–23, 2006

Bailey A, Le Couteur A, Gottesman I, et al: Autism as a strongly genetic disorder: evidence from a British twin study. Psychol Med 25:63–77, 1995

Bailey A, Phillips W, Rutter M: Autism: towards an integration of clinical, genetic, neuropsychological, and neurobiological perspectives. J Child Psychol Psychiatry 37:89–126, 1996

Baker P, Piven J, Schwartz S, et al: Brief report: duplication of chromosome 15q11–13 in two individuals with autistic disorder. J Autism Dev Disord 24:529–535, 1994

Bakker SC, van der Meulen EM, Buitelaar JK, et al: A whole-genome scan in 164 Dutch sib pairs with attention-deficit/hyperactivity disorder: suggestive evidence for linkage on chromosomes 7p and 15q. Am J Hum Genet 72:1251–1260, 2003

Barr CL, Wigg KG, Pakstis AJ, et al: Genome scan for linkage to Gilles de la Tourette syndrome. Am J Med Genet 88:437–445, 1999

Barr CL, Shulman R, Wigg K, et al: Linkage study of polymorphisms in the gene for myelin oligodendrocyte glycoprotein located on chromosome 6p and attention deficit hyperactivity disorder. Am J Med Genet 105:250–254, 2001

Bastain TM, Lewczyk CM, Sharp WS, et al: Cytogenetic abnormalities in attention-deficit/hyperactivity disorder. J Am Acad Child Adolesc Psychiatry 4:806–810, 2002

Bellodi L, Sciuto G, Diaferia G, et al: Psychiatric disorders in the families of patients with obsessive-compulsive disorder. Psychiatry Res 42:111–120, 1992

Biederman J, Munir K, Knee D, et al: A family study of patients with attention deficit disorder and normal controls. J Psychiatr Res 20:263–274, 1986

Biederman J, Faraone SV, Keenan K, et al: Family genetic and psychosocial risk factors in DSM-III attention deficit disorder. J Am Acad Child Adolesc Psychiatry 29:526–533, 1990

Biederman J, Faraone SV, Keenan K, et al: Further evidence for family genetic risk factors in attention deficit hyperactivity disorder: patterns of comorbidity in probands and relatives psychiatrically and pediatrically referred samples. Arch Gen Psychiatry 49:728–738, 1992

Billett EA, Richter MA, Sam F, et al: Investigation of dopamine system genes in obsessive-compulsive disorder. Psychiatr Genet 8:163–169, 1998

Bolton P, Macdonald H, Pickles A, et al: A case-control family history study of autism. J Child Psychol Psychiatry 35:877–900, 1994

Brown FW: Heredity in the psychoneuroses. Proc R Soc Med 35:785–790, 1942

Bryson SE, Clark BS, Smith IM: First report of a Canadian epidemiological study of autistic syndromes. J Child Psychol Psychiatry 29:433–445, 1988

Buitelaar JK: ADHD: strategies to unravel its genetic architecture. J Neural Transm Suppl 2005, pp 1–17

Bull LN, van Eijk MJ, Pawlikowska L, et al: A gene encoding a P-type ATPase mutated in two forms of hereditary cholestasis. Nat Genet 18:219–224, 1998

Bundey S, Hardy C, Vickers S, et al: Duplication of the 15q11–13 region in a patient with autism, epilepsy, and ataxia. Dev Med Child Neurol 36:736–742, 1994

Camarena B, Rinetti G, Cruz C, et al: Additional evidence that genetic variation of MAO-A gene supports a gender subtype in obsessive-compulsive disorder. Am J Med Gen B Neuropsychiatr Genet 105:279–282, 2001

Cantwell DP: Genetics of hyperactivity. J Child Psychol Psychiatry 16:261–264, 1975

Cavallini MC, Di Bella D, Pasquale L, et al: 5HT2C CYS23/SER23 polymorphism is not associated with obsessive-compulsive disorder. Psychiatry Res 77:97–104, 1998

Cavallini MC, Pasquale L, Bellodi L, et al: Complex segregation analysis for obsessive-compulsive disorder and related disorders. Am J Med Genet 88:38–43, 1999

Chabane N, Delorme R, Millet B, et al: Early onset obsessive-compulsive disorder: a subgroup with a specific clinical and familial pattern? J Child Psychol Psychiatry 46:881–887, 2005

Cohen D, Pichard N, Tordjman S, et al: Specific genetic disorders and autism: clinical contribution towards their identification. J Autism Dev Disord 35:103–16, 2005

A complete genome screen in sib pairs affected by Gilles de la Tourette syndrome. The Tourette Syndrome Association International Consortium for Genetics. Am J Hum Genet 65:1428–1436, 1999

Cook EH Jr, Courchesne RY, Cox NJ, et al: Linkage-disequilibrium mapping of autistic disorder, with 15q11–13 markers. Am J Hum Genet 62:1077–1083, 1998

Costello EJ, Mustillo S, Erkanli A, et al: Prevalence and development of psychiatric disorders in childhood and adolescence. Arch Gen Psychiatry: 60:837–844, 2003

Cruz C, Camarena B, King N, et al: Increased prevalence of the seven-repeat variant of the dopamine D4 receptor gene in patients with obsessive-compulsive disorder with tics. Neurosci Lett 231:1–4, 1997

Curran S, Mill J, Tahir E, et al: Association study of a dopamine transporter polymorphism and attention deficit hyperactivity disorder in UK and Turkish samples. Mol Psychiatry 6:425–428, 2001

Dawson G, Meltzoff AN, Osterling J, et al: Neuropsychological correlates of early symptoms of autism. Child Dev 69:1276–1285, 1998

Delorme R, Krebs MO, Chabane N, et al: Frequency and transmission of glutamate receptors GRIK2 and GRIK3 polymorphisms in patients with obsessive compulsive disorder. Neuroreport 15:699–702, 2004

De Luca V, Muglia P, Vincent JB, et al: Adrenergic alpha 2C receptor genomic organization: association study in adult ADHD. Am J Med Genet B Neuropsychiatr Genet 127:65–67, 2004

Dickel DE, Veenstra-VanderWeele J, Cox NJ, et al: Association testing of the positional and functional candidate gene SLC1A1/EAAC1 in early onset obsessive-compulsive disorder. Arch Gen Psychiatry 63:778–785, 2006

do Rosario-Campos MC, Leckman JF, Curi M, et al: A family study of early onset obsessive-compulsive disorder. Am J Med Genet B Neuropsychiatr Genet 136:92–97, 2005

Eapen V, Pauls DL, Robertson MM: Evidence for autosomal dominant transmission in Tourette's syndrome. United Kingdom cohort study. Br J Psychiatry 162:593–596, 1993

Enoch MA, Greenberg BD, Murphy DL, et al: Sexually dimorphic relationship of a 5-HT2A promoter polymorphism with obsessive-compulsive disorder. Biol Psychiatry 49:385–388, 2001

Faraone SV: Genetics of adult attention-deficit/hyperactivity disorder. Psychiatr Clin North Am 27:303–321, 2004

Faraone SV, Biederman J: Nature, nurture, and attention deficit hyperactivity disorder. Dev Rev 20:568–581, 2000

Faraone SV, Biederman J, Chen CK, et al: Segregation analysis of attention deficit hyperactivity disorder: evidence for single gene transmission. Psychiatr Genet 2:257–275, 1992

Faraone SV, Sergeant J, Gillberg C, et al: The worldwide prevalence of ADHD: is it an American condition? World Psychiatry 2:104–113, 2003

Fisher SE, Francks C, McCracken JT, et al: A genomewide scan for loci involved in attention-deficit/hyperactivity disorder. Am J Hum Genet 70:1183–1196, 2002

Folstein SE, Rosen-Sheidley B: Genetics of autism: complex aetiology for a heterogeneous disorder. Nat Rev Genet 2:943–955, 2001

Folstein S, Rutter M: Infantile autism: a genetic study of 21 twin pairs. J Child Psychol Psychiatry 18:297–321, 1977

Fombonne E: The prevalence of autism. JAMA 289:87–89, 2003

Gayan J, Willcutt EG, Fisher SE, et al: Bivariate linkage scan for reading disability and attention-deficit/hyperactivity disorder localizes pleiotropic loci. J Child Psychol Psychiatry 46:1045–1056, 2005

Gillberg C, Steffenburg S, Wahlstrom J, et al: Autism associated with marker chromosome. J Am Acad Child Adolesc Psychiatry 30:489–494, 1991

Goodman R, Stevenson J: A twin study of hyperactivity, II. The aetiological role of genes, family relationships and perinatal adversity. J Child Psychol Psychiatry 30:691–709, 1989

Gothelf D, Presburger G, Zohar AH, et al: Obsessive-compulsive disorder in patients with velocardiofacial (22q11 deletion) syndrome. Am J Med Genet B Neuropsychiatr Genet 126:99–105, 2004

Gurling H: Candidate genes and favoured loci: strategies for molecular genetic research into schizophrenia, manic depression, autism, alcoholism and Alzheimer's disease. Psychiatr Dev 4:289–309, 1986

Hanna GL, Himle JA, Curtis GC, et al: Serotonin transporter and seasonal variation in blood serotonin in families with obsessive-compulsive disorder. Neuropsychopharmacology 18:102–111, 1998

Hanna GL, Veenstra-VanderWeele J, Cox NJ, et al: Genome-wide linkage analysis of families with obsessive-compulsive disorder ascertained through pediatric probands. Am J Med Genet B Neuropsychiatr Genet 114:541–552, 2002

Hanna GL, Fingerlin TE, Himle JA, et al: Complex segregation analysis of obsessive-compulsive disorder in families with pediatric probands. Hum Hered 60:1–9, 2005

Hasstedt SJ, Leppert M, Filloux F, et al: Intermediate inheritance of Tourette syndrome, assuming assortative mating. Am J Hum Genet 57:682–689, 1995

Hebebrand J, Klug B, Fimmers R, et al: Rates for tic disorders and obsessive compulsive symptomatology in families of children and adolescents with Gilles de la Tourette syndrome. J Psychiatr Res 31:519–530, 1997

Hettema JM, Neale MC, Kendler KS: A review and meta-analysis of the genetic epidemiology of anxiety disorders. Am J Psychiatry 158:1568–1578, 2001

Hu XZ, Lipsky RH, Zhu G, et al: Serotonin transporter promoter gain-of-function genotypes are linked to obsessive-compulsive disorder. Am J Hum Genet 78:815–826, 2006

Hyde TM, Aaronson BA, Randolph C, et al: Relationship of birth weight to the phenotypic expression of Gilles de la Tourette's syndrome in monozygotic twins. Neurology 42:652–658, 1992

Jorde LB, Hasstedt SJ, Ritvo ER, et al: Complex segregation analysis of autism. Am J Hum Genet 49:932–938, 1991

Karayiorgou M, Sobin C, Blundell ML, et al: Family-based association studies support a sexually dimorphic effect of COMT and MAOA on genetic susceptibility to obsessive-compulsive disorder. Biol Psychiatry 45:1178–1189, 1999

Kent L, Green E, Hawi Z, et al: Association of the paternally transmitted copy of common Valine allele of the Val66Met polymorphism of the brain-derived neurotrophic factor (BDNF) gene with susceptibility to ADHD. Mol Psychiatry 10:939–943, 2005

Kim SJ, Veenstra-VanderWeele J, Hanna GL, et al: Mutation screening of human 5-HT(2B)receptor gene in early onset obsessive-compulsive disorder. Mol Cell Probes 14:47–52, 2000

Kinnear C, Niehaus DJ, Seedat S, et al: Obsessive-compulsive disorder and a novel polymorphism adjacent to the oestrogen response element (ERE 6) upstream from the COMT gene. Psychiatr Genet 11:85–87, 2001

Knopik VS, Sparrow EP, Madden PA, et al: Contributions of parental alcoholism, prenatal substance exposure, and genetic transmission to child ADHD risk: a female twin study. Psychol Med 35:625–635, 2005

Kringlen E: Obsessional neurotics: a long-term follow-up. Br J Psychiatry 111:709–722, 1965

Lamb JA, Parr JR, Bailey AJ, et al: Autism: in search of susceptibility genes. Neuromolecular Med 2:11–28, 2002

Larsson JO, Larsson H, Lichtenstein P: Genetic and environmental contributions to stability and change of ADHD symptoms between 8 and 13 years of age: a longitudinal twin study. J Am Acad Child Adolesc Psychiatry 43:1267–1275, 2004

Laurin N, Misener VL, Crosbie J, et al: Association of the calcyon gene (DRD1IP) with attention deficit/hyperactivity disorder. Mol Psychiatry 10:1117–1125, 2005

Leckman JF, Zhang H, Vitale A, et al: Course of tic severity in Tourette syndrome: the first two decades. Pediatrics 102:14–19, 1998

Lenane MC, Swedo SE, Leonard H, et al: Psychiatric disorders in first degree relatives of children and adolescents with obsessive compulsive disorder. J Am Acad Child Adolesc Psychiatry 29:407–412, 1990

Leonard HL, Lenane MC, Swedo SE, et al: Tics and Tourette's disorder: a 2- to 7-year follow-up of 54 obsessive-compulsive children. Am J Psychiatry 149:1244–1251, 1992

Lewis A: Problems of obsessional illness. Proc R Soc Med 29:325–336, 1935

Maher BS, Marazita ML, Moss HB, et al: Segregation analysis of attention deficit hyperactivity disorder. Am J Med Genet 88:71–78, 1999

Maher BS, Marazita ML, Ferrell RE, et al: Dopamine system genes and attention deficit hyperactivity disorder: a meta-analysis. Psychiatr Genet 12:207–215, 2002

Martin ER, Menold MM, Wolpert CM, et al: Analysis of linkage disequilibrium in gamma-aminobutyric acid receptor subunit genes in autistic disorder. Am J Med Genet 96:43–48, 2000

McMahon WM, van de Wetering BJ, Filloux F, et al: Bilineal transmission and phenotypic variation of Tourette's disorder in a large pedigree. J Am Acad Child Adolesc Psychiatry 35:672–680, 1996

Merette C, Brassard A, Potvin A, et al: Significant linkage for Tourette syndrome in a large French Canadian family. Am J Hum Genet 67:1008–1013, 2000

Mill J, Richards S, Knight J, et al: Haplotype analysis of SNAP-25 suggests a role in the aetiology of ADHD. Mol Psychiatry 9:801–810, 2004

Misener VL, Schachar R, Ickowicz A, et al: Replication test for association of the IL-1 receptor antagonist gene, IL1RN, with attention-deficit/hyperactivity disorder. Neuropsychobiology 50:231–234, 2004

Morrison JR, Stewart MA: The psychiatric status of the legal families of adopted hyperactive children. Arch Gen Psychiatry 28:888–891, 1973

Mundo E, Richter MA, Zai G, et al: 5HT1Dß receptor gene implicated in the pathogenesis of obsessive-compulsive disorder: further evidence from a family-based association study. Mol Psychiatry 7:805–809, 2002

Nestadt G, Lan T, Samuels J, et al: Complex segregation analysis provides compelling evidence for a major gene underlying obsessive-compulsive disorder and for heterogeneity by sex. Am J Hum Genet 67:1611–1616, 2000a

Nestadt G, Samuels J, Riddle M, et al: A family study of obsessive-compulsive disorder. Arch Gen Psychiatry 57:358–363, 2000b

Nicolini H, Hanna GL, Baxter L, et al: Segregation analysis of obsessive compulsive disorders: preliminary results. Ursus Medicus 1:25–28, 1991

Nicolini H, Weissbecker K, Mejia JM, et al: Family study of obsessive-compulsive disorder in a Mexican population. Arch Med Res 24:193–198, 1993

Nurmi EL, Bradford Y, Chen Y, et al: Linkage disequilibrium at the Angelman syndrome gene UBE3A in autism families. Genomics 77:105–113, 2001

Ogdie MN, Macphie IL, Minassian SL, et al: A genomewide scan for attention-deficit/hyperactivity disorder in an extended sample: suggestive linkage on 17p11. Am J Hum Genet 72:1268–1279, 2003

Ogdie MN, Fisher SE, Yang M, et al: Attention deficit hyperactivity disorder: fine mapping supports linkage to 5p13, 6q12, 16p13, and 17p11. Am J Hum Genet 75:661–668, 2004

Paschou P, Feng Y, Pakstis AJ, et al: Indications of linkage and association of Gilles de la Tourette syndrome in two independent family samples: 17q25 is a putative susceptibility region. Am J Hum Genet 75:545–560, 2004

Pauls DL: An update on the genetics of Gilles de la Tourette syndrome. J Psychosom Res 55:7–12, 2003

Pauls DL, Leckman JF: The inheritance of Gilles de la Tourette's syndrome and associated behaviors: evidence for autosomal dominant transmission. N Engl J Med 315:993–997, 1986

Pauls D, Stewart SE: Genetics of obsessive-compulsive disorder. TENS J in press

Pauls DL, Tourette Syndrome Association International Consortium on Genetics: Update on the genetics of Tourette syndrome. Adv Neurol 85:281–293, 2001

Pauls DL, Towbin KE, Leckman JF, et al: Gilles de la Tourette's syndrome and obsessive-compulsive disorder: evidence supporting a genetic relationship. Arch Gen Psychiatry 43:1180–1182, 1986

Pauls DL, Alsobrook J, II, Almasy L, et al: Genetic and epidemiological analyses of the Yale Tourette's Syndrome Family Study data. Psychiatr Genet 2:28, 1991a

Pauls DL, Raymond CL, Leckman JF, et al: A family study of Tourette's syndrome. Am J Hum Genet 48:154–163, 1991b

Pauls DL, Alsobrook JP 2nd, Goodman W, et al: A family study of obsessive-compulsive disorder. Am J Psychiatry 152:76–84, 1995

Pauls DL, Mundo E, Kennedy JL: The pathophysiology and genetics of obsessive-compulsive disorder, in Obsessive Compulsive Disorder: A Practical Guide. Edited by Fineberg F, Marazziti D, Stein D. London, Martin Dunitz, 2002, pp 61–75

Pickles A, Bolton P, Macdonald H, et al: Latent-class analysis of recurrence risks for complex phenotypes with selection and measurement error: a twin and family history study of autism. Am J Hum Genet 57:717–726, 1995

Piven J, Berthier ML, Starkstein SE, et al: Magnetic resonance imaging evidence for a defect of cerebral cortical development in autism. Am J Psychiatry 147:734–739, 1990

Price RA, Kidd KK, Cohen DJ, et al: A twin study of Tourette syndrome. Arch Gen Psychiatry 42:815–820, 1985

Purper-Ouakil D, Wohl M, Mouren MC, et al: Meta-analysis of family-based association studies between the dopamine transporter gene and attention deficit hyperactivity disorder. Psychiatr Genet 15:53–59, 2005

Rasmussen SA, Tsuang MT: Clinical characteristics and family history in DSM-III obsessive-compulsive disorder. Am J Psychiatry 143:317–322, 1986

Reddy PS, Reddy YC, Srinath S, et al: A family study of juvenile obsessive-compulsive disorder. Can J Psychiatry 46:346–351, 2001

Riddle MA, Scahill L, King R, et al: Obsessive compulsive disorder in children and adolescents: phenomenology and family history. J Am Acad Child Adolesc Psychiatry 29:766–772, 1990

Rietveld MJ, Hudziak JJ, Bartels M, et al: Heritability of attention problems in children: longitudinal results from a study of twins, age 3 to 12. J Child Psychol Psychiatry 45:577–588, 2004

Ritvo ER, Spence MA, Freeman BJ, et al: Evidence for autosomal recessive inheritance in 46 families with multiple incidences of autism. Am J Psychiatry 142:187–192, 1985

Roman T, Schmitz M, Polanczyk GV, et al: Is the alpha-2A adrenergic receptor gene (ADRA2A) associated with attention-deficit/hyperactivity disorder? Am J Med Genet B Neuropsychiatr Genet 120:116–120, 2003

Rowe DC, Stever C, Gard JM, et al: The relation of the dopamine transporter gene (DAT1) to symptoms of internalizing disorders in children. Behav Genet 28:215–225, 1998

Rutter M: Genetic studies of autism: from the 1970s into the millennium. J Abnorm Child Psychol 28:3–14, 2000

Rutter M, Bailey A, Bolton P, et al: Autism and known medical conditions: myth and substance. J Child Psychol Psychiatry 35:311–322, 1994

Santangelo SL, Folstein S: Autism: A Genetic Perspective. Boston, MA, MIT Press, 1999

Scharf J, Pauls DL: Genetics of tic disorders, in Emery & Rimoin's Principles and Practice of Medical Genetics, 5th Edition. Edited by Rimoin DL, Connor JM, Pyeritz RE, et al. Philadelphia, PA, Churchill Livingstone/Elsevier, 2007, pp 2737–2754

Schroer RJ, Phelan MC, Michaelis RC, et al: Autism and maternally derived aberrations of chromosome 15q. Am J Med Genet 76:327–336, 1998

Seuchter SA, Hebebrand J, Klug B, et al: Complex segregation analysis of families ascertained through Gilles de la Tourette syndrome. Genet Epidemiol 18:33–47, 2000

Shao Y, Raiford KL, Wolpert CM, et al: Phenotypic homogeneity provides increased support for linkage on chromosome 2 in autistic disorder. Am J Hum Genet 70:1058–1061, 2002

Shapiro AK, Shapiro ES, Young JG, et al: Gilles de la Tourette Syndrome. New York, Raven, 1988

Sheehan K, Lowe N, Kirley A, et al: Tryptophan hydroxylase 2 (TPH2) gene variants associated with ADHD. Mol Psychiatry 10:944–949, 2005

Shugart YY, Samuels J, Willour VL, et al: Genomewide linkage scan for obsessive-compulsive disorder: evidence for susceptibility loci on chromosomes 3q, 7p, 1q, 15q, and 6q. Mol Psychiatry 11:763–770, 2006

Simonic I, Gericke GS, Ott J, et al: Identification of genetic markers associated with Gilles de la Tourette syndrome in an Afrikaner population. Am J Hum Genet 63:839–846, 1998

Simonic I, Nyholt DR, Gericke GS, et al: Further evidence for linkage of Gilles de la Tourette syndrome (GTS) susceptibility loci on chromosomes 2p11, 8q22 and 11q23–24 in South African Afrikaners. Am J Med Genet 105:163–167, 2001

Smalley S, Smith M, Tanguay P: Autism and psychiatric disorders in tuberous sclerosis. Ann N Y Acad Sci 615:382–383, 1991

Smalley SL, Kustanovich V, Minassian SL, et al: Genetic linkage of attention-deficit/hyperactivity disorder on chromosome 16p13, in a region implicated in autism. Am J Hum Genet 71:959–963, 2002

Sprich S, Biederman J, Crawford MH, et al: Adoptive and biological families of children and adolescents with ADHD. J Am Acad Child Adolesc Psychiatry 39:1432–1437, 2000

Staller J, Faraone SV: Attention-deficit hyperactivity disorder in girls: epidemiology and management. CNS Drugs 20:107–123, 2006

Steffenburg S, Gillberg C, Hellgren L, et al: A twin study of autism in Denmark, Finland, Iceland, Norway, and Sweden. J Child Psychol Psychiatry 30:405–416, 1989

Stevenson J: Evidence for a genetic etiology in hyperactivity in children. Behav Genet 22:337–344, 1992

Stewart SE, Geller D, Spencer T, et al: Pediatric tics and Tourette's disorder: which therapies and when to use them. Current Psychiatry 2(10):45–56, 2003

Stewart SE, Geller DA, Jenike MA, et al: Long-term outcome of pediatric obsessive compulsive disorder: a meta-analysis and qualitative review of the literature. Acta Psychiatr Scand 110:4–13, 2004

Stewart SE, Illmann C, Geller DA, et al: A controlled family study of attention deficit hyperactivity disorder and Gilles de la Tourette's syndrome. J Am Acad Child Adolesc Psychiatry 45:1354–62, 2006

Stewart SE, Fagerness J, Jenike E, et al: Family-based association between obsessive-compulsive disorder and glutamate receptor candidate genes. Poster presented at the World Congress of Psychiatric Genetics, New York City, October 2007a

Stewart SE, Fagerness J, Platkov J, et al: Association of the SLC1A1 glutamate transporter gene and obsessive-compulsive disorder. Am J Med Genet B Neuropsychiatr Genet, September 25, 2007b (epub ahead of print)

Stewart SE, Platko J, Fagerness J, et al: A genetic family-based association study of OLIG2 in obsessive-compulsive disorder. Arch Gen Psychiatry 64:209–214, 2007c

Szatmari P, Jones MB, Tuff L, et al: Lack of cognitive impairment in first-degree relatives of children with pervasive developmental disorders. J Am Acad Child Adolesc Psychiatry 32:1264–1273, 1993

Tarnok Z, Ronai Z, Gervai J, et al: Dopaminergic candidate genes in Tourette syndrome: association between tic severity and 3′ UTR polymorphism of the dopamine transporter gene. Am J Med Genet B Neuropsychiatr Genet 144:900–905, 2007

Todd RD, Lobos EA, Sun LW, et al: Mutational analysis of the nicotinic acetylcholine receptor alpha 4 subunit gene in attention deficit/hyperactivity disorder: evidence for association of an intronic polymorphism with attention problems. Mol Psychiatry 8:103–108, 2003

Tourette Syndrome Association International Consortium for Genetics: Genome scan for Tourette disorder in affected-sibling-pair and multigenerational families. Am J Hum Genet 80:265–272, 2007

Trikalinos TA, Karvouni A, Zintzaras E, et al: A heterogeneity-based genome search meta-analysis for autism-spectrum disorders. Mol Psychiatry 11:29–36, 2006

Tsai L, Stewart MA, August G: Implication of sex differences in the familial transmission of infantile autism. J Autism Dev Disord 11:165–173, 1981

Turic D, Langley K, Mills S, et al: Follow-up of genetic linkage findings on chromosome 16p13: evidence of association of N-methyl-D-aspartate glutamate receptor 2A gene polymorphism with ADHD. Mol Psychiatry 9:169–173, 2004

van Grootheest DS, Cath DC, Beekman AT, et al: Twin studies on obsessive-compulsive disorder: a review. Twin Res Hum Genet 8:450–458, 2005

Volkmar FR, Pauls D: Autism. Lancet 362:1133–1141, 2003

Volkmar FR, Carter A, Sparrow SS, et al: Quantifying social development in autism. J Am Acad Child Adolesc Psychiatry 32:627–632, 1993

Volkmar FR, Klin A, Siegel B, et al: Field trial for autistic disorder in DSM-IV. Am J Psychiatry 151:1361–1367, 1994

Walitza S, Wewetzer C, Gerlach M, et al: Transmission disequilibrium studies in children and adolescents with obsessive-compulsive disorders pertaining to polymorphisms of genes of the serotonergic pathway. J Neural Transm 111:817–825, 2004

Walitza S, Renner TJ, Dempfle A, et al: Transmission disequilibrium of polymorphic variants in the tryptophan hydroxylase-2 gene in attention-deficit/hyperactivity disorder. Mol Psychiatry 10:1126–1132, 2005

Walkup JT, LaBuda MC, Singer HS, Brown J, Riddle MA, et al: Family study and segregation analysis of Tourette syndrome: evidence for a mixed model of inheritance. Am J Hum Genet 59:684–693, 1996

Welch JM, Lu J, Rodriguiz RM, et al: Cortico-striatal synaptic defects and OCD-like behaviours in Sapap3-mutant mice. Nature 448(7156):894–900, 2007

Wilens TE, Biederman J, Spencer TJ: Attention deficit/hyperactivity disorder across the lifespan. Annu Rev Med 53:113–131, 2002

Willour VL, Yao Shugart Y, Samuels J, et al: Replication study supports evidence for linkage to 9p24 in obsessive-compulsive disorder. Am J Hum Genet 75:508–513, 2004

Wing L, Potter D: The epidemiology of autistic spectrum disorders: is the prevalence rising? Ment Retard Dev Disabil Res Rev 8:151–161, 2002

Wohl M, Purper-Ouakil D, Mouren MC, et al: [Meta-analysis of candidate genes in attention-deficit hyperactivity disorder] (in French). Encephale 31:437–447, 2005

Xu X, Knight J, Brookes K, et al: DNA pooling analysis of 21 norepinephrine transporter gene SNPs with attention deficit hyperactivity disorder: no evidence for association. Am J Med Genet B Neuropsychiatr Genet 134:115–118, 2005

Yang L, Wang YF, Li J, et al: Association of norepinephrine transporter gene with methylphenidate response. J Am Acad Child Adolesc Psychiatry 43:1154–1158, 2004

Yoon DY, Gause CD, Leckman JF, et al: Dopaminergic polymorphisms in Tourette syndrome: association with the DAT gene (SLC6A3). Am J Med Genet B Neuropsychiatr Genet 144:605–610, 2007

Zai G, Bezchlibnyk YB, Richter MA, et al: Myelin oligodendrocyte glycoprotein (MOG) gene is associated with obsessive-compulsive disorder. Am J Med Genet B Neuropsychiatr Genet 129:64–68, 2004

Zhang H, Leckman JF, Pauls DL, et al: Genomewide scan of hoarding in sib pairs in which both sibs have Gilles de la Tourette syndrome. Am J Hum Genet 70:896–904, 2002

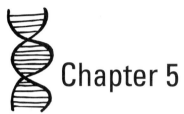

Chapter 5

Genetics of Schizophrenia and Psychotic Disorders

Anne S. Bassett, M.D., F.R.C.P.C.
Eva W. C. Chow, M.D., M.P.H., F.R.C.P.C.
Kathleen A. Hodgkinson, M.Sc.

Clinical Phenotype, Morbidity, and Epidemiology

Schizophrenia is a common psychiatric illness that typically involves lifelong but treatable changes in thinking, behavior, and emotions. The principal symptoms are psychotic in nature, including delusions (false beliefs), hallucinations (false perceptions), and thought disorder (disorganization of thought processes). In addition to these "positive" symptoms of the illness, there are also "negative" symptoms of blunted affect (reduced emotional expression), poverty of speech, anhedonia (reduced ability to feel pleasure), and amotivation, as well as disorganization of behavior and emotions. Depression, anxiety, irritability, agitation, sleep disturbance, and cognitive impairments, including changes in attention, memory, insight and judgment, are also common. Onset of schizophrenia occurs most commonly in early adulthood from 17 to 30 years of age, but onset can occur at any time from childhood (in <1% of cases) through to the elderly age range (relatively uncommon). The illness is usually lifelong–having a relapsing and remitting or a more chronic course–and is associated with substantial morbidity.

The mainstay of treatment is antipsychotic medication, and the majority of patients have some symptomatic response, if not to the initial medication tried, then to another biological treatment (Kane 1996). Adherence to treatment is an essential goal, although it is often difficult to achieve (Lieberman et al. 2005). Relapse rates approach 75% within 1 year of discontinuing treatment after initial remission of symptoms (Kane 1996). No reliable predictors of long-term outcome or treatment response have been identified. Full recovery from schizophrenia can occur but is uncommon (Lauronen et al. 2005), and impairment of social and vocational functioning is usually significant, especially in comparison to peers. In addition to functional morbidity, there is substantial medical morbidity in schizophrenia, associated with lifestyle-related factors, medication side effects, and constitutional predisposition to other disorders (Goff et al. 2005). Cardiovascular diseases contribute most to excess mortality, but respiratory diseases such as chronic obstructive pulmonary disease and pneumonia and infectious diseases such as HIV disease, hepatitis B and C, and tuberculosis also play a role (Goff et al. 2005). High rates of comorbid smoking and substance use disorders in schizophrenia contribute to these risks (Goff et al. 2005). Mortality due to suicide is also significant, having peak occurrence in the early years of the illness and involving 5%–10% of patients (Bromet et al. 2005). Medical morbidity and suicide together contribute to age-adjusted mortality rates that are increased two- to threefold over expected rates (Goff et al. 2005; Tsuang and Woolson 1977).

Schizophrenia is a common disorder with a lifetime prevalence of approximately 1% and with an incidence of 0.2–0.5 per 1,000 population per year (Jablensky 2000). The annual cost of schizophrenia in the United States in 2002 was estimated to be $62.7 billion, about one-half from direct health care and non–health care (e.g., legal) costs and one-half from indirect costs, mostly related to unemployment but also to mortality and family caregiving (Wu et al. 2005). Schizophrenia ranks among the leading causes of long-term disability; the number of disability-adjusted life years lost due to schizophrenia worldwide is similar to that for diabetes and asthma (Murray and Lopez 1997). However, in contrast to multifactorial disorders such as heart disease, asthma, or diabetes, in which environmental factors play a large role in causation, there is little variation in prevalence of schizophrenia across ethnicities or cultures (Jablensky 2000). No population has been identified that is free of schizophrenia (Jablensky 2000). Only certain genetic isolates may have higher prevalences (e.g., the large Böök pedigree [Böök 1953]). The illness affects men and women about equally, but onset may be younger and prevalence higher in men. All intellectual levels are affected, although there is a somewhat higher risk in persons at lower intellectual levels, as would be expected from a disease with cognitive disturbances.

Hypotheses About the Pathogenesis of Schizophrenia

Clinical Diagnosis

The diagnosis of schizophrenia is a clinical diagnosis, based on course of illness as well as cross-sectional symptoms. Diagnostic reliability is high when standard diagnostic criteria are used together with a thorough history and direct examination, including information from the patient, relatives, and others, to differentiate schizophrenia from other psychotic disorders. As with most neuropsychiatric disorders, there are no diagnostic tests for schizophrenia. In contrast to many neurodegenerative disorders, no characteristic neuropathology is present in schizophrenia, although in some groups of patients subtle, nonspecific changes in brain morphology are observable with various imaging techniques or by examination of postmortem brain tissue. The most common of these changes involves larger volumes of cerebrospinal fluid in ventricles and sulci and smaller gray matter volumes (Harrison 1999; Shenton et al. 2001). All brain regions, including frontal to occipital, cortical to subcortical, and cerebellar regions, have been implicated. At least some of the structural changes appear to predate onset of the illness (Pantelis et al. 2005).

Emil Kraepelin proposed neurodevelopmental origins for schizophrenia more than a century ago, and several lines of evidence, including brain imaging, premorbid clinical signs, and associations with minor dysmorphic features, indicate that early changes in neurodevelopment, together with subsequent neurodegenerative changes, may be involved in the pathogenesis of schizophrenia (Bassett et al. 2001; Rapoport et al. 2005). The early developmental changes appear greater, and the degenerative changes much less, however, than those of classic neurodegenerative diseases (Arnold et al. 2005). Similar to processes involved in normal neuronal plasticity (Kandel and Squire 2000), genetic variants that alter gene expression likely play a major role, together with stochastic and environmental effects, in the pathogenic processes leading to these neurodevelopmental abnormalities (Bassett et al. 2001). Current hypotheses about the pathogenic processes involved in schizophrenia include abnormalities of synaptic development and function, glutatmate neurotransmitter systems, and signal transduction (Arnold et al. 2005). These have somewhat superseded, but are complementary to, hypotheses related to abnormalities of the dopamine neurotransmitter system that were based on early observations of antipsychotic drug actions. More definitive clues about the etiology and pathogenesis of schizophrenia should follow advances in molecular neurobiology and molecular genetics, as they have for other adult-onset diseases such as

Huntington's disease and Alzheimer's disease (Bates 2005; Bertram and Tanzi 2005).

In schizophrenia, behavioral changes in the absence of observable physical disability, characteristic brain pathology, or a known cause have contributed to misunderstanding and stigma and have allowed fantastical theories of causation (e.g., mothers/upbringing; witchcraft/possession) to persist. This stigma, together with comorbid substance use and the changes in judgment and ability to understand that one has an illness that are associated with the neuropathological processes of schizophrenia, plays a role in poor adherence to proven treatments. Cumulatively these factors have contributed to the increasing rates of incarceration and homelessness of persons with this disease and to the concomitant lack of appropriate medical care and treatment. The elucidation of specific causes and mechanisms for schizophrenia to be expected from advances in molecular genetics and related research promises to help dispel myths and significantly reduce the stigma that continues to be associated with this disease.

Spectrum of Illness

As with most illnesses, schizophrenia likely represents the severe extreme of a spectrum of manifestations. For example, if one were to include any nonaffective psychosis in the criteria for schizophrenia, then the general population rate would be about double that of narrowly defined schizophrenia (Gottesman 1991; Gottesman and Shields 1982). Adding persons with schizotypal or paranoid personality disorders would increase the prevalence further, although prevalence estimates for this broad definition of schizophrenia, widely used in genetic studies, are largely unavailable because many such persons would not seek or require treatment. Nonaffective psychotic disorders and schizotypal and paranoid personality disorders have consistently been found to have a familial relationship to schizophrenia (Gottesman 1991; Gottesman and Shields 1982). Indeed, the original DSM-III criteria for schizotypal personality disorder (American Psychiatric Association 1980) were based on the eight features that distinguished adopted offspring of persons with schizophrenia from relatives of probands with no psychotic disorder, after excluding those with schizophrenia (Spitzer et al. 1979). There may also be a genetic relationship of at least some forms of schizophrenia to other psychiatric disorders, including mood disorders (Badner and Gershon 2002; Husted et al. 2006) and developmental disorders such as autism spectrum disorders (Sporn et al. 2004). The ultimate delineation of relationships with other disorders and alternative phenotypes will follow identification of proven mutations for schizophrenia. We are just beginning to enter the genomic era of discoveries. For individual genetic forms of the illness, this era promises to provide long-awaited answers to fundamental questions about the true extent of the schizophrenia spectrum (i.e., variable expressivity), penetrance of individual genetic changes, and interaction with nongenetic factors.

Genetic Epidemiology

General Considerations

Nearly a century of research supports the importance of genetic predisposition to schizophrenia (Gottesman 1991; Gottesman and Shields 1982). The evidence derives from family, twin, and adoption studies that provide support for the importance of genetic factors. Schizophrenia itself, however, is not a single entity. As for other common, complex illnesses, the umbrella term "schizophrenia" as used in the general population comprises a mix of etiological forms that range across a spectrum from more genetic to less genetic (see Table 5–1). Also, as for any individual disorder, each form of schizophrenia may be considered to be caused by a combination of both genetic and nongenetic factors. Single genes with high penetrance (or a set of genes in the case of chromosomal anomalies such as the 22q11.2 deletion of 22q11.2 deletion syndrome), with little influence from nongenetic factors, constitute one end of a spectrum of possibilities. The other end would be represented by environmental factors with little influence of genetic susceptibility variants. On average, in the general population, schizophrenia as an umbrella term falls closer to the more genetic end of the spectrum, as represented statistically by its high heritability (80%–87%) (Cardno et al. 1999). This value, however, reflects an average based on the as-yet-unknown specific mix of forms of schizophrenia.

Another general consideration is the degree to which "genetic" is represented by inherited factors in addition to spontaneous mutations that would usually be transmissible to a subsequent generation but not inherited from a parent. Until causal variants of schizophrenia susceptibility genes are identified, we cannot know to what extent apparently "sporadic" cases of the disorder may be caused by new mutations. From a clinical perspective, this uncertainty may be illustrated by the importance of the family history. Previously, a positive family history of schizophrenia was presumed to be the single greatest risk factor for the illness (Gottesman 1991; Gottesman and Shields 1982), and this is still the case for most persons. However, those with a deletion on chromosome 22q11.2, who rarely have a family history of schizophrenia (see Table 5–1), have a greater risk of developing schizophrenia than persons who have a first-degree relative with schizophrenia (Bassett et al. 2000) (see Figure 5–1).

TABLE 5–1. Genetic and nongenetic forms of schizophrenia in the general population

	Clinical expression		Genetic test available	Prevalence in schizophrenia population	Genes	Family history	
	Schizophrenia	Other features				Schizophrenia and related disorders	Other conditions
Genetic forms[a]							
Inherited predisposition	√	NA	None	Common	Multiple variants of small effect	Positive	NA
Spontaneous mutations	√	NA	None	Possibly and common	Variants of small or large effect	—	NA
Familial (Mendelian-like)	√	NA	None	Rare	Mutations of large effect	Highly positive	NA
Syndromic forms with chromosomal aberrations	√	√	Some	>1%–2%	Many	Usually negative; may be positive if inherited aberration	Learning disability; birth defects
22q11.2 deletion syndrome (22qDS)	√	√	√	1%	>40 in commonly deleted region	—	22qDS (uncommon)

TABLE 5–1. Genetic and nongenetic forms of schizophrenia in the general population *(continued)*

	Clinical expression		Genetic test available	Prevalence in schizophrenia population	Genes	Family history	
	Schizophrenia	Other features				Schizophrenia and related disorders	Other conditions
Genetic forms[a] *(continued)*							
Mosaic Turner syndrome	√	√	√	Very rare	Entire X chromosome	—	NA
Schizophrenia-like expression associated with other genetic disorders[b]	—[c]	√	Some	Very rare	Modifying variants	—	As for primary condition
Nongenetic forms[a]							
Secondary schizophrenia[d]	—[c]	√	NA	Very rare	NA	Negative	NA

Note. NA=not applicable.

[a]Genetic and nongenetic modifying factors, including epigenetic factors, are present for all forms, and each form could have its own pattern of variable expression, including other psychiatric disorders or features and, especially in syndromic forms, other physical disorders or features.

[b]For example, Huntington's disease (Tsuang et al. 2000).

[c]Clinical expression is likely similar to schizophrenia, but signs and symptoms do not meet the standard criteria for schizophrenia.

[d]For example, severe traumatic head injury.

Models proposed for describing genetic risk for the entire population of persons with schizophrenia have been based on aggregate data that would include many forms of schizophrenia with varying levels of genetic risk (see Figure 5–1). This mix guarantees that schizophrenia would be considered "multifactorial" (Gottesman 1991; Gottesman and Shields 1982). Advances in molecular genetics indicate that epigenetic mechanisms (modifiers of gene expression), such as methylation, could be included as one of many possible interacting factors (Bassett et al. 2001). A favored model for schizophrenia at the population level has been Risch's model of multifactorial inheritance that assumes that two to three or more genetic variants at different loci act together in an additive or multiplicative fashion to increase susceptibility (Risch 1990). Such "epistasis" is likely to be ubiquitous in nature (Moore 2005) and is probably common in many or most forms of schizophrenia. Only as schizophrenia susceptibility genes are identified and mechanisms modifying their expression elucidated will it be possible on an individual level to determine the extent to which such population-based models are applicable.

Rarely, in some families, a single major genetic mutation or few genetic variants with high penetrance may increase susceptibility for an individual to express schizophrenia (Hodgkinson et al. 2001). This expression could present clinically as a pedigree showing multiple individuals affected with schizophrenia, in which a more Mendelian inheritance pattern (autosomal recessive or autosomal dominant) appears to be operating. Population-based recurrence risks are unlikely to be accurate for such a family (Hodgkinson et al. 2001). Unlike mature-onset diabetes of the young or familial Alzheimer's disease, schizophrenia has no readily identifiable familial forms in the general population, but in the mix of patients with schizophrenia, there will likely be rare persons with familial forms of the illness. These persons are from families whose participation in linkage studies is likely to be most valuable. Unlike many other diseases, however, earlier age at onset is associated with only a modest increased risk in schizophrenia (Husted et al. 2006; Nicolson and Rapoport 1999). Thus, this easily observable clinical clue has not proved as useful for identifying genetically useful subtypes as it has for the younger-onset subtypes of familial Alzheimer's disease or diabetes mellitus, for which gene discoveries have been made (Bertram and Tanzi 2005; Permutt et al. 2005). On the other hand, a syndromic form of schizophrenia–22q11.2 deletion syndrome (22qDS)–exists that can be identified clinically and confirmed with a clinically available test (Bassett and Chow 1999).

Incomplete penetrance in schizophrenia, as in most disorders, is common (Hodgkinson et al. 2001). This finding is supported by studies of offspring of discordant monozygotic twins, in which offspring of both affected

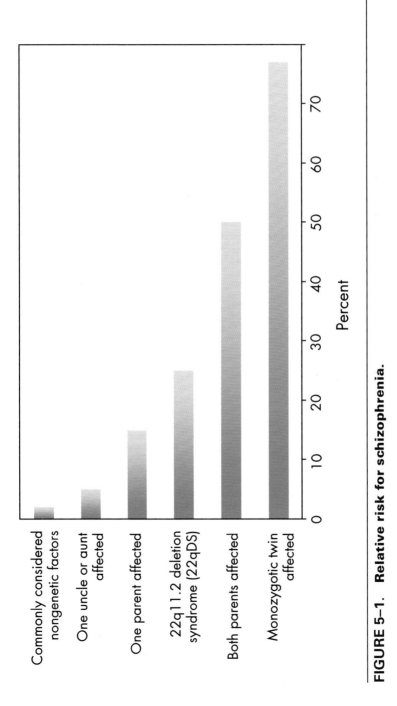

FIGURE 5–1.   Relative risk for schizophrenia.

and unaffected monozygotic co-twins have shown similar rates of schizophrenia (Gottesman and Bertelsen 1989; Kringlen and Cramer 1989). The
most common clinical example would be a family in which an aunt (or
uncle) and the proband have schizophrenia but the parent through which
the affected persons are related does not have schizophrenia. This pattern
may be observable in families where there is a single major genetic mutation or several genes with variants of small or moderate effect (Hodgkinson
et al. 2001).

Spontaneous Mutations

The long-standing clinical observation of reduced reproductive fitness in
schizophrenia, which is a more prominent feature in men than women,
supports the likelihood that recurrent spontaneous mutations account for
some forms of schizophrenia (Bassett et al. 1996). This phenomenon is evident in the 22qDS subtype of schizophrenia (see section "Syndromic Forms
of Schizophrenia–22q11.2 Deletion Syndrome"), where low copy repeat
sequences predispose to the occurrence of a deletion during gametogenesis. For other forms of schizophrenia, the observation of a small but significantly increased risk with advanced paternal age also supports the likelihood that new mutations are important (Hodgkinson et al. 2001).

Molecular Genetics of Schizophrenia

Search for Candidate Genes

Genetic linkage studies have localized several regions of the genome likely
to contain schizophrenia susceptibility genes (Badner and Gershon 2002;
Lewis et al. 2003), and several plausible candidate genes have been identified (see Table 5–2) (Kirov et al. 2005). However, as yet there are no functional variants (mutations) (Kirov et al. 2005) and therefore no impact of
these findings on clinical practice. Moving from localizations to candidate
genes has been challenging because of the broad areas of linkage in most
studies and the fact that many proposed candidate genes are not under significant linkage peaks (Hennah et al. 2004). The field of molecular genetics
is rapidly advancing, however, suggesting that much of what appears in the
literature today may well be found to be inadequate or incorrect in 5 years'
time. For schizophrenia, in contrast to Alzheimer's disease (Bertram and
Tanzi 2005), there are no readily identifiable familial forms in the general
population to aid in gene discovery, and no genetic variant associated with
as high a relative risk as the epsilon 4 allele of the apolipoprotein E gene
(*APOE*). However, the underrecognized genetic syndrome 22qDS represents a form of schizophrenia for which genetic testing is available and for

which important differences in management exist, compared with other forms of schizophrenia (see Tables 5–3 and 5–4; Figures 5–2 and 5–3).

Syndromic Forms of Schizophrenia — 22q11.2 Deletion Syndrome

Before the availability of advanced molecular cytogenetic methods such as fluorescence in situ hybridization (FISH) (see Figure 5–3) in the mid-1990s, no genetic syndromes or chromosomal abnormalities had been identified that had broad clinical relevance to clinicians who treated patients with schizophrenia. To be meaningful, a genetic syndrome or chromosomal anomaly should be relatively prevalent in the general population and there should be elevated rates of schizophrenia in persons with the syndrome and elevated rates of the syndrome in patients with schizophrenia (Bassett et al. 2000). Many associations of schizophrenia with chromosomal anomalies have been reported in case reports or surveys (Bassett et al. 2000). Some of these anomalies, such as mosaic Turner syndrome, may be important to persons who are affected and to the management of their syndrome; these issues may be addressed in genetic counseling (Bassett et al. 2000; Hodgkinson et al. 2001), and some have pointed to potential candidate genes for schizophrenia (Blackwood et al. 2001). However, most have limited broader clinical significance. An understanding of the principles of identification of genetic syndromes and the practical significance of a genetic syndromic diagnosis, however, could be helpful to clinicians who treat patients with schizophrenia (Table 5–3).

The chromosomal abnormality with the strongest evidence for association with schizophrenia in the general population is a deletion on chromosome 22q11.2 that involves more than 40 genes (Bassett and Chow 1999; Bassett et al. 2000, 2005). The genetic syndrome associated with this deletion is known as 22qDS and is also known as velocardiofacial syndrome, DiGeorge syndrome, or conotruncal anomaly face syndrome. 22q11.2 deletion syndrome has a prevalence in the general population of approximately 1 in 4,000 live births, although this is likely an underestimate (Bassett et al. 2005). Characteristic features of this highly variable condition include learning difficulties, subtle and variable facial features, palatal anomalies, cardiac and other birth defects, and later-onset conditions including psychiatric illnesses, most commonly schizophrenia (Bassett and Chow 1999; Bassett et al. 2005; Murphy et al. 1999) (see Table 5–3). Variability of features in 22qDS is observed even within families and between monozygotic twins.

Several studies have confirmed that 22qDS accounts for approximately 1% of all cases of schizophrenia (Horowitz et al. 2005; Karayiorgou et al. 1995; Wiehahn et al. 2004), comparable to the relative prevalence of schizo-

TABLE 5–2. Replicated linkage and association findings for schizophrenia (as of 2007)

Locus	Candidate genes			Associated chromosomal aberration	Linkage peak	Gene association	Meta-analysis support
	Gene	Name	Functions[a]	Phenotype			
1q22–q23	NOS1AP (CAPON)	Nitric oxide synthase 1 (neuronal) adaptor protein	Scaffolding protein; glutamate neurotransmission; signal transduction; synaptogenesis	SZ/SA	NA	Narrow[b,c]	Brzustowicz et al. 2004; Rosa et al. 2002; Zheng et al. 2005	Lewis et al. 2003
1q42	DISC1	Disrupted in schizophrenia 1	Cytoskeletal regulation	Very broad; many psychiatric disorders	Balanced translocation (Blackwood et al. 2001)	NA	Ekelund et al. 2004; Hodgkinson et al. 2004	NA
6p22	DTNBP1	Dysbindin; dystrobrevin-binding protein 1	Synaptic structure and function; glutamate neurotransmission	SZ	NA	Broad	Straub et al. 1995, 2002	Lewis et al. 2003
8p21–22	NRG1	Neuregulin 1	Synaptogenesis; myelination; neurotransmission	SZ	NA	Broad	Petryshen et al. 2005; Stefansson et al. 2002	Lewis et al. 2003

TABLE 5–2. Replicated linkage and association findings for schizophrenia (as of 2007) *(continued)*

Locus	Candidate genes			Phenotype	Associated chromosomal aberration	Linkage peak	Gene association	Meta-analysis support
	Gene	Name	Functions[a]					
13q32–34	*DAOA*	D–Amino acid oxidase activator/ G72/G30	Oxidation of D-serine Glutamate neuro- transmission	SZ	NA	Broad	Blouin et al. 1998; Mulle et al. 2005	Badner and Gershon 2002
22q11.2	>40 genes			SZ; other disorders	22q11.2 deletion (Bassett et al. 2005; Murphy et al. 1999)	NA	NA	Badner and Gershon 2002; Lewis et al. 2003

Note. NA=Not applicable; SZ=schizophrenia; SA=schizoaffective disorder.

[a]Multiple functions are common for individual proteins; selected functions are displayed.

[b]Meeting the criteria for genomewide significance at the highly significant level (lod>5.5) (Lander and Kruglyak 1995).

[c]Brzustowicz et al. 2000.

TABLE 5–3. Index of suspicion for syndromic forms of schizophrenia

Feature[a]	Genetic syndromes in general	22q11.2 deletion syndrome as a specific example[b]
Cognitive, developmental	Developmental delay Learning difficulties Specific learning disorder Mental retardation	Speech delay Learning difficulties (especially in arithmetic)* Borderline intellect (~50%) or mild mental retardation (~33%)* Any level of mental retardation* and average intellect are possible
Medical history	Birth defects	Velopharyngeal insufficiency and other palatal anomalies (~40–50%)* Congenital cardiac defects (~30%)* Birth defects involving any other system (including athymus)*
	Later-onset conditions	Multiple medical problems, including: Hypocalcemia (~65%)* Seizures (~40%; 5% with epilepsy) Recurrent infections (childhood infections, e.g., otitis media; pneumonia)
Growth	Abnormal growth parameters	Short stature (~20%) Obesity (~35%) Microcephaly (~6%)

TABLE 5–3. Index of suspicion for syndromic forms of schizophrenia *(continued)*

Feature[a]	Genetic syndromes in general	22q11.2 deletion syndrome as a specific example[b]
Physical examination	Dysmorphic facies	Characteristic but variable 22q11.2 deletion syndrome dysmorphic facies*
	Speech deficits	Hypernasal speech*
	Evidence of birth defects and/or their surgical treatment	Evidence of birth defects and/or their surgical treatment
Psychiatric phenotype	Schizophrenia	Schizophrenia
	Any other psychiatric/behavioral disorder	Emotional outbursts in some cases
Family history[c]	Possibly schizophrenia	Usually no schizophrenia
	Some occurrence of mental retardation or learning difficulties	Rarely, mental retardation or learning difficulties
	Some occurrence of recurrent miscarriages, stillbirth, early infant death	Rarely, recurrent miscarriages, stillbirth, early infant death

[a]The more severe and numerous the features, the greater the index of suspicion (Bassett and Chow 1999; Bassett et al. 2005).
[b]Bassett and Chow 1999; Bassett et al. 2005.
[c]Chromosomal anomalies often occur as de novo (spontaneous) mutations and would then have no particular family history.
*Features used in clinical screening criteria for adults with 22q11.2 deletion syndrome (Bassett and Chow 1999).

TABLE 5–4. Clinical recommendations for the 22q11.2 deletion syndrome form of schizophrenia

Genetic counseling

Risk of transmitting 22q11.2 deletion to offspring	Risk is 50%. Deletion is transmitted as an autosomal dominant trait, but severity of expression of any feature of 22qDS is not predictable (e.g., average intellect to severe mental retardation; life-threatening congenital cardiac defect to no defect).
Risk of schizophrenia in offspring	In offspring with 22q11.2 deletion, risk is ~25%.
	In offspring with no 22q11.2 deletion, risk is ~ general population rate (~1%), or higher if there is a family history of schizophrenia in other than the proband with 22qDS.
	Note: Fertility of individuals with 22qDS is usually unaffected.
Risk of 22q11.2 deletion in parents	Risk is 5%–10%. All parents of newly diagnosed patients with 22qDS should be tested for the deletion and receive counseling about de novo and transmitted 22q11.2 deletion.
Risk of 22q11.2 deletion in siblings	Testing for a 22q11.2 deletion would be recommended for siblings with features of 22qDS, or if a parent carries the deletion or is unavailable for testing.
Counseling about medical and psychiatric conditions	Endocrinological and other treatable disorders are common, e.g., hypoparathyroidism, hypothyroidism.
	Lifelong monitoring, anticipatory care, and follow-up are necessary.

Medical conditions

Risk for medical comorbidity and treatment	Differs from other forms of schizophrenia, e.g., high rate of hypoparathyroidism/ hypocalcemia requiring vitamin D and calcium supplements.
	Consider possible drug interactions, e.g., calcium supplements can interfere with absorption of other medications.
	Unknown effect but possibly elevated mortality

TABLE 5–4. Clinical recommendations for the 22q11.2 deletion syndrome form of schizophrenia *(continued)*

Medical conditions *(continued)*

Investigations at diagnosis and selected monitoring thereafter	Multiple standard recommendations, including abdominal ultrasound (renal agenesis, splenomegaly, fatty liver, and cholelithiasis are relatively common), echocardiogram, pH-corrected ionized calcium, parathyroid hormone, thyroid-stimulating hormone.
Appropriate referrals and treatment	Endocrinology, congenital cardiac care for adults, and other specialty care as needed. A multidisciplinary team experienced with 22qDS is optimal.

Psychiatric care

Medications	Standard psychotropic medications, but consider: Increased risk of seizures and other neurological side effects May need anticonvulsant therapy Increased rate of thrombocytopenia Increased rate of leukopenia Increased risk of obesity High rate of hypocalcemia and attendant fatigue, neuropsychiatric symptoms, and prolonged QT interval
Therapy	Standard supportive, educational, family-based, and cognitive-behavioral therapy, but consider: Learning difficulties Family involvement usually essential
Supports	Standard community supports, but consider: Possible financial and other competency issues Family involvement usually essential

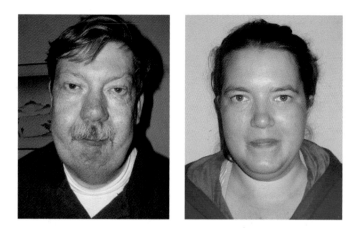

FIGURE 5–2.   Two individuals with 22q11.2 deletion syndrome showing typical facial features.

phrenia in the general population (see Figure 5–4). The features of schizophrenia, including symptoms and age at onset, in 22qDS are typical and appear to be unrelated to general intellectual level (Bassett et al. 2003). The prevalence of schizophrenia in 22qDS is 23%–25% (Bassett et al. 2005; Murphy et al. 1999), indicating that persons with this syndrome are at high risk for developing schizophrenia. Other nonpsychotic illnesses, including anxiety disorders, major depression, and attention-deficit disorder (in childhood), however, are also collectively common in 22qDS (Bassett et al. 2005; Murphy et al. 1999), suggesting the psychiatric phenotype is as variable as the physical phenotype in 22qDS.

The 22q11.2 deletion syndrome is associated with a microdeletion on chromosome 22q11.2 (see Figure 5–5) of variable length and, in some cases, variable position within this region. Neither deletion length nor position appears to have a relationship with major features of the syndrome, including schizophrenia (Weksberg et al. 2007). These deletions are too small for detection using routine karyotype analysis. The specialized cytogenetic technique of FISH, available in clinical laboratories, is necessary for molecular diagnosis. The standard 22q11.2 probes (D22S75 or TUPLE1) used will detect most deletions in this region (see Figure 5–5). Most deletions occur as spontaneous (de novo) mutations. Only 5%–10% of cases are inherited from transmitting parents, who often have a less severe phenotype (Cohen et al. 1999).

With a high index of suspicion for syndromic forms of schizophrenia (see Table 5–3), a clinician would initiate a comprehensive diagnostic workup of the patient, including a thorough developmental, medical, and family history and physical examination by a clinician experienced in ge-

Individual without deletion (critical region present on both copies of chromosome 22)

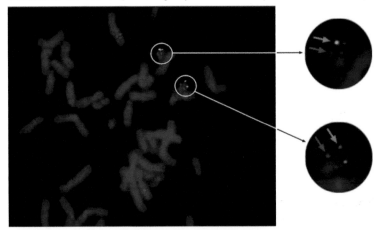

Individual with deletion (critical region missing from one copy of chromosome 22)

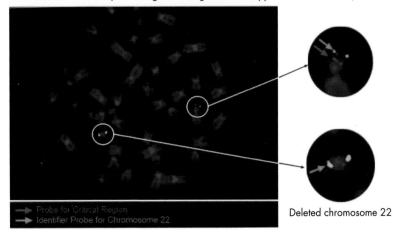

Probe for Critical Region
Identifier Probe for Chromosome 22

Deleted chromosome 22

FIGURE 5–3.   Fluorescence in situ hybridization (FISH) for common deletion in 22q11.2 deletion syndrome.

Source.   Reprinted from Bassett A, Chow E, Brzustowicz L: "The Genetics of Schizophrenia." *Neuroscience News* 4:20–26, 2001. Used with permission.

netic syndromes and dysmorphology. Family members should be seen, and, if possible, family photographs should be examined. Genetic testing would follow if sufficient features were present in the identified patient to support a clinical diagnosis of a syndrome such as 22qDS. Testing would usually include a standard karyotype and FISH for a 22q11.2 deletion. Be-

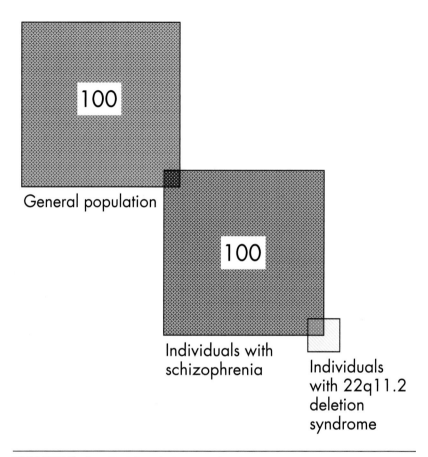

FIGURE 5–4.   Epidemiology of schizophrenia.

cause the phenotype is often subtle and relatively few clinicians have yet become aware of 22qDS, this condition is underrecognized, especially in adults (Cohen et al. 1999). A diagnosis of a 22qDS subtype of schizophrenia, however, has important clinical implications (Bassett and Chow 1999; Bassett et al. 2005; Hodgkinson et al. 2001), as summarized in Table 5–4.

For the psychiatrist treating a patient with 22qDS, there are also management implications, as summarized in Table 5–4. As is common in patients with schizophrenia, the psychiatrist is often the primary physician for the patient and may therefore provide primary care for the accompanying medical conditions or have the responsibility for arranging appropriate investigations and follow-up. Careful attention to the commonly accompanying endocrinological and neurological features in particular may be helpful in the psychiatric management of patients with 22qDS (Bassett et al. 2005).

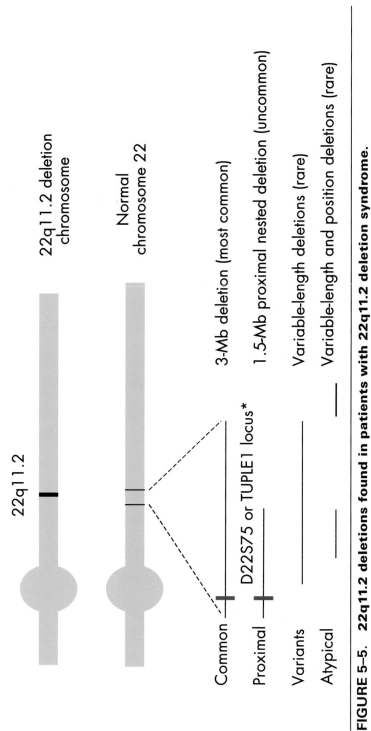

FIGURE 5–5. 22q11.2 deletions found in patients with 22q11.2 deletion syndrome.

*Probes at these loci are commonly used in clinical fluorescence in situ hybridization (FISH) testing for 22q11.2 deletions.

Genetic Counseling

Initial Information Gathering, Risk Assessment, and Counseling

In any genetic counseling session, the first steps would be to obtain a detailed family history on both sides of the subject's family, as well as a medical history and a psychiatric history, in order to determine the psychiatric diagnosis and decide whether the history suggests a syndromic subtype of schizophrenia such as 22qDS or, in rare cases, a schizophrenia-like psychosis, such as that associated with adult-onset Huntington's disease (Hodgkinson et al. 2001; Tsuang et al. 2000) (see Table 5–1). Risk assessment and genetic counseling would follow very different paths for these cases than for the far more common cases in which the history suggests a multifactorial form of schizophrenia (Bassett et al. 2005; Hodgkinson et al. 2001).

Syndromic Schizophrenia and 22q11.2 Deletion Syndrome

If 22qDS or another syndromic form of schizophrenia is suspected from the subject's history and the family history (see Table 5–3), a referral to a genetics specialist would usually be recommended for diagnostic assessment. In the case of a person with a previous diagnosis of the 22qDS form of schizophrenia, genetic counseling would include discussion of the risks for associated medical conditions and recommendations for investigations and follow-up in a multidisciplinary clinic where available, as well as for counseling about the 50% risk of transmitting the deletion (see Table 5–4) (Hodgkinson et al. 2001).

Also, parents of someone who has 22qDS are routinely tested for the deletion. In 5%–10% of cases, the deletion may be inherited from one parent, who may have a mild presentation of the syndrome (Cohen et al. 1999; McDonald-McGinn et al. 2001; Ryan et al. 1997). A comprehensive family history can help to determine if there are other persons (e.g., siblings) who may be eligible for genetic testing for the deletion. In the majority of newly diagnosed cases of 22qDS, however, the deletion has occurred as a de novo mutation. Counseling regarding the nature of these mutations, which appear to occur during gametogenesis, and the related predisposing repeat sequences, is often helpful. By helping the family to understand the association between the chromosomal abnormality and the psychiatric and multiple other features of the syndrome, the clinician provides an explanation of what may have long been suspected. Particularly with respect to the condition's behavioral manifestations, this may relieve parents of guilt or inappropriate blame (Hodgkinson et al. 2001).

Multifactorial Schizophrenia

In the more common instance of one case of schizophrenia within a family that appears to be of multifactorial (i.e., unknown) genetic origin, genetic counseling would follow standard practice (Hodgkinson et al. 2001). Some of the issues commonly discussed in genetic counseling are outlined in Table 5–5. Counseling about the lack of genetic or diagnostic testing is often an important component. Empiric recurrence risks shown in Table 5–6 are those commonly in use and are most relevant for simple pedigree situations (e.g., a single first- or second-degree relative with the condition). These empiric risks are derived from the observed frequencies of the condition of interest in relatives of a person who has the condition, such as those by Gottesman (1991) and Vogel and Motulsky (1997). Risks for first-degree relatives range from 6% to 13% and for second-degree relatives from 2% to 4%. The risk estimate for third-degree relatives is approximately 2%, but this figure is based on few studies and is less likely to be accurate. One must also consider the age of the person seeking counseling. Modification of risk information may be appropriate for those who are beyond the most common age range of presentation. Another factor to consider is the presence of psychiatric symptoms or history of a related psychiatric disorder in the person who is inquiring about risk; if such symptoms or history is present, more detailed psychiatric assessment may be warranted (Hodgkinson et al. 2001).

In the case of more complex family structures with schizophrenia and/or other psychiatric disorder(s) in several members, the available empiric risk statistics may be less useful. Relative risk increases dramatically in the rare case of a person where both parents have schizophrenia (see Figure 5–1 and Table 5–6). However, there are no available empiric risk estimates for the more common instances of aunts or uncles or other relatives on both sides of the family having schizophrenia. Also, the empiric risks do not take into account disorders other than narrowly defined schizophrenia.

Family members who are concerned about the recurrence of schizophrenia in themselves or other family members (e.g., children) may benefit from a discussion regarding early signs and symptoms to be alert for, together with encouragement to seek a psychiatric evaluation if they have significant concerns. Timely diagnosis of a treatable condition such as schizophrenia has the potential to alter the prognosis of the disorder. Also, an effective treatment for one family member may be a predictor of effective treatment for other family members (Hodgkinson et al. 2001). Thus, history of treatment trials, future treatment options, and proneness to certain side effects may also be discussed in the genetic counseling session.

Parents With Schizophrenia: Complications in Offspring and Parents

Another special area of genetic counseling involves women with schizophrenia, as they tend for many reasons to have high-risk pregnancies. Psychosis may worsen during pregnancy, and risk of relapse is significantly elevated post partum (Howard 2005). In general, the risks of antipsychotic treatment appear to be less than the risks to the mother and fetus of not treating schizophrenia during pregnancy (Howard 2005). The general health and nutrition of persons with schizophrenia are often poor; they have high rates of smoking, substance use, and gestational diabetes; and rates of fetal and infant mortality in offspring are double that in the general population (Howard 2005). There is an elevated risk of pregnancy complications (Sacker et al. 1996), including the rare complication placental abruption (Jablensky et al. 2005). Rates of death of offspring in childhood are also elevated, as are rates of losing custody of children, possibly due to parenting difficulties associated with severe mental illness, together with limited supports (Howard 2005). A thorough assessment for genetic syndromes and other malformation syndromes, including 22qDS, would be recommended for any fetus or infant with birth defects or developmental delay and for any prospective or expectant mother with schizophrenia and features suggesting such a syndrome (see Table 5–3) (Bassett and Chow 1999; Bassett et al. 2005).

Nongenetic Risk Factors and Early Intervention

Many nongenetic factors have been proposed, but none have more than modest effect on risk for schizophrenia (Rapoport et al. 2005). Few studies have examined the interaction between genetic and nongenetic factors, biologically the most plausible scenario (Bassett et al. 2001; Tsuang et al. 2001). In contrast to obesity in type 2 diabetes, for example, there is no major environmental factor detected that globally influences incidence. Some have suggested that there is no evidence to support preclinical treatment or related prevention programs (Jablensky 2000). In contrast, there is strong justification for early intervention in incipient first-episode psychosis (i.e., after symptoms develop). In this case, long-term outcome is improved, with better response to treatment and greater likelihood of remission, with a shorter duration of untreated psychosis (Perkins et al. 2005). This finding may be related to a progressive pathological process that is well developed by the time the frank psychopathology of schizophrenia emerges (Perkins et al. 2005).

Preventing or Delaying Schizophrenia

The absence of environmental factors of large effect for schizophrenia means that there is little one can do, take, or avoid to alter risk for developing the illness. The mechanism of most possible risk factors is so uncertain at this point, their roles so minimal, and the ability to control them modest in most cases, that they do not bear much consideration. Having said this, there may be some general measures that may decrease risk to some extent (see Table 5–5).

In addition to avoiding substance use, particularly early marijuana use, lifelong general health measures, including good nutrition and mental and physical exercise, may be helpful. There is some evidence that environmental enrichment can delay onset and slow progression of neurodegenerative diseases such as Huntington's disease and Alzheimer's disease (Spires and Hannan 2005). The proposed mechanisms include induction of synaptogenesis and/or neurogenesis (Spires and Hannan 2005). Although no direct evidence exists for schizophrenia, an enriched environment may be helpful. Such an environment would include social interactions; physical activity; a healthy diet, including fish, folate-rich foods, and fresh fruits and vegetables; and mental stimulation such as puzzles. Preliminary evidence suggests that parents' use of a clear communication style may also be helpful in prevention of schizophrenia (Wahlberg et al. 2004). Most important, however, would be recognizing early signs of illness and promptly seeking expert help in diagnosis and effective treatment. Relatives and caregivers could potentially have the greatest impact by recognizing the early stages of illness.

Early changes that may herald the onset of schizophrenia include increasing anxiety or worrying, avoiding people, irritability, changed sleep patterns, depression, suspiciousness, preoccupations, and worsening academic or work performance (Beiser et al. 1993; Singh et al. 2005).

Future Considerations

There is much to look forward to in the fast-paced field of genetics, including research to help elucidate the genetics of schizophrenia. Identification of rare single-gene forms of schizophrenia remains possible and could contribute to understanding of molecular pathogenesis. Considering 22qDS and other identifiable syndromic forms of schizophrenia in the mix of patient samples studied may improve homogeneity of samples and increase the power of studies. Recently discovered structural genomic variants that are common in the general population could prove important for delineating the genetic etiology of schizophrenia (Feuk et al. 2006). Other evolving

TABLE 5–5. General recommendations for measures that may reduce risk for persons with an elevated risk of schizophrenia

Life stage[a]	Recommendation
Preconception	Maintain good nutrition and physical activity
	Optimize mental and physical health (e.g., consider HIV and other infections, obesity, diabetes)
	Take folate supplements (0.4 mg/day; 0.8–5 mg/day if diabetes, epilepsy, or family history of neural tube defects is present)
	Obtain genetic counseling (maternal and paternal contributions for both the woman and her partner) and individualized risk assessment
	Discuss options with partner, family members, health professionals
	Plan possible pregnancy medication strategies (e.g., change anticonvulsant) (consult http://www.motherisk.org)
During pregnancy	Maintain good nutrition and physical activity
	Maintain optimal mental and physical health
	Obtain antenatal care and monitoring, including planning for use of specialized unit at delivery if necessary and available
	Take folate and iron supplements
	Avoid smoking, alcohol, and street drugs
	Obtain genetic counseling (maternal and paternal contributions for both the woman and her partner), if not previously available or obtained
	Discuss options with partner, family members, health professionals
	Optimize psychiatric care, including medications, for mother and fetus, and partner if necessary

TABLE 5–5. **General recommendations for measures that may reduce risk for persons with an elevated risk of schizophrenia** *(continued)*

Life stage[a]	Recommendation
Postpartum period	Obtain psychiatric care and monitoring for the mother, and partner if necessary
	Ensure that sufficient supports are available, including appropriate housing
	Obtain contraceptive advice and follow-up
	Ensure adequacy of care and safety of infant
	Maintain good nutrition and physical activity
	Address need for infant care and stimulation; make use of specialized programs if developmental delays observed
	Avoid smoking and substance use (by mother and partner and in the home environment)
Childhood, adolescence, adult years	Become aware of possible early signs of schizophrenia (change in sleep pattern, emotional state, behavior, thinking)
	Obtain prompt referral for assessment and effective treatment as necessary
	Maintain an adequate social network, supports, educational opportunities, and stimulation
	Obtain genetic counseling if not previously available or obtained
	Avoid substance use (including alcohol; marijuana use in adolescence especially may increase risk of schizophrenia)

[a]At all stages, and in both parents, the possibility of a genetic syndrome should be considered (see Table 5–3). A diagnosis of a genetic syndrome can significantly change management and planning, including decisions about specialized care and supports.

TABLE 5–6. Empiric risks for schizophrenia for relatives of individuals with the illness

Relationship to affected individual	Lifelong risk, % (range)
First-degree relative	
Offspring with two parents with schizophrenia	46
Offspring with one parent with schizophrenia	13 (9–16)
Sibling	10 (8–14)
Parent	6 (5–10)
Second-degree relative	
Half-sibling	4
Grandchild	4 (2–8)
Nephew or niece	3 (1–4)
Uncle or aunt	2
Third-degree relative	
First cousin	2 (2–6)
General population	1

Source. Adapted from Gottesman 1991; Vogel and Motulsky 1997; Hodgkinson et al. 2001.

areas of research include noncoding RNA, epigenetics (e.g., methylation, imprinting), expression microarrays, pharmacogenomics, stem cells, viral changes of genetic expression during development (Fatemi et al. 2005), and gene therapy. Together with the clinical advances that have already been made, these emerging areas of research hold the promise of increasing our understanding of the genetics and pathophysiology of the collection of conditions known as schizophrenia. We can hope that this understanding will foster a significant decrease in the stigma associated with this serious brain disease and allow exciting treatment developments.

References

American Psychiatric Association: Diagnostic and Statistical Manual of Mental Disorders, 3rd Edition. Washington, DC, American Psychiatric Association, 1980

Arnold SE, Talbot K, Hahn CG: Neurodevelopment, neuroplasticity, and new genes for schizophrenia. Prog Brain Res 147:319–345, 2005

Badner JA, Gershon ES: Meta-analysis of whole-genome linkage scans of bipolar disorder and schizophrenia. Mol Psychiatry 7:405–411, 2002

Bassett AS, Chow EWC: 22q11 deletion syndrome: a genetic subtype of schizophrenia. Biol Psychiatry 46:882–891, 1999

Bassett AS, Bury A, Hodgkinson KA, et al: Reproductive fitness in familial schizophrenia. Schizophr Res 21:151–160, 1996

Bassett AS, Chow EWC, Weksberg R: Chromosomal abnormalities and schizophrenia. Am J Med Genet (Semin Med Genet) 97:45–51, 2000

Bassett AS, Chow EWC, O'Neill S, et al: Genetic insights into the neurodevelopmental hypothesis of schizophrenia. Schizophr Bull 27:417–430, 2001

Bassett AS, Chow EWC, AbdelMalik P, et al: The schizophrenia phenotype in 22q11 deletion syndrome. Am J Psychiatry 160:1580–1586, 2003

Bassett AS, Chow EWC, Husted J, et al: Clinical features of 78 adults with 22q11 deletion syndrome. Am J Med Genet A 138:307–313, 2005

Bates GP: History of genetic disease: the molecular genetics of Huntington disease—a history. Nat Rev Genet 6:766–773, 2005

Beiser M, Erickson D, Fleming JA, et al: Establishing the onset of psychotic illness. Am J Psychiatry 150:1349–1354, 1993

Bertram L, Tanzi RE: The genetic epidemiology of neurodegenerative disease. J Clin Invest 115:1449–1457, 2005

Blackwood DH, Fordyce A, Walker MT, et al: Schizophrenia and affective disorders—cosegregation with a translocation at chromosome 1q42 that directly disrupts brain-expressed genes: clinical and P300 findings in a family. Am J Hum Genet 69:428–433, 2001

Blouin JL, Dombroski BA, Nath SK, et al: Schizophrenia susceptibility loci on chromosomes 13q32 and 8p21. Nat Genet 20:70–73, 1998

Böök JA: Schizophrenia as a gene mutation. Acta Genetica 4:133–139, 1953

Bromet EJ, Naz B, Fochtmann LJ, et al: Long-term diagnostic stability and outcome in recent first-episode cohort studies of schizophrenia. Schizophr Bull 31:639–649, 2005

Brzustowicz LM, Hodgkinson KA, Chow EWC, et al: Location of a major susceptibility locus for familial schizophrenia on chromosome 1q21-q22. Science 288:678–682, 2000

Brzustowicz L, Simone J, Mohseni P, et al: Linkage disequilibrium mapping of schizophrenia susceptibility to the CAPON region of chromosome 1q22. Am J Hum Genet 74:1057–1063, 2004

Cardno AG, Marshall EJ, Coid B, et al: Heritability estimates for psychotic disorders: the Maudsley twin psychosis series. Arch Gen Psychiatry 56:162-168, 1999

Cohen E, Chow EWC, Weksberg R, et al: Phenotype of adults with the 22q11 deletion syndrome: a review. Am J Med Genet 86:359–365, 1999

Ekelund J, Hennah W, Hiekkalinna T, et al: Replication of 1q42 linkage in Finnish schizophrenia pedigrees. Mol Psychiatry 9:1037–1041, 2004

Fatemi SH, Pearce DA, Brooks AI, et al: Prenatal viral infection in mouse causes differential expression of genes in brains of mouse progeny: a potential animal model for schizophrenia and autism. Synapse 57:91–99, 2005

Feuk L, Carson AR, Scherer SW: Structural variation in the human genome. Nat Rev Genet 7:85–97, 2006

Goff DC, Cather C, Evins AE, et al: Medical morbidity and mortality in schizophrenia: guidelines for psychiatrists. J Clin Psychiatry 66:183–194, 2005

Gottesman I: Schizophrenia Genesis: The Origins of Madness. New York, WH Freeman, 1991

Gottesman II, Bertelsen A: Confirming unexpressed genotypes for schizophrenia. Arch Gen Psychiatry 46:867–872, 1989

Gottesman I, Shields J: Schizophrenia: The Epigenetic Puzzle. Cambridge, UK, Cambridge University Press, 1982

Harrison PJ: The neuropathology of schizophrenia: a critical review of the data and their interpretation. Brain 122:593–624, 1999

Hennah W, Varilo T, Paunio T, et al: Haplotype analysis and identification of genes for a complex trait: examples from schizophrenia. Ann Med 36:322–331, 2004

Hodgkinson CA, Goldman D, Jaeger J, et al: Disrupted in schizophrenia 1 (DISC1): association with schizophrenia, schizoaffective disorder, and bipolar disorder. Am J Hum Genet 75:862–872, 2004

Hodgkinson K, Murphy J, O'Neill S, et al: Genetic counselling for schizophrenia in the era of molecular genetics. Can J Psychiatry 46:123–130, 2001

Horowitz A, Shifman S, Rivlin N, et al: A survey of the 22q11 microdeletion in a large cohort of schizophrenia patients. Schizophr Res 73:263–267, 2005

Howard LM: Fertility and pregnancy in women with psychotic disorders. Eur J Obstet Gynecol Reprod Biol 119:3–10, 2005

Husted J, Greenwood CM, Bassett AS: Heritability of schizophrenia and major affective disorder as a function of age, in the presence of strong cohort effects. Eur Arch Psychiatry Clin Neurosci 256:222–229, 2006

Jablensky A: Prevalence and incidence of schizophrenia spectrum disorders: implications for prevention. Aust N Z J Psychiatry 34:s26–s34, 2000

Jablensky AV, Morgan V, Zubrick SR, et al: Pregnancy, delivery, and neonatal complications in a population cohort of women with schizophrenia and major affective disorders. Am J Psychiatry 162:79–91, 2005

Kandel ER, Squire LR: Neuroscience: breaking down scientific barriers to the study of brain and mind. Science 290:1113–1120, 2000

Kane JM: Schizophrenia. N Engl J Med 334:34–41, 1996

Karayiorgou M, Morris MA, Morrow B, et al: Schizophrenia susceptibility associated with interstitial deletions of chromosome 22q11. Proc Natl Acad Sci USA 92:7612–7616, 1995

Kirov G, O'Donovan M C, Owen MJ: Finding schizophrenia genes. J Clin Invest 115:1440–1448, 2005

Kringlen E, Cramer G: Offspring of monozygotic twins discordant for schizophrenia. Arch Gen Psychiatry 46:873–877, 1989

Lander E, Kruglyak L: Genetic dissection of complex traits: guidelines for interpreting and reporting linkage results. Nat Genet 11:241–247, 1995

Lauronen E, Koskinen J, Veijola J, et al: Recovery from schizophrenic psychoses within the northern Finland 1966 Birth Cohort. J Clin Psychiatry 66:375–383, 2005

Lewis CM, Levinson DF, Wise LH, et al: Genome scan meta-analysis of schizophrenia and bipolar disorder, part II: schizophrenia. Am J Hum Genet 73:34–48, 2003

Lieberman JA, Stroup TS, McEvoy JP, et al: Effectiveness of antipsychotic drugs in patients with chronic schizophrenia. N Engl J Med 353:1209–1223, 2005

McDonald-McGinn DM, Tonnesen MK, Laufer-Cahana A, et al: Phenotype of the 22q11.2 deletion in individuals identified through an affected relative: cast a wide FISHing net! Genet Med 3:23–29, 2001

Moore JH: A global view of epistasis. Nat Genet 37:13–14, 2005

Mulle JG, Chowdari KV, Nimgaonkar V, et al: No evidence for association to the G72/G30 locus in an independent sample of schizophrenia families. Mol Psychiatry 10:431–433, 2005

Murphy KC, Jones LA, Owen MJ: High rates of schizophrenia in adults with velo-cardio-facial syndrome. Arch Gen Psychiatry 56:940–945, 1999

Murray CJ, Lopez AD: Global mortality, disability, and the contribution of risk factors: global burden of disease study. Lancet 349:1436–1442, 1997

Nicolson R, Rapoport JL: Childhood-onset schizophrenia: rare but worth studying. Biol Psychiatry 46:1418–1428, 1999

Pantelis C, Yucel M, Wood SJ, et al: Structural brain imaging evidence for multiple pathological processes at different stages of brain development in schizophrenia. Schizophr Bull 31:672–696, 2005

Perkins DO, Gu H, Boteva K, et al: Relationship between duration of untreated psychosis and outcome in first-episode schizophrenia: a critical review and meta-analysis. Am J Psychiatry 162:1785–1804, 2005

Permutt MA, Wasson J, Cox N: Genetic epidemiology of diabetes. J Clin Invest 115:1431–1439, 2005

Petryshen TL, Middleton FA, Kirby A, et al: Support for involvement of neuregulin 1 in schizophrenia pathophysiology. Mol Psychiatry 10:366–374, 328, 2005

Rapoport JL, Addington AM, Frangou S, et al: The neurodevelopmental model of schizophrenia: update 2005. Mol Psychiatry 10:434–449, 2005

Risch N: Linkage strategies for genetically complex traits: I: multilocus models. Am J Hum Genet 46:222–228, 1990

Rosa A, Fananas L, Cuesta MJ, et al: 1q21-q22 locus is associated with susceptibility to the reality-distortion syndrome of schizophrenia spectrum disorders. Am J Med Genet 114:516–518, 2002

Ryan AK, Goodship JA, Wilson DI, et al: Spectrum of clinical features associated with interstitial chromosome 22q11 deletions: a European collaborative study. J Med Genet 34:798–804, 1997

Sacker A, Done DJ, Crow TJ: Obstetric complications in children born to parents with schizophrenia: a meta-analysis of case-control studies. Psychol Med 26:279–287, 1996

Shenton ME, Dickey CC, Frumin M, et al: A review of MRI findings in schizophrenia. Schizophr Res 49:1–52, 2001

Singh SP, Cooper JE, Fisher HL, et al: Determining the chronology and components of psychosis onset: the Nottingham Onset Schedule (NOS). Schizophr Res 80:117–130, 2005

Spires TL, Hannan AJ: Nature, nurture and neurology: gene-environment interactions in neurodegenerative disease. FEBS J 272:2347–2361, 2005

Spitzer RL, Endicott J, Gibbon M: Crossing the border into borderline personality and borderline schizophrenia. Arch Gen Psychiatry 36:17–24, 1979

Sporn AL, Addington AM, Gogtay N, et al: Pervasive developmental disorder and childhood-onset schizophrenia: comorbid disorder or a phenotypic variant of a very early onset illness? Biol Psychiatry 55:989–994, 2004

Stefansson H, Sigurdsson E, Steinthorsdottir V, et al: Neuregulin 1 and susceptibility to schizophrenia. Am J Hum Genet 71:877–892, 2002

Straub RE, MacLean CJ, O'Neill FA, et al: A potential vulnerability locus for schizophrenia on chromosome 6p24-22: evidence for genetic heterogeneity. Nat Genet 11:287–293, 1995

Straub RE, Jiang Y, MacLean CJ, et al: Genetic variation in the 6p22.3 gene DTNBP1, the human ortholog of the mouse dysbindin gene, is associated with schizophrenia. Am J Hum Genet 71:337–348, 2002

Tsuang D, Almqvist EW, Lipe H, et al: Familial aggregation of psychotic symptoms in Huntington's disease. Am J Psychiatry 157:1955–1959, 2000

Tsuang MT, Woolson RF: Mortality in patients with schizophrenia, mania, depression and surgical conditions. A comparison with general population mortality. Br J Psychiatry 130:162–166, 1977

Tsuang MT, Stone WS, Faraone SV: Genes, environment and schizophrenia. Br J Psychiatry 2001:s18–s24, 2001

Vogel F, Motulsky AG: Human Genetics: Problems and Approaches, 3rd ed. Berlin, Springer-Verlag, 1997

Wahlberg KE, Wynne LC, Hakko H, et al: Interaction of genetic risk and adoptive parent communication deviance: longitudinal prediction of adoptee psychiatric disorders. Psychol Med 34:1531–1541, 2004

Weksberg R, Stachon AC, Squire JA, et al: Molecular characterization of deletion breakpoints in adults with 22q11 deletion syndrome. Hum Genet 120:837–845, 2007

Wiehahn GJ, Bosch GP, du Preez RR, et al: Assessment of the frequency of the 22q11 deletion in Afrikaner schizophrenic patients. Am J Med Genet B (Neuropsychiatr Genet) 129:20–22, 2004

Wu EQ, Birnbaum HG, Shi L, et al: The economic burden of schizophrenia in the United States in 2002. J Clin Psychiatry 66:1122–1129, 2005

Zheng Y, Li H, Qin W, et al: Association of the carboxyl-terminal PDZ ligand of neuronal nitric oxide synthase gene with schizophrenia in the Chinese Han population. Biochem Biophys Res Commun 328:809–815, 2005

Chapter 6

Genetics of Mood and Anxiety Disorders

Jordan W. Smoller, M.D., Sc.D.

Mood and anxiety disorders are, in the aggregate, the most common psychiatric disorders in the United States. The toll of these disorders, in terms of both economic costs and human suffering, is staggering. The annual costs associated with mood and anxiety disorders have been estimated to exceed \$100 billion (Uhl and Grow 2004). Bipolar disorder, major depression, and anxiety disorders are associated with substantial disability, medical morbidity, and even mortality (from associated medical illness, suicide, and other sequelae). In this chapter I review the current state of knowledge about the genetic epidemiology and molecular genetic basis of mood and anxiety disorders. The body of research in these areas is vast; the aim in this chapter is to provide a succinct overview of the evidence, highlighting findings that are the most robust and, where possible, emphasizing information that may be of interest to clinicians.

Bipolar Disorder

Clinical Features and Epidemiology

The defining feature of bipolar disorder is the occurrence of a manic episode. Mania is characterized by a week or more of abnormally and persistently elevated, expansive, or irritable mood accompanied by three or more associated symptoms (or at least four if mood is only irritable). The associated symptoms include inflated self-esteem, decreased need for sleep, increased or pressured speech, racing thoughts, distractibility, increased goal-directed activity or psychomotor agitation, and excessive involvement in pleasurable but risky activities (e.g., spending sprees) (American Psychiatric Association 2000). In the vast majority of cases, individuals with bipolar disorder also experience episodes of depression (defined in the next section). The official classification of bipolar disorder evolved with DSM-IV (American Psychiatric Association 1994) to include bipolar II disorder. Bipolar II disorder is characterized by hypomanic (as opposed to manic) episodes in addition to recurrent depressive episodes. Hypomania differs from mania in that symptoms are not severe enough to cause marked impairment in social or occupational functioning or to require hospitalization, and there are no psychotic features (American Psychiatric Association 2000).

The lifetime prevalence of bipolar disorder is typically reported to be between 1% and 3%, although recent population-based estimates for bipolar I disorder together with bipolar II disorder from the National Comorbidity Survey are as high as 3.9% (Kessler et al. 2005a). Although rates of illness do not differ substantially by gender (Kessler et al. 1997), women have a somewhat higher risk of illness, and men have been reported to have an earlier age at onset (Kennedy et al. 2005a). The median age at onset of bipolar disorder is 25 years, although there is evidence for a bimodal age distribution with a smaller later incidence peak around age 40 years (Kennedy et al. 2005b). The most common comorbid disorders among individuals with bipolar disorder are substance use disorders and anxiety disorders (Kessler et al. 2005b; Simon et al. 2004). Suicidality is a serious and frequent complication of bipolar disorder, with lifetime risk as high as 20% (Goldberg and Harrow 2004).

Genetic Epidemiology

Since 1960, 18 family studies have examined the risk of bipolar disorder among first-degree relatives of affected individuals (Smoller and Finn 2003). Despite methodological differences among them, these studies consistently reported excess risks of bipolar disorder among first-degree relatives of bipolar probands. Overall, a summary estimate of familial risk, in which studies were weighted by the number of relatives at risk, indicates that the recurrence risk of bipolar disorder for first-degree relatives of bipolar probands is 8.7% and the risk for unipolar depression is 14.1%. Table 6–1 lists estimates of familial risk of mood disorders in methodologically sophisticated family studies that included comparison (control) individuals and their relatives.

Table 6–2 shows absolute and relative risks (expressed as odds ratios [ORs]) of bipolar disorder and major depressive disorder among relatives of affected individuals and control subjects based on the controlled family studies. Although the relative risk of bipolar disorder is greater than that for major depressive disorder among relatives of probands with bipolar disorder, the absolute risk of major depressive disorder is higher. That is, relatives of individuals with bipolar disorder are more likely to be affected with major depressive disorder than with bipolar disorder, even though their relative risk of bipolar disorder is higher. Because major depressive disorder is a more common disorder, even a 2- to 3-fold increased risk of major depressive disorder translates into a larger absolute risk than a 10-fold increased risk of bipolar disorder. In the genetic counseling context, this example illustrates the importance of providing both types of risk information.

Earlier onset of bipolar disorder in probands has been associated with greater familial risk of mood disorder in several studies that used age cutoff points of 20 years (Pauls et al 1992), 25 years (Grigoroiu-Serbanescu et al. 2001; Somanath et al. 2002), 30 years (James 1977; Taylor and Abrams 1981), and even 50 years (Angst et al. 1980). In addition, there is evidence that pediatric or prepubertal bipolar disorder may represent a distinct form of the disorder and that it may be genetically related to disruptive behavior disorders, particularly attention-deficit/hyperactivity disorder (ADHD) (Spencer et al. 2001; Todd 2002). In general, early-onset disorder appears to represent a more severe subtype with stronger genetic loading (Schurhoff et al. 2000; Strober et al. 1988). Segregation analyses incorporating age at onset have been consistent with the existence of a single major gene influencing the early-onset subtype (Grigoroiu-Serbanescu et al. 2001; Rice et al. 1987). In a controlled family study, Geller and colleagues (2006) found that the prevalence of bipolar disorder among first-degree relatives of probands with prepubertal/early adolescent–onset bipolar disorder was substantially higher (28.2%) than among relatives of probands with ADHD (11.2%) or healthy control probands (3.8%). The prevalence of either bipolar I disorder or recurrent major depressive disorder was as high as 46.5% among first-degree relatives of probands with prepubertal/early adolescent–onset bipolar disorder. In addition, relatives with ADHD were at increased risk for bipolar disorder; this finding is consistent with the results of other studies suggesting that comorbid bipolar disorder and ADHD is a familial phenotype (Faraone et al. 2003).

Family studies have provided some evidence that bipolar II disorder is a distinct entity. Risks of bipolar II disorder have tended to be highest among relatives of probands with bipolar II disorder, as opposed to those with bipolar I disorder or unipolar depression (Andreasen et al. 1987; Cor-

TABLE 6–1. Morbid risk estimates of bipolar and unipolar mood disorders from controlled family studies

Study	Proband group	Relatives at risk: bipolar/unipolar[a]	Morbid risk, first-degree relatives (%)[a]	
			Bipolar disorder	Unipolar disorder
Gershon et al. 1975	Bipolar I disorder, bipolar II disorder	341/264	3.5[b] (3.8[c])	8.7
	Unipolar MDD	96/77	0[b] (2.1[c])	14.2
	Control subjects	518/411	0.2[b] (0.2[c])	0.7
Tsuang et al. 1980	Bipolar disorder	169	5.3	12.4
	Unipolar MDD	362	3.0	15.2
	Control subjects	345	0.3	7.5
Gershon et al. 1982	Bipolar I disorder	441/422	4.5[b] (8.6[c])	14.0
	Bipolar II disorder	157/150	2.6[b] (8.1[c])	17.3
	Unipolar MDD	138/133	1.5[b] (3.0[c])	16.6
	Control subjects	217/208	0[b] (0.5[c])	5.8
Weissman et al. 1984a	Unipolar mood disorder[d]	287	0.8[b] (2.0[c])	18.4
	Control subjects	521	0.2[b] (1.3[c])	5.9

TABLE 6–1. Morbid risk estimates of bipolar and unipolar mood disorders from controlled family studies *(continued)*

Study	Proband group	Relatives at risk: bipolar/unipolar[a]	Morbid risk, first-degree relatives (%)[a] Bipolar disorder	Morbid risk, first-degree relatives (%)[a] Unipolar disorder
Weissman et al. 1993	Unipolar MDD (onset < age 30 yrs)	209	Not reported	21.0
	Control subjects	255	Not reported	5.5
Maier et al. 1993	Bipolar disorder	389	7.0	21.9
	Unipolar mood disorder	697	1.8	21.6
	Unscreened control subjects	419	1.8	10.6

Note. MDD=major depressive disorder.
[a]Number at risk and rates are not age-corrected.
[b]Risk of bipolar I disorder.
[c]Risk of bipolar I disorder and bipolar II disorder combined.
[d]Includes some probands from the study by Gershon et al. (1982).

TABLE 6–2. Recurrence risks and odds ratios for mood disorders from controlled family studies of bipolar disorder

| | First-degree relatives | | | |
| | Bipolar disorder | | Unipolar MDD | |
Probands	Recurrence risk	OR	Recurrence risk	OR
Bipolar	6.7%	10.8*	15.4%	3.3*
Unipolar MDD	2.2%	3.4*	18.7%	4.2*
Control subjects	0.7%	1	5.2%	1

Note. MDD=major depressive disorder; OR=odds ratio (vs. control subjects).
*$P<0.001$.
Source. Adapted from Smoller and Finn 2003.

yell et al. 1984; Endicott et al. 1985; Gershon et al. 1982; Heun and Maier 1993; Simpson et al. 1993). However, the observations that familial risks of unipolar disorder are similar across these proband groups and (in some studies) that risk of bipolar I disorder is also elevated in relatives of probands with bipolar II disorder suggest that these affective disorders are not completely etiologically distinct (Andreasen et al. 1987; Gershon et al. 1982; Heun and Maier 1993). It seems likely that bipolar II disorder is a heterogeneous entity in which some cases are more closely related to bipolar I disorder, some are more closely related to unipolar depression, and others may represent a genetically distinct disorder that breeds true (Blacker and Tsuang 1992; Heun and Maier 1993).

Twin studies have demonstrated that genes account for most of the familial aggregation of bipolar disorder. Table 6–3 shows concordance rates and heritability estimates from the largest recent twin studies of bipolar disorder. The study by Kieseppa and colleagues (2004) included a small number of twin-pairs but had the advantage that the twin-pairs in the study consisted of a representative sample from a nationwide cohort of all Finnish twins born from 1940 to 1957. The risk of bipolar disorder in the identical twin of an affected individual was approximately 40%–45%, and the disorder was highly heritable (~80%). As reviewed in Chapter 1 ("Psychiatric Genetics: A Primer"), it is important to recall that heritability is a measure of how much genes contribute to variation in risk in the population; a heritability of 80% does not mean that 80% of an individual's bipolar dis-

TABLE 6–3. Twin studies of bipolar disorder

	Monozygotic twins		Dizygotic twins		Estimated heritability (h^2)
	Number of twin-pairs[a]	Concordance	Number of twin-pairs[a]	Concordance	
Bertelsen et al. 1977	34	62%	37	8.0%	59%
Kendler et al. 1993c, 1995a	13	38.5%	22	4.5%	79%
McGuffin et al. 2003	30	40%	37	5.4%	85%
Kieseppa et al. 2004	7	43%	18	5.6%	93%

[a]Number of pairs with a bipolar disorder proband.

order is due to genes. The two adoption studies that have used a modern definition of bipolar disorder (Mendlewicz and Rainer 1977; Wender et al. 1986) were too small to support clear conclusions about the heritability of bipolar disorder itself.

Molecular Genetic Studies

More than 40 linkage studies of bipolar disorder have been reported. Suggestive evidence of linkage has been reported for almost all chromosomes, but few genomewide significant results have emerged. Three meta-analyses combining results of bipolar disorder genome scans have appeared, with conflicting results (Badner and Gershon 2002; McQueen et al. 2005; Segurado et al. 2003). The most recent and comprehensive meta-analysis combined genotype data from the 11 largest whole genome linkage studies and identified genomewide significant evidence for linkage on chromosomes 6q (for bipolar I disorder) and 8q (for bipolar I disorder and bipolar II disorder) (McQueen et al. 2005). This provides strong evidence for the locations of at least two susceptibility genes for bipolar disorder. Other regions with strong evidence of linkage include 12q, 13q, and chromosome 18 (Craddock and Forty 2006; Craddock et al. 2005). Evidence from linkage and cytogenetic studies have pointed to the 22q11 region as another genomic location for one or more susceptibility genes. As discussed in Chapters 5 and 8, velocardiofacial/DiGeorge syndrome, which results from a microdeletion of 1.5–3 million base pairs from 22q11, confers a high risk of psychotic disorders. An excess risk of bipolar spectrum disorders has also been reported among individuals with velocardiofacial syndrome (Papolos et al. 1996). The deleted region contains approximately 30 genes, some of which (e.g., the catechol-O-methyltransferase gene [$COMT$]) are plausible candidates for involvement in bipolar disorder.

A large and ever-growing number of association studies have examined association between specific genes and bipolar disorder. Candidate gene association studies of bipolar disorder have had the same limitations that genetic studies of other psychiatric disorder have had: most have been too small to provide convincing results, few variants have been examined within each gene, selection of candidate genes has been limited by our incomplete understanding of the biology of the disorder, and multiple testing of many genes and phenotypes has produced a large number of findings that have been difficult to replicate. Nevertheless, several specific genes have been associated with bipolar disorder in independent samples or metaanalyses, including disrupted in schizophrenia 1 ($DISC1$), the dopamine transporter ($SLC6A3$), brain-derived neurotrophic factor ($BDNF$), the N-methyl-D-aspartate glutamate receptor subunit 2B ($GRIN2B$), d-amino acid oxidase activator (*DAOA*, aka *G72*), the serotonin transporter (*SLC6A4*), tryptophan hydroxylase–2 (*TPH2*), and *COMT* (Craddock and Forty 2006; De Luca et al. 2005; Fallin et al. 2005; Martucci et al. 2006; Van Den Bogaert et al. 2006). In particular, multiple studies or meta-analyses of association studies have supported a role for *SLC6A4* (Lasky-Su et al. 2005), *BDNF* (Kremeyer et al. 2006; Neves-Pereira et al. 2002; Sklar et al. 2002), *DAOA* (Detera-Wadleigh and McMahon 2006) and the gene encoding 5,10-methylenetetrahydrofolate reductase (*MTHFR*) (Gilbody et al. 2007). However, to date, no gene has been established as a bipolar disorder susceptibility gene. One approach to reducing the complexity of the phenotype for association studies has been to focus on phenotypic subtypes (e.g., early-onset or rapid-cycling bipolar disorder) that may be more genetically homogeneous. This approach has suggested that, for example, *BDNF* may influence rapid-cycling bipolar disorder (Green et al. 2006; Muller et al. 2006).

Several large-scale whole genome association studies of bipolar disorder are under way and may provide more definitive evidence of the involvement of specific genetic variants. As of this writing, two such studies have been published. In the first, Baum and colleagues (2007) analyzed 550,000 single nucleotide polymorphisms (SNPs) in samples of European origin. Their strongest result implicated *DGKH,* the gene encoding diacylglycerol kinase eta, on chromosome 13q14. This gene is of interest because its product is involved in the phosphatidyl inositol pathway through which lithium may exert some of its mood-stabilizing effects. A second, larger study was conducted as part of the Wellcome Trust Case Control Consortium (WTCCC) (2007) in a report on seven major diseases. A sample of 1,868 case subjects and 3,000 U.K. control subjects were genotyped at 500,000 SNPs. The strongest result in the primary analysis was for a SNP (rs420259) on chromosome 16p12, which gave a genotypic P value of 6.3×10^{-8}, exceeding the prespecified significance threshold of 5×10^{-7}, and an odds ratio of approximately 2.1 for both heterozygotes and homozygotes. This SNP falls in a region near several genes that might be plausible candidates for bipolar disorder, including *PALB2* (involved in the stability of key nuclear structures, including chromatin), *NDUFAB1* (which encodes a component of the mitochondrial respiratory chain), and *DCTN5* (which interacts with *DISC1*). Of note, there was no significant evidence to support association with leading candidate genes, including *BDNF, DAOA, DTNBP1, DISC1,* or *NRG1* (neuregulin).

An intriguing theme emerging from family, twin, and molecular genetic studies of bipolar disorder has been the possibility that genetic influences on the disorder overlap with those contributing to other psychiatric disorders. The relationship between bipolar disorder and unipolar major depressive disorder has received a great deal of attention. As shown in Table 6–2, the risk of major depressive disorder is elevated among relatives of probands with bipolar disorder. To a lesser extent, the risk of bipolar disorder is also elevated among relatives of probands with major depressive disorder. Evidence from twin studies has suggested that some of the genetic liability to bipolar disorder and major depressive disorder is overlapping (McGuffin et al. 2003). However, no reliable features of latent bipolarity among depressed relatives of bipolar disorder probands have been identified (Blacker et al. 1996).

Evidence also suggests that comorbid bipolar disorder and panic disorder represents a familial subtype of bipolar disorder. Data from independent family sets suggest that risk for panic disorder in families segregating bipolar disorder is a familial trait (Doughty et al. 2004; MacKinnon et al. 1997, 2002). Relatives of probands with comorbid bipolar disorder and panic disorder were also more likely to have bipolar II disorder rather than bipolar I disorder. The presence of panic disorder comorbidity in families segregating bipolar disorder has also been associated with rapid mood switching in individuals affected with bipolar disorder (MacKinnon et al. 2003). Linkage and association analyses have provided some support for the hypothesis that the bipolar disorder/panic disorder phenotype is genetically influenced (Cheng et al. 2006; MacKinnon et al. 1998; Rotondo et al. 2002).

A variety of studies have suggested that bipolar disorder is also genetically related to psychotic disorders (i.e., schizophrenia, schizoaffective disorder) (Taylor et al. 1993; Tsuang et al. 1980; Valles et al. 2000), although results have been mixed (Gershon et al. 1975, 1982; Maier et al. 1993a; Weissman et al. 1984a). Data from twin studies have supported a genetic relationship between bipolar disorder and psychotic disorders. Cardno and colleagues (2002a), applying nonhierarchical diagnostic definitions such that twins could be assigned lifetime diagnoses for more than one of these disorders, reported significant correlations in genetic liability among the three syndromes; the genetic correlations were 0.68 for schizophrenic and manic syndromes and 0.88 for schizoaffective and manic syndromes. The genetic liability to schizoaffective disorder was entirely shared with the two other syndromes. One possibility raised by these studies is that genes actually influence psychosis, a phenotypic feature common to schizophrenia and a subset of probands with bipolar disorder. Consistent with this possibility, family studies have demonstrated that psychotic symptoms define a familial phenotype within bipolar disorder families (Potash et al. 2001, 2003a; Schurhoff et al. 2003, 2005), and twin studies in schizophrenia, bipolar disorder, Alzheimer's disease, and non-ill control subjects have indicated that psychosis itself is heritable (Bacanu et al. 2005; Cardno et al. 2002a, 2002b; Gambini et al. 1997; Jacobs et al. 2005; Jang et al. 2005).

Molecular genetic studies have supported the hypothesis of overlapping genetic influences on bipolar disorder and psychotic disorders. The phenotype of psychotic bipolar disorder has been linked to specific chromosomal regions (Kerner et al 2007; Park et al. 2004; Potash et al. 2003b; Sklar et al. 2004). Some of the regions with the strongest linkage evidence for schizophrenia (e.g., 6q, 13q, 22q) are also among the regions most strongly linked to bipolar disorder (Badner et al. 2002; Craddock et al. 2006a; McQueen et al. 2005). The balanced translocation (1; 11) (q42;q14.3) that disrupts *DISC1* was first identified from its co-segregation with a broad phenotype comprising schizophrenia, bipolar disorder, and recurrent major depressive disorder (Blackwood et al. 2001), and the 22q11 microdeletion responsible for velocardiofacial syndrome appears to confer increased risk of both psychotic and mood disorders (Bassett et al. 2003, 2005) and encompasses genes (e.g., *COMT*) that have been associated with both mood and psychotic disorders (Craddock et al. 2006b; Kirov et al. 1998; Papolos et al. 1998; Shifman et al. 2004). Other genes have been associated with both schizophrenia and bipolar disorder in multiple studies, including neuregulin 1 (*NRG1*), dysbindin (*DTNBP1*), *DISC1, SLC6A4, DAOA,* and *MTHFR* (Craddock et al. 2006a; Gilbody et al. 2007).

Implications for Genetic Counseling

Although genetic counseling may not be relevant for many patients and families, in appropriate circumstances and when conducted by informed clinicians, education and counseling about familial and genetic aspects of bipolar disorder can be helpful (Finn and Smoller 2006). The American Psychiatric Association guidelines for the treatment of bipolar disorder suggest that genetic counseling may be helpful for patients who are considering having children (American Psychiatric Association 2002) As described by Peay and Rosen Sheidley in Chapter 2 ("Principles of Genetic Counseling") of this volume, individuals and families may seek genetic counseling for a variety of reasons in addition to gathering information prior to having or adopting children (e.g., to assess personal risk of illness in the setting of having affected family members). Individuals may also inquire about the availability of genetic testing. General issues involved in providing genetic counseling and discussing quantitative risk information are reviewed in Chapter 2 and Chapter 3 ("Risk Communication: Simple Tools to Foster Understanding") of this volume and will not be reiterated here. I will focus instead on issues relevant to discussions about familial and genetic factors in bipolar disorder specifically.

In the absence of established susceptibility genes, disease risk estimation for bipolar disorder is limited to data from family studies (which, as noted, cannot distinguish genetic and nongenetic risk factors). As is the case for other disorders, empiric risk estimates may be difficult to apply directly to an individual family because these estimates are derived from the particular families that were ascertained for the family studies on which they are based. For a given family, patterns of comorbidities, ages at onset of affected members, the number of affected individuals, and other family-specific features of illness may substantially alter risk likelihoods. Nevertheless, the available evidence does support some inferences and principles relevant to genetic counseling.

First, the fact that genes contribute strongly to bipolar disorder can be an important element of psychoeducation. Some families carry the burden of misconceptions about the etiology of bipolar disorder than can engender feelings of guilt and shame—for example, the idea that poor parenting or other features of family life are the primary cause of the disorder. At the same time, some individuals may understand that bipolar disorder is heritable but have misconceptions about the nature of inheritance. In light of these misconceptions, it is helpful to explain the distinction between classic single-gene inheritance (as seen in Huntington's disease and cystic fibrosis) and the complex multifactorial inheritance that characterizes common psychiatric disorders. Multiple genes (likely with small individual effects) contribute to the disorder and may need to interact with each other or with environmental factors to show their effects. This complexity is reflected in the fact that the concordance rate for bipolar disorder for genetically identical (monozygotic [MZ]) twin pairs is only about 40%.

Second, available empiric risk estimates, when presented with the appropriate caveats about their applicability to the consultand's family, can provide useful information about recurrence risks. These estimates suggest that first-degree relatives of affected individuals have a roughly 10% risk of the disorder. This represents up to a 10-fold greater risk of the disorder compared with the general population but also means that the probability of being unaffected is approximately 90%. More limited data are available on risks for second-degree relatives of bipolar disorder probands, but they suggest that the risks of bipolar disorder and major depressive disorder are not substantially elevated above population risks (Smoller and Finn 2003). Although it is not possible to precisely individualize risk estimates for a given patient or family, some data exist that can be used to inform such estimates. For example, the median age at onset of bipolar disorder is 25 years, and only 10% of cases have onset after age 50 years. Thus, whereas the overall risk of bipolar disorder for a woman whose brother is affected might be 10%, that risk would be lower if she is 55 years old with no history of mood disorder. Other factors, however, may increase risk for relatives. For example, early-onset bipolar disorder is associated with greater familial risk (Kennedy et al.

2005b); thus, all other things being equal, an individual whose parent developed bipolar disorder in childhood or adolescence would be at greater risk than someone whose parent had an onset after age 30 years.

Empiric risks from family studies indicate that the absolute risk of major depressive disorder among first-degree relatives of bipolar disorder probands (~15%–20%) is more than twofold higher than the risk for bipolar disorder (~7%–10%). Data from family and high-risk studies suggest that other disorders may co-segregate with bipolar disorder. For example, children of parents with bipolar disorder have been reported to be at increased risk for ADHD and overanxious disorder (Hirshfeld-Becker et al. 2006). Indeed, studies of children at risk for bipolar disorder (i.e., those with parents affected with the disorder) have found elevated risks of a broad range of psychopathology, including disruptive behavior disorders, anxiety disorders, and depression (DelBello and Geller 2001; Henin et al. 2005; Hirshfeld-Becker et al. 2006; Lapalme et al. 1997). In a recent controlled study of young (mean age=7 years) offspring of bipolar disorder parents, Hirshfeld-Becker and colleagues (2006) found a fivefold increased risk of ADHD (23.5%) and a sixfold increased risk of anxiety disorder (44.1%), compared with offspring of non-ill parents.

In some cases, individuals may overestimate familial risks. Quaid and colleagues (2001) reported that bipolar disorder patients estimated a "moderate" risk of illness in siblings (mean risk estimate=35.2%) and high risk in children (mean=44.6%). They also overestimated the general population prevalence of bipolar disorder (28.1%). Family and epidemiological studies have indicated that the risk is closer to 10% for first-degree relatives of affected individuals (Smoller and Finn 2003) and 1%–4% in the general population (Kessler et al. 2005c; Weissman et al. 1996). In another survey, the risk of bipolar disorder to a child when one parent has the disorder was overestimated by both patients with bipolar disorder (mean estimate= 46.7%) and their spouses (mean estimate=41.4%) (Trippitelli et al. 1998). To the extent that recurrence risk estimates have been overestimated by consultands who seek genetic counseling, more accurate information may provide reassurance.

Genetic testing is not currently available for bipolar disorder, and given the complexity of the disorder, it is not clear whether highly predictive testing will ever be feasible. Nevertheless, surveys of patients and health professionals indicate that there might be substantial demand for genetic tests for bipolar disorder (Finn et al. 2005; Trippitelli et al. 1998). Note that the high heritability of a disorder such as bipolar disorder does not necessarily mean that the development of genetic testing will be straightforward, because heritability reflects the additive effects of all contributing genes. Heritability estimates do not provide information about the genetic architecture of the disorder. For example, an overall heritability of 80% could reflect the influence of 100 genes of small effect, a few genes of large effect, or some combination of these. The number and penetrance of the genes involved are more important than the heritability in determining the utility of predictive tests. For example, the population heritability of breast cancer, for which highly predictive genetic tests for major genes are available, has been estimated at less than 30% (Lichtenstein et al. 2000). For mood and anxiety disorders, there is little evidence of effects of a single major gene. In association studies implicating specific genetic variants in risk for bipolar disorder, effect sizes have been modest (e.g., OR<1.5). By itself, a test based on such a variant would be of limited value in the absence of other information; given a baseline risk of 2% for bipolar disorder, carrying such a risk allele would increase an individual's risk to 3%. Although the prospect of genetic testing for common forms of bipolar disorder is uncertain, it should be noted that in rare cases, patients presenting with bipolar disorder symptoms may have underlying medical genetic disorders (e.g., velocardiofacial syndrome) for which tests are available (see Chapters 2, 5 ["Genetics of Schizophrenia and Psychotic Disorders"], and 8 ["Neuropsychiatric Aspects of Genetic Disorders"] for further discussion).

Major Depressive Disorder

Clinical Features and Epidemiology

Major depressive disorder is a common disorder characterized by one or more major depressive episodes that are not better accounted for by bereavement, substance use, or a general medical condition (American Psychiatric Association 2000). A major depressive episode is defined by 2 weeks or more of persistent depressed mood and/or loss of interest in usual activities that is accompanied by three or more additional symptoms comprising significant changes in appetite/weight, insomnia or hypersomnia, psychomotor agitation or retardation, fatigue or decreased energy, feelings of worthlessness or excessive guilt, impaired concentration or indecisiveness, and recurrent thoughts of death or suicide. Recognized risk factors for major depressive disorder include family history of mood disorder, childhood adversity and parental loss, and stressful life events in adolescence and adulthood (Kendler et al. 2002, 2006b). The estimated lifetime prevalence of major depressive disorder from the National Comorbidity Survey Replication study is 16.2%, and the rate is 1.7-fold higher in women than in men (Kessler et al. 2003). The most common lifetime comorbidities associated with depression are anxiety disorders, substance use disorders, and impulse-control disorders (Kessler et al. 2003).

The burden of disease associated with depression is tremendous. At the start of this century, major depressive disorder was identified as the leading cause of years lived with disability worldwide and the fourth leading cause of disease burden (Ustun et al. 2004). The direct and indirect costs of major depressive disorder exceed $80 billion annually (Greenberg et al. 2003). In addition to the disability associated with major depressive disorder, the risk of mortality due to suicide is substantial, with lifetime risk estimates as high as 15%–20% (Ebmeier et al. 2006).

Genetic Epidemiology

A substantial body of evidence has established that major depressive disorder is a familial phenotype (Smoller and Perlis 2004). In case-control family studies, the risk of depression to relatives of depressed probands has been significantly higher than the risk to relatives of unaffected control subjects, with relative risks ranging from approximately twofold to ninefold (Bland et al. 1986; Farmer et al. 2000; Gershon et al. 1982; Kutcher and Marton 1991; Warner et al. 1995; Weissman et al. 1984a, 1993). In a meta-analysis of high-quality family studies, Sullivan et al. (2000) found that the prevalence of major depressive disorder was threefold higher in the relatives of affected probands, compared with the relatives of unaffected control subjects (summary OR=2.84; 95% confidence interval [CI]: 2.31–3.49). More limited data have suggested that other depressive disorders also show familial aggregation. Dysthymic disorder, characterized by chronic lower-level depressive symptoms lasting at least 2 years, also appears to aggregate in families (Klein et al. 1995, 2004). Forty et al. (2006) reported that postpartum depression occurring within 2 months of delivery is also familial.

Twin studies of major depression have provided consistent evidence that genes account for a substantial proportion of the familial aggregation of major depression. In almost all of the more recent twin studies, concordance rates for MZ twins have exceeded those for dizygotic (DZ) twins (Sullivan et al. 2000; Tsuang and Faraone 1990). For studies published since 1985, the MZ concordance rates have typically been in the range of 30% to 50%, and DZ concordance rates have typically ranged from 12% to 40%, with somewhat higher rates seen in female twin-pairs, compared with male twin-pairs (Sullivan et al. 2000; Tsuang and Faraone 1990). Estimates of heritability in these studies ranged from 17% to 78%. Combining data from these studies, Sullivan et al. (2000) estimated the summary heritability at 37% (95% CI: 33%–42%), with a larger share of the variance explained by individual-specific environment (63%; 95% CI: 58%–67%). The absence of a significant effect of shared family environment suggests that the familial aggregation of major depression is due mostly or entirely to genetic influences. These estimates are consistent with those of the largest and most recent twin study comprising more than 15,000 Swedish twin-pairs, in which the heritability of major depressive disorder was estimated at 42% for women and 29% for men (Kendler et al. 2006c).

A number of clinical features of depression have been identified as markers of familial risk. The most widely studied has been age at onset. Several studies have indicated that early-onset depression (up to age 30 years) is associated with increased familiality. For example, whereas the major depressive disorder recurrence risk ratio for first-degree relatives is about three overall, relatives of probands with major depressive disorder onset before age 20 have an approximately eightfold increased risk (Weissman et al. 1984c). Early-onset depression may itself be a familial subtype such that relatives of probands with early-onset depression are more likely to have early-onset than late-onset depression (Weissman et al. 1993). The greatest risk appears to be associated with early-onset recurrent depression (Bland et al. 1986; Warner et al. 1995). Chronicity of depression is also a marker of increased familial risk of major depressive disorder and appears to be transmitted in families (Klein et al. 2004; Mondimore et al. 2006). In one family study, the risk of major depressive disorder among relatives of probands with chronic major depressive disorder (43.2%) or probands with dysthymia (38.4%) was significantly higher than the risk among relatives of probands with episodic major depressive disorder (29.4%) or relatives of healthy control subjects (21.9%) (Klein et al. 2004). Other proband features that have been associated with increased recurrence risk of major depressive disorder include suicidal depression, severe depression, and history of anxiety disorder or alcoholism (Gershon et al. 1986; Kendler et al. 1999a, 2000; Weissman et al. 1986).

As is the case for bipolar disorder, family and twin studies have suggested that familial and genetic influences on major depressive disorder overlap with those influencing several other disorders. The familial/genetic relationship between bipolar disorder and major depressive disorder was discussed earlier in the section on bipolar disorder. Several family, twin, and molecular studies have suggested a shared diathesis underlying major depressive disorder and alcoholism in at least a subset of individuals (Grant et al. 1996; Kendler et al. 1997; Nurnberger et al. 2001; Winokur and Coryell 1992). The frequent lifetime comorbidity of anxiety and depressive disorders and the fact that antidepressant medications are effective treatments for both groups of disorders have raised the possibility of a shared diathesis (Brier et al. 1985). In fact, data from twin studies suggest that the genetic factors underlying major depressive disorder and generalized anxiety disorder are almost completely overlapping (Kendler et al. 1992b;

Kendler et al. 1993b, 1995b; Roy et al. 1995). On the other hand, family studies of panic disorder probands have generally not shown increased familial rates of major depressive disorder in the absence of comorbid major depressive disorder in the proband (Crowe et al. 1983; Goldstein et al. 1994; Harris et al. 1983; Mannuzza et al. 1994/1995; Mendlewicz et al. 1993; Noyes et al. 1986; Weissman et al. 1993), although there have been exceptions (Maier et al. 1993b, 1995; Munjack and Moss 1981). Family studies of depressed probands have suggested that panic occurring secondary to depression is associated with familial risk of major depressive disorder but not panic disorder (Coryell et al. 1988, 1992; Leckman et al. 1983; Price et al. 1987; Weissman et al. 1984b). Studies of children at risk for anxiety or depressive disorders have yielded somewhat conflicting results, with the findings from some studies suggesting that children of depressed parents are at increased risk for anxiety disorders (Biederman et al. 2001; Breslau et al. 1987) and others indicating an increased risk of depression but not anxiety disorders (Biederman et al. 1991; Weissman et al. 1984b). In a 20-year follow-up study, Weissman et al. (2006) found that offspring of the depressed parents had a threefold increased risk of anxiety disorders, depression, and substance dependence, compared with offspring of nondepressed parents.

Molecular Genetic Studies

Genetic linkage studies of major depressive disorder have implicated several chromosome regions as harboring susceptibility genes, including 1p (McGuffin et al. 2005; Zubenko et al. 2002a, 2002b, 2002c), 2q (Zubenko et al. 2003), 12q (Abkevich et al. 2003; McGuffin et al. 2005), and 15q (Holmans et al. 2004; McGuffin et al. 2005), although these findings await confirmation. A recent large linkage study of families with recurrent early-onset major depressive disorder provided strong support for the 15q region (Holmans et al. 2007; Levinson et al. 2007), and fine mapping of the region indicated that a 15q25–q26 locus increases risk to siblings by as much as 20% (Levinson et al. 2007). Of the many candidate genes examined, the most widely studied has been *SLC6A4* on chromosome 17, which is the gene encoding the serotonin transporter, the therapeutic target of selective serotonin reuptake inhibitor antidepressants. In particular, a common polymorphism in the promoter of the serotonin transporter gene (the serotonin transporter length polymorphic region, 5-HTTLPR) has been the focus of association studies in mood disorders and other mood disorder phenotypes (Levinson 2005). Two common alleles exist and are distinguishable by the insertion ("long" allele) or deletion ("short" allele) of a 44-base pair sequence (Heils et al. 1996; Lesch et al. 1996). The short allele has been associated with reduced expression of the serotonin transporter. Several meta-analyses of association studies of this polymorphism in major depressive disorder have been reported, with mixed results (Anguelova et al. 2003; Furlong et al. 1998; Lotrich and Pollock 2004). More consistent results have been obtained in studies that have incorporated analyses of gene–environment interaction. In a landmark study, Caspi and colleagues (2003) examined the 5-HTTLPR polymorphism in a longitudinal birth cohort of 847 individuals. These authors found that the short allele was associated with risk for major depressive disorder, depressive symptoms, and suicidality among individuals who experienced stressful life events.

At least 11 subsequent studies have examined 5-HTTLPR–environment interactions and depression (Eley et al. 2004; Gillespie et al. 2005; Grabe et al. 2005; Kaufman et al. 2004; Kendler et al. 2005; Scheid et al. 2006; Sjoberg et al. 2006; Surtees et al. 2006; Taylor et al. 2006; Wilhelm et al. 2006; Zalsman et al. 2006), with most supporting an effect on depressive episodes or depressive symptoms, although the two largest studies (Gillespie et al. 2005; Surtees et al. 2006) had negative findings. There is also evidence that environmental influences can counteract genetic and environmental risk factors for depression. Kaufman et al. (2004, 2006) reported that among children with both genetic (5-HTTLPR short alleles) and environmental vulnerabilities (childhood maltreatment), positive environmental factors (i.e., social support) exerted a protective effect on risk of depressive symptoms.

Evidence from functional neuroimaging studies has suggested that the short allele may exert its effect on negative affectivity by enhancing amygdala reactivity to threat, perhaps through reduced cortical inhibition of the amygdala (Pezawas et al. 2005). A second common polymorphism in intron 2 of *SLC6A4* has also been widely studied, although its functional relevance and role in major depressive disorder are as yet unclear (Levinson 2005).

Numerous other genes have been associated with risk of depression in multiple studies, although, as with the serotonin transporter, conflicting results have been reported. Brain-derived neurotrophic factor (BDNF) has been implicated as a mediator of the etiological effects of stress on depression (Duman and Monteggia 2006). As noted in the section on bipolar disorder, *BDNF* has been associated with bipolar disorder in several studies, however. Recent studies have also implicated this gene in major depressive disorder and childhood-onset mood disorder (Schumacher et al. 2005; Strauss et al. 2004, 2005), although conflicting results have also been reported. The gene encoding tryptophan hydroxylase–2 (*TPH2*) has also been associated with major depressive disorder (De Luca et al. 2005; Van Den Bogaert et al. 2006; Zhang et al. 2005; Zill et al. 2004). A recent meta-analysis of studies of 18 genes found statistically significant evidence of association for six: *APOE, DRD4, GNB3, MTHFR, SLC6A3,* and *SLC6A4* (Lopez-Leon et al. 2007).

Implications for Genetic Counseling

The general considerations raised earlier in the section on bipolar disorder also apply to genetic counseling and psychoeducation regarding major depressive disorder. These considerations include the importance of acknowledging the limitations of empiric risk estimates and the importance of presenting quantitative risks in both absolute and relative terms (also see Chapters 2 and 3 for further discussion).

Empiric risk estimates derived from family studies of major depressive disorder suggest that first-degree relatives of affected individuals have a two- to threefold increased risk of the disorder. Given the population prevalence of major depressive disorder (approximately 15%), a risk of approximately 30%–45% exists for first-degree relatives. An important point to note in discussing familial risks of major depressive disorder is that because the lifetime prevalence of major depressive disorder is high, many if not most families in the population will include at least one member with the disorder. It is noteworthy that in family studies of major depressive disorder, the lifetime risk of the disorder in first-degree relatives of control probands has typically been about 5%–10%–lower than population estimates from recent epidemiologic surveys (e.g., 16.6% in the National Comorbidity Survey Replication study; Kessler et al. 2005a). A threefold increased risk of major depressive disorder for relatives in these family studies translates to an absolute risk of approximately 15%–30%. Thus, the overall risk of major depressive disorder in the first-degree relative of an affected individual may be on the order of 15%–30%. Again, however, individualizing risks for a particular consultand or family can be challenging because the influence of variables such as the density and configuration of affected families, the presence of co-segregating comorbidities, and clinical features of major depressive disorder that may be present in a given family (e.g., age at onset) are not well captured in these general estimates. As noted, recurrent, severe, chronic, and/or early-onset major depressive disorder is associated with increased familial risk for relatives of affected probands. For example, the risk of major depressive disorder in the first-degree relative of a proband with recurrent, early-onset major depressive disorder may be two to three times higher than that for relatives of probands with single-episode, later-onset major depressive disorder.

The only three-generation family study of major depressive disorder conducted to date illustrates the importance of documenting a three-generation pedigree in assessing risks. Weissman et al. (2005) reported a 20-year follow-up of families in which three generations were assessed for psychiatric disorders, beginning with the grandparental generation, which included depressed and nondepressed probands. Because the mean age of the grandchildren was only 12 years, most had not passed through the period of risk for major depressive disorder and other disorders. Thus, their lifetime risk of major depressive disorder and other psychopathology could not be defined. Nevertheless, nearly 60% of grandchildren who had a parent and grandparent with major depressive disorder were already affected with a psychiatric disorder. Risks of psychiatric disorders in offspring of depressed parents were moderated by the presence or absence of depression in the grandparental generation. In particular, depression in the parental generation conferred no increased risk of psychiatric disorders in the youngest generation unless there was also a history of depression in at least one grandparent. For example, among children with a depressed grandparent, there was more than a fivefold increased risk of anxiety disorder or any psychiatric disorder in those with a depressed parent, compared with those with nondepressed parents. Furthermore, in offspring with depressed grandparents, the severity of depression in parents was a predictor of mood disorder. Thus, risk differed according to both familial loading and severity of parental depression; the individuals in the highest-risk group were grandchildren with a depressed grandparent and with a parent having moderate to severe depression. Thirty percent of these children met the criteria for a mood disorder, and 45% met the criteria for an anxiety disorder.

Other family, twin, and molecular studies have suggested that depression shares familial and genetic determinants with anxiety disorders, alcoholism, and eating disorders (Camp et al. 2005; Hudson et al. 2003; Kendler et al. 1993a, 2006a; Koenen et al. 2003; Nurnberger et al. 2004; Weissman et al. 1993a, 2005). Thus, relatives of probands affected with major depressive disorder may also be at increased risk for these disorders, although the magnitudes of these risks have not been well defined. Finally, some data suggest that patients with major depressive disorder with a family history of bipolar disorder may be at increased risk of antidepressant-induced mania/hypomania (Wada et al. 2006), but the available evidence is limited.

Anxiety Disorders

The primary anxiety disorders defined in DSM-IV-TR (American Psychiatric Association 2000) are listed in Table 6–4, along with their core clinical features. Anxiety disorders not shown are separation anxiety disorder (an anxiety disorder of childhood), anxiety disorder due to a general medical condition, substance-induced anxiety disorder, and acute stress disorder (a posttraumatic stress syndrome limited to the first month following a traumatic event). The current configuration of anxiety disorders was first defined relatively recently, in DSM-III (American Psychiatric Association 1980). Effective treatments for anxiety disorders include antidepressant and benzodiazepine medications and behavioral or cognitive-behavioral therapy. The following discussion focuses on the disorders about which we know the most from a genetic standpoint. The genetics of obsessive-compulsive disorder are covered in Chapter 4, "Genetics of Childhood-Onset Psychiatric Disorders."

TABLE 6–4. Core features of major anxiety disorders

Disorder	Defining feature(s)
Panic disorder	Recurrent unexpected panic attacks; anticipatory anxiety about attacks; altered behavior due to attacks
With agoraphobia	Fear and avoidance of situations associated with panic attacks
Agoraphobia without a history of panic disorder	Agoraphobia and panic-like symptoms without recurrent unexpected panic attacks
Social phobia	Fear and avoidance of social and/or performance situations
Generalized subtype	Fears include most social situations
Specific phobia	Fear and avoidance of specific objects or situations
Animal, natural environment, blood-injection-injury, situational, other	Focus of fear
Generalized anxiety disorder	Uncontrollable worry, excessive anxiety associated with symptoms of physiological arousal
Obsessive-compulsive disorder	Recurrent, intrusive obsessions; repetitive compulsive behaviors or mental rituals
Posttraumatic stress disorder	Psychic trauma followed by reexperiencing of trauma, avoidance of associated stimuli, emotional numbing, hyperarousal

Panic Disorder

Clinical Features and Epidemiology

In its current definition in DSM-IV-TR, panic disorder includes recurrent, unexpected panic attacks accompanied by persistent worry about having additional attacks or about the consequences of the attacks, and/or a significant change in behavior related to the attacks. Panic attacks are defined as discrete episodes of intense fear or discomfort accompanied by at least 4 of 13 cognitive (e.g., fear of dying, fear of losing control) or somatic (e.g., palpitations, shortness of breath, chest pain) anxiety symptoms that develop abruptly and peak within 10 minutes. Panic attacks themselves can occur as part of other anxiety disorders (including phobic disorders, obsessive-compulsive disorder, and posttraumatic stress disorder [PTSD]) and are a necessary but not specific feature of the diagnosis. Panic attacks are relatively common, occurring in the absence of panic disorder in approximately 23% of the U.S. population (Kessler et al. 2006).

The relationship between panic disorder and agoraphobia has been somewhat controversial. In DSM-IV, agoraphobia is defined by anxiety about and avoidance of situations in which panic attacks or panic-like symptoms may occur. In individuals within clinical settings, agoraphobia is usually felt to be a complication of panic disorder, although epidemiological studies have indicated that agoraphobia frequently occurs in the absence of panic disorder (Wittchen et al. 1998).

Recent estimates place the lifetime prevalence of panic disorder (with or without agoraphobia) at 4.7% (Kessler et al. 2006), with a twofold higher prevalence among women, compared with men. Like other anxiety disorders, panic disorder tends to be a chronic disorder. The complexity of defining the core features and boundaries of the panic disorder diagnosis present particular challenges to genetic studies of this phenotype (Smoller and Tsuang 1998).

Genetic Epidemiology

In a meta-analysis of controlled family studies, Hettema et al. (2001) found that the summary OR (analogous to the recurrence risk ratio) for panic disorder was 5. That is, first-degree relatives of probands with panic disorder have an approximately fivefold increased risk of panic disorder (range= 3.4–15.6). Early-onset panic disorder appears to confer increased risk of the disorder for relatives. Goldstein et al. (1997) found a 17-fold increased risk of panic disorder in first-degree relatives of probands with onset by age 20 years but only a sixfold increase when the proband's onset was after age 20 years. Twin studies have suggested that genes influence the familial aggregation of panic disorder. In their meta-analysis, Hettema et al. (2001) estimated a summary heritability of 0.43 for panic disorder. The specificity of familial and genetic influences on panic disorder is unclear. Family studies of panic disorder have provided support for specific influences. For example, relatives of probands with panic disorder appear to be at greatest risk for panic disorder rather than other anxiety or mood disorders (Smoller and Tsuang 1998). On the other hand, twin studies have provided evidence that genes influencing panic disorder overlap with those influencing generalized anxiety disorder, phobic disorders, PTSD, and depression (Chantarujikapong et al. 2001; Hettema et al. 2005; Scherrer et al. 2000).

Molecular Genetic Studies

Whole genome linkage analyses of panic disorder have implicated several chromosomal regions, including 1q (Gelernter et al. 2001), 2q (Fyer et al. 2006) 7p (Crowe et al. 2001; Knowles et al. 1998), 9q (Thorgeirsson et al. 2003), 12q (Smoller et al. 2001), 13q (Hamilton et al. 2003; Weissman et al. 2000), 15q (Fyer et al. 2006), and 22q (Hamilton et al. 2003). Strong evidence for the 13q locus was found when the phenotype was defined as a syndrome that included panic disorder as well as several other medical conditions (mitral valve prolapse, serious headaches, and/or thyroid problems) (Hamilton et al. 2003; Weissman et al. 2000). A large number of candidate gene studies of panic disorder have been reported, but as with other complex disorders, there have been few replications of significant findings in independent samples. Genes that have been reported to be associated with panic disorder in more than one sample include *COMT* (Domschke et al. 2004; Hamilton et al. 2002; Rothe et al. 2006; Woo et al. 2004), adenosine$_{2A}$ receptor (*ADORA2A*) (Deckert et al. 1998; Hamilton et al. 2004), cholecystokinin (*CCK*) (Hattori et al. 2001; Maron et al. 2005; Wang et al. 1998), CCK-B receptor (*CCKBR*) (Kennedy et al. 1999), serotonin$_{2A}$ receptor (*HTR2A*) (Inada et al. 2003; Maron et al. 2005), and monoamine oxidase A (*MAOA*) (Deckert et al. 1999; Maron et al. 2004; Samochowiec et al. 2004). However, in some cases, different alleles of these genes have been associated in different studies, negative findings in studies of these genes have also been reported, and none has been established as panic disorder susceptibility genes.

Phobic Disorders

Clinical Features and Epidemiology

The phobic disorders defined in DSM-IV are agoraphobia without a history of panic, social phobia (social anxiety disorder), and specific phobias (e.g., animal phobias, situational phobias such as claustrophobia, blood-injection-injury phobia, and others). The key feature of these disorders is excessive, irrational fear and avoidance of the phobic stimulus. In agoraphobia without a history of panic, the fear is of developing panic-like symptoms in situations from which escape might be difficult or embarrassing. Individuals with social phobia avoid social or performance situations because of excessive fears of embarrassment or negative evaluation by others. In the generalized subtype of social phobia, these fears extend to most social situations (e.g., initiating or maintaining conversations, attending parties, interactions at work, dating, etc). Specific phobias involve impairing fears and avoidance of specific objects or situations. The four subtypes of specific phobias differ by the focus of fear and avoidance: animals, natural environment (e.g., storms, heights), blood-injection-injury, and situational (e.g., flying, closed spaces). As shown in Table 6–5, phobic disorders are quite common, and tend to have onset at an early age.

Genetic Epidemiology

Family studies have demonstrated that phobic disorders aggregate in families. The familial risk of social phobia is approximately 3- to 10-fold higher among relatives of affected probands than among relatives of control subjects (Fyer et al. 1993, 1995; Stein et al. 1998). Stein et al. (1998) found that first-degree relatives of probands with generalized social phobia had a nearly 10-fold increased risk of the generalized type of social phobia, while nongeneralized or discrete social phobias did not show familial transmission. Specific phobias also show evidence of familial aggregation, with first-degree relatives of affected probands being three to four times more likely to be affected than relatives of control subjects (Fyer et al. 1990, 1995). In their meta-analysis of controlled studies, Hettema et al. (2001) reported that the risk of phobic disorders in first-degree relatives of affected probands ranged from 10% to 31%, with a summary OR of 4.1 (95% CI: 2.7–6.1). Twin studies have documented that genes contribute to the familiality of phobic disorders, with a heritability of approximately 10%–39% (Hettema et al. 2001, 2005). Higher heritabilities (50%–60%) were reported in a twin study that including repeated measures and corrected for the unreliability of the assessments (Kendler et al. 1999b). Modeling of variance components from twin data suggests that individual-specific environmental experiences appear to be the most important influence on the development of phobic disorders, a finding consistent with conditioning models of phobias (Kendler et al. 1992a).

TABLE 6–5. Summary of genetic epidemiology of mood and anxiety disorders

Disorder	Lifetime prevalence[a]	Median age at onset[a] (90th %ile)	FDR risk	Relative risk ratio	h²	Linkage regions[b]	Gene associations[c]
Bipolar disorder	1%–4%	25 (50)	4%–13%	9–10	80%	6q, 8q, 12q, 13q, 18q, 22q	*NRG1, DAOA/G72, BDNF, MTHFR, SLC6A4*
MDD	16%	32 (56)	15%–30%	2–3	40%	1p, 2q, 12q, 15q	*SLC6A4, MTHFR, TPH2*
Panic disorder	4%–5%	24 (51)	8%–17%	5	40%	9q, 13q, 22q	*ADORA2A, MAOA, COMT, CCK*
SAD	11%	13 (23)	16%–26%	3–10	30%	16q	—
Specific phobia	11%	7 (23)	31%	3–4	30%	14q	—
GAD	6%	31 (58)	9%–20%	6	30%	—	—
OCD	2%	19 (48)	3%–12%	4	30%–45%	3q, 9p	*COMT, SLC1A1, SLC6A4*
PTSD	7%	23 (53)	Undefined	—	35%	—	—

Note. Lifetime prevalence, FDR risk, recurrence risk ratio, and h² are approximate values.
FDR risk=approximate risk to first-degree relatives of affected probands reported in controlled family studies; GAD=generalized anxiety disorder; h²=heritability; MDD=major depressive disorder; OCD=obsessive-compulsive disorder; PTSD=posttraumatic stress disorder; SAD=social anxiety disorder.
[a]Kessler et al. 2005a.
[b]Strongest evidence for linkage.
[c]Examples of genes with association reported in more than two samples or meta-analyses.

Molecular Genetics

Gelernter and colleagues conducted whole genome linkage analyses of phobic disorders in a set of pedigrees ascertained for panic disorder and reported evidence implicating chromosome 3q for agoraphobia (Gelernter et al. 2001), 14q for specific phobia (Gelernter et al. 2003), and 16q for social phobia (Gelernter et al. 2004). Few candidate gene studies of phobic disorders have appeared, although reports of association with *COMT* (McGrath et al. 2004) and *MAOA* (Samochowiec et al. 2004) and with the dopamine transporter gene (*DAT1*) (Rowe et al. 1998) have appeared. As of this writing, however, no genes have been associated with phobias in independent samples.

Generalized Anxiety Disorder

Clinical Features and Epidemiology

Generalized anxiety disorder first appeared as a diagnostic category in DSM-III, and it is the anxiety disorder whose diagnostic criteria have changed the most since then. The key feature of generalized anxiety disorder, in its current form, is excessive, persistent anxiety and worry about multiple events or activities. For the diagnosis to be present, the worry must extend to multiple events or activities, be difficult to control, and be associated with at least three additional symptoms that include restlessness, fatigability, irritability, difficulty concentrating, muscle tension, and disturbed sleep.

The lifetime prevalence of generalized anxiety disorder is 5.7%, with a median age at onset of 31 years (Kessler et al. 2005a).

Genetic Epidemiology

Generalized anxiety disorder has received relatively little attention from a genetic standpoint, perhaps in part because the diagnostic criteria have changed substantially since DSM-III, making the diagnosis something of a "moving target." Findings from family studies of generalized anxiety disorder suggest that first-degree relatives have a 8.9% to 19.5% risk of developing the disorder, and the OR (which approximates the recurrence risk ratio) is approximately 6 (Hettema et al. 2001; Newman and Bland 2006). However, in a recent population-based family study of DSM-III generalized anxiety disorder, results showed a lower OR for first-degree relatives (1.4–1.8, or 2.1–2.8 for offspring of affected probands) (Newman and Bland 2006). In twin studies, the estimated heritability of generalized anxiety disorder ranged from 20% to 30% (Hettema et al. 2001, 2005). As for the other anxiety disorders, most of the population phenotypic variance in generalized anxiety disorder appears to be attributable to individual-specific environment. As discussed later in this chapter, several twin studies have suggested that the genetic determinants of generalized anxiety disorder overlap substantially with those influencing major depressive disorder.

Molecular Genetics

No linkage and few association studies have addressed generalized anxiety disorder. There have been sporadic reports of association between generalized anxiety disorder and variants in several of the most widely studied mood and anxiety disorder candidate genes (e.g., *MAOA* and *SLC6A4*) (Peroutka et al. 1998; Tadic et al. 2003; You et al. 2005), but none of these findings have been replicated.

Posttraumatic Stress Disorder

Clinical Features and Epidemiology

Posttraumatic stress disorder is unique among the mood and anxiety disorders in that a specific environmental exposure (trauma) is a prerequisite for the diagnosis. According to DSM-IV-TR, the traumatic event must have been personally experienced or witnessed and involve actual or threatened death, serious injury, or a threat to the physical integrity of the victim (American Psychiatric Association 2000).

The key clinical feature of PTSD is the subsequent development of three classes of posttraumatic symptoms: reexperiencing (e.g., flashbacks, nightmares, intrusive memories), avoidance/numbing (e.g., amnesia for aspects of the trauma, constricted affect, avoidance of reminders of the trauma), and increased arousal (e.g., exaggerated startle reactions, hypervigilance, insomnia, irritability). When these symptoms develop within the first month after the trauma, a diagnosis of acute stress disorder is made; PTSD is diagnosed when the duration of illness exceeds 1 month.

Results of the National Comorbidity Survey showed that more than 50% of Americans report exposure to at least one traumatic event (Kessler et al. 1995), but most will not develop PTSD. The lifetime prevalence of PTSD has been estimated at 6.8% (Kessler et al. 2005a). Two meta-analyses of the PTSD literature (Brewin et al. 2000; Ozer et al. 2003) have identified several risk factors for the development of PTSD, including female gender, premorbid psychological adjustment, family history of psychopathology, and peritraumatic dissociative symptoms. Research on the role of genetic contributions to PTSD has been complicated by the need to match affected and unaffected individuals on trauma exposure.

Genetic Epidemiology

Although data are limited, study findings indicate that relatives of probands with PTSD are at higher risk of the disorder, compared with relatives of trauma-exposed probands who did not develop PTSD. For example, in one study, offspring of Cambodian refugees with PTSD were found to be at higher risk of PTSD (Sack et al. 1995). In a twin study of Vietnam-era veterans, the estimated heritability for PTSD symptom clusters ranged from 13% to 30% for reexperiencing, 30% to 34% for avoidance, and 28% to 32% for increased arousal symptoms (True et al. 1993). Among twin-pairs who did not serve in Vietnam, the heritability of these symptom clusters was even higher, ranging from 32% to 45%. Similar estimates of heritability of symptom clusters (30%–40%) were obtained in a twin study that included both men and women exposed to noncombat trauma (Stein et al. 2002). It is interesting to note that these studies have also shown that genes contribute to whether or not a twin is exposed to trauma, possibly reflecting genetic effects on personality traits.

Molecular Genetics

Genetic studies of PTSD are made difficult by the need to compare family members or cases with control subjects who have experienced similar trauma. Although no linkage studies of PTSD have appeared, several candidate genes have been examined. These genes have primarily been the "usual suspects"–namely, candidate loci from biological systems implicated in the biology and treatment of mood and anxiety disorders (e.g., serotonergic and dopaminergic genes). As with other anxiety disorders, most studies have been limited to examination of one polymorphism and have been underpowered. A few positive associations have been reported (dopamine receptor 2 [*DRD2*], FK506 binding protein [*FKBP5*], *SLC6A3*, *SLC6A4*) (Comings et al. 1996; Koenen et al. 2005b; Lee et al. 2005; Segman et al. 2002), but none has been established.

Complex Genetic Boundaries of Anxiety Disorders and Anxiety Proneness

Perhaps more than other groups of psychiatric disorders, the anxiety disorders appear to have overlapping familial and genetic determinants. Although the results of some family studies of panic and phobic disorders suggest that these phenotypes "breed true," other family, twin, and molecular studies suggest shared genetic influences on anxiety disorders and between anxiety disorders and major depressive disorder (Smoller and Tsuang 1998). Twin studies have documented overlap between genetic determinants of panic disorder and phobic anxiety disorders (Kendler et al. 1995b), social phobia, agoraphobia, and specific phobias (Kendler et al.

1992a), panic disorder and generalized anxiety disorder (Scherrer et al. 2000), and PTSD and alcohol, nicotine, and drug dependence (Koenen et al. 2005a; McLeod et al. 2001; Xian et al. 2000), and major depressive disorder (Koenen et al. 2003). In a twin analysis comprising more than 5,000 twins, Hettema et al. (2005) examined genetic and environmental influences on anxiety disorders using structural equation modeling. They identified two genetic factors underlying the disorders: one factor primarily predisposing to panic disorder, agoraphobia, and generalized anxiety disorder, and the second factor primarily influencing specific phobias. Social phobia was influenced by both broad factors.

The epidemiological evidence that genetic effects on anxiety transcend diagnostic boundaries is supported by molecular genetic studies (Kaabi et al. 2006; Smoller et al. 2001). For example, in a genome scan linkage study, Kaabi et al. (2006) observed significant linkage on chromosome 4q for a phenotype comprising panic disorder, agoraphobia, social phobia, and specific phobia. In addition, several candidate genes (e.g., *COMT, MAOA*) have been associated with both panic and phobic anxiety (Deckert et al. 1999; Domschke et al. 2004; McGrath et al. 2004; Samochowiec et al. 2004; Woo et al. 2002). The glutamic acid decarboxylase 1 gene (*GAD1*) was recently reported to show association with a genetic liability underlying panic disorder, generalized anxiety disorder, phobias, major depressive disorder, and the anxiety-related personality trait of neuroticism (Hettema et al. 2006).

As noted earlier, the frequent lifetime comorbidity of anxiety and depressive disorders and the fact that antidepressant medications are effective treatments for both groups of disorders have raised the possibility that they also reflect a shared diathesis (Brier et al. 1985). There is mixed evidence on this issue. Some family studies suggest that anxiety disorders segregate independently of major depressive disorder in the absence of comorbid major depressive disorder in the proband (Goldstein et al. 1994; Klein et al. 2003; Noyes et al. 1987; Stein et al. 1998), although others show shared familial risk (Fyer et al. 1993; Merikangas et al. 1998). Similarly, studies of children at risk for anxiety or depressive disorders have yielded somewhat conflicting results, with some studies suggesting that children of depressed parents are at increased risk for anxiety disorders (Biederman et al. 2001; Breslau et al. 1987), and others finding an increased risk of depression but not anxiety disorders (Biederman et al. 1991; Weissman et al. 1984a). On the other hand, twin studies have found that the genetic basis of generalized anxiety disorder and depression is substantially the same (Kendler et al. 2006a; Roy et al. 1995).

The complexity and overlapping genetic influences on anxiety phenotypes have led some researchers to examine intermediate phenotypes that may be more proximal expressions of the underlying genes and thus more amenable to genetic dissection. This strategy has also been exploited in the study of mood disorders. For the anxiety disorders, intermediate phenotypes may include temperamental anxiety proneness and characteristic patterns noted with neuroimaging measures of brain function. For example, association studies have implicated specific genes with heritable anxiety-related temperament and personality traits, including behavioral inhibition to the unfamiliar (Smoller et al. 2005), neuroticism (Sen et al. 2004), and harm avoidance (Munafo et al. 2005). The use of neuroimaging phenotypes is exemplified by studies demonstrating association between the 5-HTTLPR short allele and amygdala reactivity to threatening faces (Hariri et al. 2006).

Implications for Genetic Counseling

Recurrence risk estimates derived from family studies of the anxiety disorders are shown in Table 6–5. Overall, first-degree relatives of affected probands have an approximately four- to sixfold increased risk of the anxiety disorder present in the proband. The same caveats discussed with regard to the mood disorders apply here as well, of course. The modest heritabilities associated with anxiety disorders (generally <40%) indicate that nongenetic factors explain most of the risk of illness for common forms of these disorders. In families densely affected with anxiety disorders, recurrence risks are expected to be higher, although providing individualized risks is difficult in such instances. Age at onset and age of relatives provide some basis for modifying risk estimates. Greater familial risk has been associated with early-onset disorder for panic disorder and OCD (do Rosario-Campos et al. 2005; Goldstein et al. 1997). Unaffected relatives who have passed through the typical period of risk (see Table 6-5 for 90th percentile for age at onset) have correspondingly lower risks of developing anxiety disorders.

No genetic tests for anxiety disorders are available. Given the complexity of these disorders and expected lack of major gene effects, it is not clear if the development of clinically useful genetic tests will be feasible. Anxiety is sometimes a feature of certain medical genetic disorders for which genetic testing exists. For example, social phobia may be more common in women carrying the fragile X mutation or premutation (Franke et al. 1998), and generalized anxiety disorder and phobias are common among individuals with Williams syndrome (Dykens 2003; Leyfer et al. 2006). However, anxiety is unlikely to justify genetic testing for these conditions.

Anxiety disorders are commonly comorbid, and comorbidity with other psychiatric disorders (particularly major depressive disorder and substance abuse/dependence) is also common (Kessler et al. 2005b). This finding highlights the importance of obtaining a complete psychiatric history for the proband and, to the extent possible, a three-generation pedigree. For example, panic disorder in a proband may be one manifestation of a susceptibility to multiple anxiety disorders or alcohol abuse that may be segregating in the family.

Conclusions

Mood and anxiety disorders are common, chronic, and often disabling disorders. Family studies have established that these disorders are familial, and twin studies have provided compelling evidence that genes contribute to this familial aggregation. Although no specific susceptibility genes have been established, several genes have been associated with these disorders in independent samples. The increasing trend toward large-scale studies and the availability of high-throughput genotyping and gene expression methods should permit the identification of true susceptibility genes while reducing the probable large number of false-positive findings that have appeared in the literature. At present, genetic counseling for mood and anxiety disorders relies on empiric risks derived from family studies. These data can provide useful information but must be placed in the context of the limitations of the available evidence.

References

Abkevich V, Camp NJ, Hensel CH, et al: Predisposition locus for major depression at chromosome 12q22–12q23.2. Am J Hum Genet 73:1271–1281, 2003

American Psychiatric Association: Diagnostic and Statistical Manual of Mental Disorders, 3rd Edition. Washington, DC, American Psychiatric Association, 1980

American Psychiatric Association: Diagnostic and Statistical Manual of Mental Disorders, 4th edition. Washington, DC, American Psychiatric Association, 1994

American Psychiatric Association: Diagnostic and Statistical Manual of Mental Disorders, 4th Edition, Text Revision. Washington, DC, American Psychiatric Association, 2000

American Psychiatric Association: Practice guideline for the treatment of patients with bipolar disorder (revision). Am J Psychiatry 159:1–50, 2002

Andreasen NC, Rice J, Endicott J, et al: Familial rates of affective disorder: a report from the National Institute of Mental Health Collaborative Study. Arch Gen Psychiatry 44:461–469, 1987

Angst J, Frey R, Lohmeyer B, et al: Bipolar manic-depressive psychoses: results of a genetic investigation. Hum Genet 55:237–254, 1980

Anguelova M, Benkelfat C, Turecki G: A systematic review of association studies investigating genes coding for serotonin receptors and the serotonin transporter: II. suicidal behavior. Mol Psychiatry 8:646–653, 2003

Bacanu SA, Devlin B, Chowdari KV, et al: Heritability of psychosis in Alzheimer disease. Am J Geriatr Psychiatry 13:624–627, 2005

Badner JA, Gershon ES: Meta-analysis of whole-genome linkage scans of bipolar disorder and schizophrenia. Mol Psychiatry 7:405–411, 2002

Bassett AS, Chow EW, AbdelMalik P, et al: The schizophrenia phenotype in 22q11 deletion syndrome. Am J Psychiatry 160:1580–1586, 2003

Bassett AS, Chow EW, Husted J, et al: Clinical features of 78 adults with 22q11 deletion syndrome. Am J Med Genet A 138:307–313, 2005

Baum AE, Akula N, Cabanero M, et al: A genome-wide association study implicates diacylglycerol kinase eta (DGKH) and several other genes in the etiology of bipolar disorder. Mol Psychiatry May 8, 2007 (epub ahead of print)

Bertelsen A, Harvald B, Hauge M: A Danish twin study of manic-depressive disorders. Br J Psychiatry 130:330–351, 1977

Biederman J, Rosenbaum J, Bolduc E, et al: A high risk study of young children of parents with panic disorder and agoraphobia with and without comorbid major depression. Psychiatry Res 37:333–348, 1991

Biederman J, Faraone SV, Hirshfeld-Becker DR, et al: Patterns of psychopathology and dysfunction in high-risk children of parents with panic disorder and major depression. Am J Psychiatry 158:49–57, 2001

Blacker D, Tsuang M: Contested boundaries of bipolar disorder and the limits of categorical diagnosis in psychiatry. Am J Psychiatry 149:1473–1483, 1992

Blacker D, Faraone SV, Rosen AE, et al: Unipolar relatives in bipolar pedigrees: a search for elusive indicators of underlying bipolarity. Am J Med Genet 67:445–454, 1996

Blackwood DH, Fordyce A, Walker MT, et al: Schizophrenia and affective disorders—cosegregation with a translocation at chromosome 1q42 that directly disrupts brain-expressed genes: clinical and P300 findings in a family. Am J Hum Genet 69:428–433, 2001

Bland RC, Newman SC, Orn H: Recurrent and nonrecurrent depression: a family study. Arch Gen Psychiatry 43:1085–1089, 1986

Breslau N, Davis GC, Prabucki K: Searching for evidence on the validity of generalized anxiety disorder: psychopathology in children of anxious mothers. Psychiatry Res 20:285–297, 1987

Brewin CR, Andrews B, Valentine JD: Meta-analysis of risk factors for posttraumatic stress disorder in trauma-exposed adults. J Consult Clin Psychol 68:748–766, 2000

Brier A, Charney D, Heninger G: The diagnostic validity of anxiety disorders and their relationship to depressive illness. Am J Psychiatry 142:787–797, 1985

Camp NJ, Lowry MR, Richards RL, et al: Genome-wide linkage analyses of extended Utah pedigrees identifies loci that influence recurrent, early onset major depression and anxiety disorders. Am J Med Genet B Neuropsychiatr Genet 135:85–93, 2005

Cardno AG, Sham PC, Murray RM, et al: Twin study of symptom dimensions in psychoses. Br J Psychiatry 179:39–45, 2001

Cardno AG, Rijsdijk FV, Sham PC, et al: A twin study of genetic relationships between psychotic symptoms. Am J Psychiatry 159:539–545, 2002a

Cardno AG, Sham PC, Farmer AE, et al: Heritability of Schneider's first-rank symptoms. Br J Psychiatry 180:35–38, 2002b

Caspi A, Sugden K, Moffitt TE, et al: Influence of life stress on depression: moderation by a polymorphism in the 5-HTT gene. Science 301:386–389, 2003

Chantarujikapong SI, Scherrer JF, Xian H, et al: A twin study of generalized anxiety disorder symptoms, panic disorder symptoms and post-traumatic stress disorder in men. Psychiatry Res 103:133–145, 2001

Cheng R, Juo SH, Loth JE, et al: Genome-wide linkage scan in a large bipolar disorder sample from the National Institute of Mental Health genetics initiative suggests putative loci for bipolar disorder, psychosis, suicide, and panic disorder. Mol Psychiatry 11:252–260, 2006

Comings DE, Muhleman D, Gysin R: Dopamine D2 receptor (DRD2) gene and susceptibility to posttraumatic stress disorder: a study and replication. Biol Psychiatry 40:368–372, 1996

Coryell W, Endicott J, Reich T, et al: A family study of bipolar II disorder. Br J Psychiatry 145:49–54, 1984

Coryell W, Endicott J, Andreasen N, et al: Depression and panic attacks: the significance of overlap as reflected in follow-up and family study data. Am J Psychiatry 145:293–300, 1988

Coryell W, Endicott J, Winokur G: Anxiety syndromes as epiphenomena of primary major depression: outcome and familial psychopathology. Am J Psychiatry 149:100–107, 1992

Craddock N, Forty L: Genetics of affective (mood) disorders. Eur J Hum Genet 14:660–668, 2006

Craddock N, O'Donovan MC, Owen MJ: The genetics of schizophrenia and bipolar disorder: dissecting psychosis. J Med Genet 42:193–204, 2005

Craddock N, O'Donovan MC, Owen MJ: Genes for schizophrenia and bipolar disorder? Implications for psychiatric nosology. Schizophr Bull 32:9–16, 2006a

Craddock N, Owen MJ, O'Donovan MC: The catechol-*O*-methyl transferase (COMT) gene as a candidate for psychiatric phenotypes: evidence and lessons. Mol Psychiatry 11:446–458, 2006b

Crowe RR, Noyes R, Pauls DL, et al: A family study of panic disorder. Arch Gen Psychiatry 40:1065–1069, 1983

Crowe RR, Goedken R, Samuelson S, et al: Genomewide survey of panic disorder. Am J Med Genet 105:105–109, 2001

Deckert J, Nothen M, Franke P, et al: Systematic mutation screening and association study of the A_1 and A_{2a} adenosine receptor genes in panic disorder suggest a contribution of the A_{2a} gene to the development of disease. Mol Psychiatry 3:81–85, 1998

Deckert J, Catalano M, Syagailo YV, et al: Excess of high activity monoamine oxidase A gene promoter alleles in female patients with panic disorder. Hum Mol Genet 8:621–624, 1999

DelBello MP, Geller B: Review of studies of child and adolescent offspring of bipolar parents. Bipolar Disord 3:325–334, 2001

De Luca V, Likhodi O, Van Tol HH, et al: Tryptophan hydroxylase 2 gene expression and promoter polymorphisms in bipolar disorder and schizophrenia. Psychopharmacology (Berl) 183:378–382, 2005

Detera-Wadleigh SD, McMahon FJ: G72/G30 in schizophrenia and bipolar disorder: review and meta-analysis. Biol Psychiatry 60:106–114, 2006

Domschke K, Freitag CM, Kuhlenbaumer G, et al: Association of the functional V158M catechol-*O*-methyl-transferase polymorphism with panic disorder in women. Int J Neuropsychopharmacol 7:183–188, 2004 do Rosario-Campos MC, Leckman JF, Curi M, et al: A family study of early onset obsessive-compulsive disorder. Am J Med Genet B Neuropsychiatr Genet 136: 92–97, 2005

Doughty CJ, Wells JE, Joyce PR, et al: Bipolar-panic disorder comorbidity within bipolar disorder families: a study of siblings. Bipolar Disord 6:245–252, 2004

Duman RS, Monteggia LM: A neurotrophic model for stress-related mood disorders. Biol Psychiatry 59:1116-1127, 2006

Dykens EM: Anxiety, fears, and phobias in persons with Williams syndrome. Dev Neuropsychol 23:291–316, 2003

Ebmeier KP, Donaghey C, Steele JD: Recent developments and current controversies in depression. Lancet 367:153–167, 2006

Eley TC, Sugden K, Corsico A, et al: Gene-environment interaction analysis of serotonin system markers with adolescent depression. Mol Psychiatry 9:908–915, 2004

Endicott J, Nee J, Andreasen N, et al: Bipolar II. Combine or keep separate? J Affect Disord 8:17–28, 1985

Fallin MD, Lasseter VK, Avramopoulos D, et al: Bipolar I disorder and schizophrenia: a 440-single-nucleotide polymorphism screen of 64 candidate genes among Ashkenazi Jewish case-parent trios. Am J Hum Genet 77:918–936, 2005

Faraone SV, Glatt SJ, Tsuang MT: The genetics of pediatric-onset bipolar disorder. Biol Psychiatry 53:970–977, 2003

Farmer A, Harris T, Redman K, et al: Cardiff depression study. A sib-pair study of life events and familiality in major depression. Br J Psychiatry 176:150–155, 2000

Finn CT, Smoller JW: Genetic counseling in psychiatry. Harv Rev Psychiatry 14:109–121, 2006

Finn CT, Wilcox MA, Korf BR, et al: Psychiatric genetics: a survey of psychiatrists' knowledge, opinions, and practice patterns. J Clin Psychiatry 66:821–830, 2005

Forty L, Jones L, Macgregor S, et al: Familiality of postpartum depression in unipolar disorder: results of a family study. Am J Psychiatry 163:1549–1553, 2006

Franke P, Leboyer M, Gansicke M, et al: Genotype-phenotype relationship in female carriers of the premutation and full mutation of FMR-1. Psychiatry Res 80:113–127, 1998

Furlong RA, Ho L, Walsh C, et al: Analysis and meta-analysis of two serotonin transporter gene polymorphisms in bipolar and unipolar affective disorders. Am J Med Genet 81:58–63, 1998

Fyer A, Mannuzza S, Gallops S, et al: Familial transmission of simple phobias and fears. Arch Gen Psychiatry 47:252–256, 1990

Fyer A, Mannuzza S, Chapman T, et al: A direct interview family study of social phobia. Arch Gen Psychiatry 50:286–293, 1993

Fyer AJ, Mannuzza S, Chapman TF, et al: Specificity in familial aggregation of phobic disorders. Arch Gen Psychiatry 52:564–573, 1995

Fyer AJ, Hamilton SP, Durner M, et al: A third-pass genome scan in panic disorder: evidence for multiple susceptibility loci. Biol Psychiatry 60:388–401, 2006

Gambini O, Campana A, Macciardi F, et al: A preliminary report of a strong genetic component for thought disorder in normals. A twin study. Neuropsychobiology 36:13–18, 1997

Gelernter J, Bonvicini K, Page G, et al: Linkage genome scan for loci predisposing to panic disorder or agoraphobia. Am J Med Genet 105:548–557, 2001

Gelernter J, Page GP, Bonvicini K, et al: A chromosome 14 risk locus for simple phobia: results from a genomewide linkage scan. Mol Psychiatry 8:71–82, 2003

Gelernter J, Page GP, Stein MB, et al: Genome-wide linkage scan for loci predisposing to social phobia: evidence for a chromosome 16 risk locus. Am J Psychiatry 161:59–66, 2004

Geller B, Tillman R, Bolhofner K, et al: Controlled, blindly rated, direct-interview family study of a prepubertal and early adolescent bipolar I disorder phenotype: morbid risk, age at onset, and comorbidity. Arch Gen Psychiatry 63:1130–1138, 2006

Gershon ES, Mark A, Cohen N, et al: Transmitted factors in the morbid risk of affective disorders: a controlled study. J Psychiat Res 12:283–299, 1975

Gershon ES, Hamovit J, Guroff JJ, et al: A family study of schizoaffective, bipolar I, bipolar II, unipolar, and normal control probands. Arch Gen Psychiatry 39:1157–1167, 1982

Gershon ES, Weissman MM, Guroff JJ, et al: Validation of criteria for major depression through controlled family study. J Affect Disord 11:125–131, 1986

Gilbody S, Lewis S, Lightfoot T: Methylenetetrahydrofolate reductase (MTHFR) genetic polymorphisms and psychiatric disorders: a HuGE review. Am J Epidemiol 165:1–13, 2007

Gillespie NA, Whitfield JB, Williams B, et al: The relationship between stressful life events, the serotonin transporter (5-HTTLPR) genotype and major depression. Psychol Med 35:101–111, 2005

Goldberg JF, Harrow M: Consistency of remission and outcome in bipolar and unipolar mood disorders: a 10-year prospective follow-up. J Affect Disord 81:123–131, 2004

Goldstein RB, Weissman MM, Adams PB, et al: Psychiatric disorders in relatives of probands with panic disorder and/or major depression. Arch Gen Psychiatry 51:383–394, 1994

Goldstein R, Wickramaratne P, Horwath E, et al: Familial aggregation and phenomenology of "early"-onset (at or before age 20 years) panic disorder. Arch Gen Psychiatry 542:71–278, 1997

Grabe HJ, Lange M, Wolff B, et al: Mental and physical distress is modulated by a polymorphism in the 5-HT transporter gene interacting with social stressors and chronic disease burden. Mol Psychiatry 10:220–224, 2005

Grant BF, Hasin DS, Dawson DA: The relationship between DSM-IV alcohol use disorders and DSM-IV major depression: examination of the primary-secondary distinction in a general population sample. J Affect Disord 38:113–128, 1996

Green EK, Raybould R, Macgregor S, et al: Genetic variation of brain-derived neurotrophic factor (BDNF) in bipolar disorder: case-control study of over 3000 individuals from the UK. Br J Psychiatry 188:21–25, 2006

Greenberg PE, Kessler RC, Birnbaum HG, et al: The economic burden of depression in the United States: how did it change between 1990 and 2000? J Clin Psychiatry 64:1465–1475, 2003

Grigoroiu-Serbanescu M, Martinez M, Nothen MM, et al: Different familial transmission patterns in bipolar I disorder with onset before and after age 25. Am J Med Genet 105:765–773, 2001

Hamilton SP, Slager SL, Heiman GA, et al: Evidence for a susceptibility locus for panic disorder near the catechol-*O*-methyltransferase gene on chromosome 22. Biol Psychiatry 51:591–601, 2002

Hamilton SP, Fyer AJ, Durner M, et al: Further genetic evidence for a panic disorder syndrome mapping to chromosome 13q. Proc Natl Acad Sci U S A 100:2550–2555, 2003

Hamilton SP, Slager SL, De Leon AB, et al: Evidence for genetic linkage between a polymorphism in the adenosine 2A receptor and panic disorder. Neuropsychopharmacology 29:558–565, 2004

Hariri AR, Drabant EM, Weinberger DR: Imaging genetics: perspectives from studies of genetically driven variation in serotonin function and corticolimbic affective processing. Biol Psychiatry 59:888–897, 2006

Harris EL, Noyes R, Jr., Crowe RR, et al: Family study of agoraphobia: report of a pilot study. Arch Gen Psychiatry 40:1061–1064, 1983

Hattori E, Ebihara M, Yamada K, et al: Identification of a compound short tandem repeat stretch in the 5′-upstream region of the cholecystokinin gene, and its association with panic disorder but not with schizophrenia. Mol Psychiatry 6:465–470, 2001

Heils A, Teufel A, Petri S, et al: Allelic variation of human serotonin transporter gene expression. J Neurochem 66:2621–2624, 1996

Henin A, Biederman J, Mick E, et al: Psychopathology in the offspring of parents with bipolar disorder: a controlled study. Biol Psychiatry 58:554–561, 2005

Hettema JM, Neale MC, Kendler KS: A review and meta-analysis of the genetic epidemiology of anxiety disorders. Am J Psychiatry 158:1568–1578, 2001

Hettema JM, Prescott CA, Myers JM, et al: The structure of genetic and environmental risk factors for anxiety disorders in men and women. Arch Gen Psychiatry 62:182–189, 2005

Hettema JM, An SS, Neale MC, et al: Association between glutamic acid decarboxylase genes and anxiety disorders, major depression, and neuroticism. Mol Psychiatry 11:752–762, 2006

Heun R, Maier W: The distinction of bipolar II disorder from bipolar I and recurrent unipolar depression: results of a controlled family study. Acta Psychiatr Scand 87:279–284, 1993

Hirshfeld-Becker DR, Biederman J, Henin A, et al: Psychopathology in the young offspring of parents with bipolar disorder: a controlled pilot study. Psychiatry Res 145:155–167, 2006

Holmans P, Zubenko GS, Crowe RR, et al: Genomewide significant linkage to recurrent, early onset major depressive disorder on chromosome 15q. Am J Hum Genet 74:1154–1167, 2004

Holmans P, Weissman MM, Zubenko GS, et al: Genetics of recurrent early onset major depression (GenRED): final genome scan report. Am J Psychiatry 164:248–258, 2007

Hudson JI, Mangweth B, Pope HG Jr, et al: Family study of affective spectrum disorder. Arch Gen Psychiatry 60:170–177, 2003

Inada Y, Yoneda H, Koh J, et al: Positive association between panic disorder and polymorphism of the serotonin 2A receptor gene. Psychiatry Res 118:25–31, 2003

Jacobs N, Myin-Germeys I, Derom C, et al: Deconstructing the familiality of the emotive component of psychotic experiences in the general population. Acta Psychiatr Scand 112:394–401, 2005

James NM: Early and late-onset bipolar affective disorder. A genetic study. Arch Gen Psychiatry 34:715–717, 1977

Jang KL, Woodward TS, Lang D, et al: The genetic and environmental basis of the relationship between schizotypy and personality: a twin study. J Nerv Ment Dis 193:153–159, 2005

Kaabi B, Gelernter J, Woods SW, et al: Genome scan for loci predisposing to anxiety disorders using a novel multivariate approach: strong evidence for a chromosome 4 risk locus. Am J Hum Genet 78:543–553, 2006

Kaufman J, Yang BZ, Douglas-Palumberi H, et al: Social supports and serotonin transporter gene moderate depression in maltreated children. Proc Natl Acad Sci U S A 101:17316–17321, 2004

Kaufman J, Yang BZ, Douglas-Palumberi H, et al: Brain-derived neurotrophic factor-5-HTTLPR gene interactions and environmental modifiers of depression in children. Biol Psychiatry 59:673–680, 2006

Kendler KS, Neale MC, Kessler RC, et al: The genetic epidemiology of phobias in women. Arch Gen Psychiatry 49:273–281, 1992a

Kendler KS, Neale MC, Kessler RC, et al: Major depression and generalized anxiety disorder: same genes, (partly) different environments? Arch Gen Psychiatry 49:716–722, 1992b

Kendler KS, Heath AC, Neale MC, et al: Alcoholism and major depression in women: a twin study of the causes of comorbidity. Arch Gen Psychiatry 50:690–698, 1993a

Kendler K, Neale M, Kessler R, et al: Major depression and phobias: the genetic and environmental sources of comorbidity. Psychol Med 23:361–371, 1993b

Kendler KS, Pedersen N, Johnson L, et al: A pilot Swedish twin study of affective illness, including hospital- and population-ascertained subsamples. Arch Gen Psychiatry 50:699–700, 1993c

Kendler KS, Pedersen NL, Neale MC, et al: A pilot Swedish twin study of affective illness including hospital- and population-ascertained subsamples: results of model fitting. Behav Genet 25:217–232, 1995a

Kendler KS, Walter EE, Neale MC, et al: The structure of the genetic and environmental risk factors for six major psychiatric disorders in women. Arch Gen Psychiatry 52:374–383, 1995b

Kendler KS, Davis CG, Kessler RC: The familial aggregation of common psychiatric and substance use disorders in the National Comorbidity Survey: a family history study. Br J Psychiatry 170:541–548, 1997

Kendler K, Gardner C, Prescott C: Clinical characteristics of major depression that predict risk of depression in relatives. Arch Gen Psychiatry 56:322–327, 1999a

Kendler KS, Karkowski LM, Prescott CA: Fears and phobias: reliability and heritability. Psychol Med 29:539–553, 1999b

Kendler KS, Gardner CO, Prescott CA: Corrections to 2 prior published articles. Arch Gen Psychiatry 57:94–95, 2000

Kendler KS, Gardner CO, Prescott CA: Toward a comprehensive developmental model for major depression in women. Am J Psychiatry 159:1133–1145, 2002

Kendler KS, Kuhn JW, Vittum J, et al: The interaction of stressful life events and a serotonin transporter polymorphism in the prediction of episodes of major depression: a replication. Arch Gen Psychiatry 62:529–535, 2005

Kendler KS, Gardner CO, Gatz M, et al: The sources of co-morbidity between major depression and generalized anxiety disorder in a Swedish national twin sample. Psychol Med:1–10, 2006a

Kendler KS, Gardner CO, Prescott CA: Toward a comprehensive developmental model for major depression in men. Am J Psychiatry 163:115–124, 2006b

Kendler KS, Gatz M, Gardner CO, et al: A Swedish national twin study of lifetime major depression. Am J Psychiatry 163:109–114, 2006c

Kennedy JL, Bradwejn J, Koszycki D, et al: Investigation of cholecystokinin system genes in panic disorder. Mol Psychiatry 4:284–285, 1999

Kennedy N, Boydell J, Kalidindi S, et al: Gender differences in incidence and age at onset of mania and bipolar disorder over a 35-year period in Camberwell, England. Am J Psychiatry 162:257–262, 2005a

Kennedy N, Everitt B, Boydell J, et al: Incidence and distribution of first-episode mania by age: results from a 35-year study. Psychol Med 35:855–863, 2005b

Kerner B, Brugman DL, Freimer NB: Evidence of linkage to psychosis on chromosome 5q33–34 in pedigrees ascertained for bipolar disorder. Am J Med Genet B Neuropsychiatr Genet 144:74–78, 2007

Kessler R, Sonnega A, Bromet E, et al: Posttraumatic stress disorder in the National Comorbidity Survey. Arch Gen Psychiatry 52:1048–1060, 1995

Kessler RC, Rubinow DR, Holmes C, et al: The epidemiology of DSM-III-R bipolar I disorder in a general population survey. Psychol Med 27:1079–1089, 1997

Kessler RC, Berglund P, Demler O, et al: The epidemiology of major depressive disorder: results from the National Comorbidity Survey Replication (NCS-R). JAMA 289:3095–3105, 2003

Kessler RC, Berglund P, Demler O, et al: Lifetime prevalence and age-of-onset distributions of DSM-IV disorders in the National Comorbidity Survey Replication. Arch Gen Psychiatry 62:593–602, 2005a

Kessler RC, Chiu WT, Demler O, et al: Prevalence, severity, and comorbidity of 12-month DSM-IV disorders in the National Comorbidity Survey Replication. Arch Gen Psychiatry 62:617–627, 2005b

Kessler RC, Demler O, Frank RG, et al: Prevalence and treatment of mental disorders, 1990 to 2003. N Engl J Med 352:2515–2523, 2005c

Kessler RC, Chiu WT, Jin R, et al: The epidemiology of panic attacks, panic disorder, and agoraphobia in the National Comorbidity Survey replication. Arch Gen Psychiatry 63:415–424, 2006

Kieseppa T, Partonen T, Haukka J, et al: High concordance of bipolar I disorder in a nationwide sample of twins. Am J Psychiatry 161:814–821, 2004

Kirov G, Murphy KC, Arranz MJ, et al: Low activity allele of catechol-O-methyltransferase gene associated with rapid cycling bipolar disorder. Mol Psychiatry 3:342–345, 1998

Klein DN, Riso LP, Donaldson SK, et al: Family study of early onset dysthymia: mood and personality disorders in relatives of outpatients with dysthymia and episode major depression and normal controls. Arch Gen Psychiatry 52:487–496, 1995

Klein DN, Lewinsohn PM, Rohde P, et al: Family study of co-morbidity between major depressive disorder and anxiety disorders. Psychol Med 33:703–714, 2003

Klein DN, Shankman SA, Lewinsohn PM, et al: Family study of chronic depression in a community sample of young adults. Am J Psychiatry 161:646–653, 2004

Knowles JA, Fyer AJ, Vieland VJ, et al: Results of a genome-wide genetic screen for panic disorder. Am J Med Genet 81:139–147, 1998

Koenen KC, Lyons MJ, Goldberg J, et al: A high risk twin study of combat-related PTSD comorbidity. Twin Res 6:218–226, 2003

Koenen KC, Hitsman B, Lyons MJ, et al: A twin registry study of the relationship between posttraumatic stress disorder and nicotine dependence in men. Arch Gen Psychiatry 62:1258–1265, 2005a

Koenen KC, Saxe G, Purcell S, et al: Polymorphisms in FKBP5 are associated with peritraumatic dissociation in medically injured children. Mol Psychiatry 10:1058–1059, 2005b

Kremeyer B, Herzberg I, Garcia J, et al: Transmission distortion of BDNF variants to bipolar disorder type I patients from a South American population isolate. Am J Med Genet B Neuropsychiatr Genet 141:435–439, 2006

Kutcher S, Marton P: Affective disorders in first-degree relatives of adolescent onset bipolars, unipolars, and normal controls. J Am Acad Child Adolesc Psychiatry 30:75–78, 1991

Lapalme M, Hodgins S, LaRoche C: Children of parents with bipolar disorder: a meta-analysis of risk for mental disorders. Can J Psychiatry 42:623–631, 1997

Lasky-Su JA, Faraone SV, Glatt SJ, et al: Meta-analysis of the association between two polymorphisms in the serotonin transporter gene and affective disorders. Am J Med Genet B Neuropsychiatr Genet 133:110–115, 2005

Leckman J, Weissman M, Merikangas K, et al: Panic disorder and major depression: increased risk of depression, alcoholism, panic, and phobic disorders in families of depressed probands with panic disorder. Arch Gen Psychiatry 40:1055–1060, 1983

Lee HJ, Lee MS, Kang RH, et al: Influence of the serotonin transporter promoter gene polymorphism on susceptibility to posttraumatic stress disorder. Depress Anxiety 21:135–139, 2005

Lesch K-P, Bengel D, Heils A, et al: Association of anxiety-related traits with a polymorphism in the serotonin transporter gene regulatory region. Science 274:1527–1531, 1996

Levinson DF: The genetics of depression: a review. Biol Psychiatry 60:84–92, 2005

Levinson DF, Evgrafov OV, Knowles JA, et al: Genetics of recurrent early onset major depression (GenRED): significant linkage on chromosome 15q25–q26 after fine mapping with single nucleotide polymorphism markers. Am J Psychiatry 164:259–264, 2007

Leyfer OT, Woodruff-Borden J, Klein-Tasman BP, et al: Prevalence of psychiatric disorders in 4- to 16-year-olds with Williams syndrome. Am J Med Genet B Neuropsychiatr Genet 141:615–622, 2006

Lichtenstein P, Holm NV, Verkasalo PK, et al: Environmental and heritable factors in the causation of cancer–analyses of cohorts of twins from Sweden, Denmark, and Finland. N Engl J Med 343:78–85, 2000

López-León S, Janssens AC, González-Zuloeta Ladd AM, et al: Meta-analyses of genetic studies on major depressive disorder. Mol Psychiatry October 16, 2007 (epub ahead of print)

Lotrich FE, Pollock BG: Meta-analysis of serotonin transporter polymorphisms and affective disorders. Psychiatr Genet 14:121–129, 2004

MacKinnon DF, McMahon FJ, Simpson SG, et al: Panic disorder with familial bipolar disorder. Biol Psychiatry 42:90–95, 1997

MacKinnon DF, Xu J, McMahon FJ, et al: Bipolar disorder and panic disorder in families: an analysis of chromosome 18 data. Am J Psychiatry 155:829–831, 1998

MacKinnon DF, Zandi PP, Cooper J, et al: Comorbid bipolar disorder and panic disorder in families with a high prevalence of bipolar disorder. Am J Psychiatry 159:30–35, 2002

MacKinnon DF, Zandi PP, Gershon ES, et al: Association of rapid mood switching with panic disorder and familial panic risk in familial bipolar disorder. Am J Psychiatry 160:1696–1698, 2003

Maier W, Lichtermann D, Minges J, et al: Continuity and discontinuity of affective disorders and schizophrenia: results of a controlled family study. Arch Gen Psychiatry 50:871–883, 1993a

Maier W, Lichtermann D, Minges J, et al: A controlled family study in panic disorder. J Psychiat Res 27(suppl 1):79–87, 1993b

Maier W, Minges J, Lichtermann D: The familial relationship between panic disorder and unipolar depression. J Psychiatr Res 29:375–388, 1995

Mannuzza S, Chapman TF, Klein DF, et al: Familial transmission of panic disorder: effect of major depression comorbidity. Anxiety 1:180–185, 1994/1995

Maron E, Tasa G, Toru I, et al: Association between serotonin-related genetic polymorphisms and CCK-4-induced panic attacks with or without 5-hydroxytryptophan pretreatment in healthy volunteers. World J Biol Psychiatry 5:149–154, 2004

Maron E, Nikopensius T, Koks S, et al: Association study of 90 candidate gene polymorphisms in panic disorder. Psychiatr Genet 15:17–24, 2005

Martucci L, Wong AH, De Luca V, et al: N-methyl-D-aspartate receptor NR2B subunit gene GRIN2B in schizophrenia and bipolar disorder: polymorphisms and mRNA levels. Schizophr Res 84(2–3):214–221, 2006

McGrath M, Kawachi I, Ascherio A, et al: Association between catechol-O-methyltransferase and phobic anxiety. Am J Psychiatry 161:1703–1705, 2004

McGuffin P, Rijsdijk F, Andrew M, et al: The heritability of bipolar affective disorder and the genetic relationship to unipolar depression. Arch Gen Psychiatry 60:497–502, 2003

McGuffin P, Knight J, Breen G, et al: Whole genome linkage scan of recurrent depressive disorder from the depression network study. Hum Mol Genet 14:3337–3345, 2005

McLeod DS, Koenen KC, Meyer JM, et al: Genetic and environmental influences on the relationship among combat exposure, posttraumatic stress disorder symptoms, and alcohol use. J Trauma Stress 14:259–275, 2001

McQueen MB, Devlin B, Faraone SV, et al: Combined analysis from eleven linkage studies of bipolar disorder provides strong evidence of susceptibility loci on chromosomes 6q and 8q. Am J Hum Genet 77:582–595, 2005

Mendlewicz J, Rainer J: Adoption study supporting genetic transmission in manic-depressive illness. Nature 268:326–329, 1977

Mendlewicz J, Papdimitriou G, Wilmotte J: Family study of panic disorder: comparison with generalized anxiety disorder, major depression and normal subjects. Psychiatr Genet 3:73–78, 1993

Merikangas K, Stevens D, Fenton B, et al: Co-morbidity and familial aggregation of alcoholism and anxiety disorders. Psychol Med 28:773–778, 1998

Mondimore FM, Zandi PP, Mackinnon DF, et al: Familial aggregation of illness chronicity in recurrent, early onset major depression pedigrees. Am J Psychiatry 163:1554–1560, 2006

Muller DJ, de Luca V, Sicard T, et al: Brain-derived neurotrophic factor (BDNF) gene and rapid-cycling bipolar disorder: family-based association study. Br J Psychiatry 189:317–323, 2006

Munafo MR, Clark T, Flint J: Does measurement instrument moderate the association between the serotonin transporter gene and anxiety-related personality traits? A meta-analysis. Mol Psychiatry 10:415–419, 2005

Munjack D, Moss H: Affective disorder and alcoholism in families of agoraphobics. Arch Gen Psychiatry 38:869–871, 1981

Neves-Pereira M, Mundo E, Muglia P, et al: The brain-derived neurotrophic factor gene confers susceptibility to bipolar disorder: evidence from a family-based association study. Am J Hum Genet 71:651–655, 2002

Newman SC, Bland RC: A population-based family study of DSM-III generalized anxiety disorder. Psychol Med 36:1275–1281, 2006

Noyes R Jr, Crowe RR, Harris EL, et al: Relationship between panic disorder and agoraphobia: a family study. Arch Gen Psychiatry 43:227–232, 1986

Noyes R Jr, Clarksohn C, Crowe RR, et al: A family study of generalized anxiety disorder. Am J Psychiatry 144:1019–1024, 1987

Nurnberger JI Jr, Foroud T, Flury L, et al: Evidence for a locus on chromosome 1 that influences vulnerability to alcoholism and affective disorder. Am J Psychiatry 158:718–724, 2001

Nurnberger JI Jr, Wiegand R, Bucholz K, et al: A family study of alcohol dependence: coaggregation of multiple disorders in relatives of alcohol-dependent probands. Arch Gen Psychiatry 61:1246–1256, 2004

Ozer EJ, Best SR, Lipsey TL, et al: Predictors of posttraumatic stress disorder and symptoms in adults: a meta-analysis. Psychol Bull 129:52–73, 2003

Papolos DF, Faedda GL, Veit S, et al: Bipolar spectrum disorders in patients diagnosed with velo-cardio-facial syndrome: does a hemizygous deletion of chromosome 22q11 result in bipolar affective disorder? Am J Psychiatry 153:1541–1547, 1996

Papolos DF, Veit S, Faedda GL, et al: Ultra-ultra rapid cycling bipolar disorder is associated with the low activity catecholamine-O-methyltransferase allele. Mol Psychiatry 3:346–349, 1998

Park N, Juo SH, Cheng R, et al: Linkage analysis of psychosis in bipolar pedigrees suggests novel putative loci for bipolar disorder and shared susceptibility with schizophrenia. Mol Psychiatry 9:1091–1099, 2004

Pauls DL, Morton LA, Egeland JA: Risks of affective illness among first-degree relatives of bipolar I old-order Amish probands. Arch Gen Psychiatry 49:703–708, 1992

Peroutka S, Price S, Wilhoit T, et al: Comorbid migraine with aura, anxiety, and depression is associated with dopamine D2 receptor (DRD2) NcoI alleles. Mol Med 4:14–21, 1998

Pezawas L, Meyer-Lindenberg A, Drabant EM, et al: 5-HTTLPR polymorphism impacts human cingulate-amygdala interactions: a genetic susceptibility mechanism for depression. Nat Neurosci 8:828–834, 2005

Potash JB, Willour VL, Chiu YF, et al: The familial aggregation of psychotic symptoms in bipolar disorder pedigrees. Am J Psychiatry 158:1258–1264, 2001

Potash JB, Chiu YF, MacKinnon DF, et al: Familial aggregation of psychotic symptoms in a replication set of 69 bipolar disorder pedigrees. Am J Med Genet B Neuropsychiatr Genet 116:90–97, 2003a

Potash JB, Zandi PP, Willour VL, et al: Suggestive linkage to chromosomal regions 13q31 and 22q12 in families with psychotic bipolar disorder. Am J Psychiatry 160:680–686, 2003b

Price RA, Kidd KK, Weissman MM: Early onset (under age 30 years) and panic disorder as markers for etiologic homogeneity in major depression. Arch Gen Psychiatry 44:434–440, 1987

Quaid KA AS, Smiley CL, Nurnberger JI: Perceived genetic risks for bipolar disorder in a patient population: an exploratory study. J Genet Couns 10:41–51, 2001

Rice J, Reich T, Andreasen NC, et al: The familial transmission of bipolar illness. Arch Gen Psychiatry 44:441–447, 1987

Rothe C, Koszycki D, Bradwejn J, et al: Association of the Val158Met catechol-O-methyltransferase genetic polymorphism with panic disorder. Neuropsychopharmacology 31:2237–2242, 2006

Rotondo A, Mazzanti C, Dell'Osso L, et al: Catechol-O-methyltransferase, serotonin transporter, and tryptophan hydroxylase gene polymorphisms in bipolar disorder patients with and without comorbid panic disorder. Am J Psychiatry 159:23–29, 2002

Rowe D, Stever C, Gard J, et al: The relation of the dopamine transporter gene (DAT1) to symptoms of internalizing disorders in children. Behav Genet 28:215–225, 1998

Roy MA, Neale MC, Pedersen NL, et al: A twin study of generalized anxiety disorder and major depression. Psychol Med 25:1037–1049, 1995

Sack WH, Clarke GN, Seeley J: Posttraumatic stress disorder across two generations of Cambodian refugees. J Am Acad Child Adolesc Psychiatry 34:1160–1166, 1995

Samochowiec J, Hajduk A, Samochowiec A, et al: Association studies of MAO-A, COMT, and 5-HTT genes polymorphisms in patients with anxiety disorders of the phobic spectrum. Psychiatry Res 128:21–26, 2004

Scheid JM, Holzman CB, Jones N, et al: Depressive symptoms in mid-pregnancy, lifetime stressors and the 5-HTTLPR genotype. Genes Brain Behav 6:453–464, 2006

Scherrer JF, True WR, Xian H, et al: Evidence for genetic influences common and specific to symptoms of generalized anxiety and panic. J Affect Disord 57:25–35, 2000

Schumacher J, Jamra RA, Becker T, et al: Evidence for a relationship between genetic variants at the brain-derived neurotrophic factor (BDNF) locus and major depression. Biol Psychiatry 58:307–314, 2005

Schurhoff F, Bellivier F, Jouvent R, et al: Early and late onset bipolar disorders: two different forms of manic-depressive illness? J Affect Disord 58:215–221, 2000

Schurhoff F, Szoke A, Meary A, et al: Familial aggregation of delusional proneness in schizophrenia and bipolar pedigrees. Am J Psychiatry 160:1313–1319, 2003

Schurhoff F, Laguerre A, Szoke A, et al: Schizotypal dimensions: continuity between schizophrenia and bipolar disorders. Schizophr Res 80:235–242, 2005

Segman RH, Cooper-Kazaz R, Macciardi F, et al: Association between the dopamine transporter gene and posttraumatic stress disorder. Mol Psychiatry 7:903–907, 2002

Segurado R, Detera-Wadleigh SD, Levinson DF, et al: Genome scan meta-analysis of schizophrenia and bipolar disorder, Part III: bipolar disorder. Am J Hum Genet 73:49–62, 2003

Sen S, Burmeister M, Ghosh D: Meta-analysis of the association between a serotonin transporter promoter polymorphism (5-HTTLPR) and anxiety-related personality traits. Am J Med Genet B Neuropsychiatr Genet 127:85–89, 2004

Shifman S, Bronstein M, Sternfeld M, et al: COMT: a common susceptibility gene in bipolar disorder and schizophrenia. Am J Med Genet B Neuropsychiatr Genet 128:61–64, 2004

Simon NM, Otto MW, Wisniewski SR, et al: Anxiety disorder comorbidity in bipolar disorder patients: data from the first 500 participants in the Systematic Treatment Enhancement Program for Bipolar Disorder (STEP-BD). Am J Psychiatry 161:2222–2229, 2004

Simpson SG, Folstein SE, Meyers DA, et al: Bipolar II: the most common bipolar phenotype? Am J Psychiatry 150:901–903, 1993

Sjoberg RL, Nilsson KW, Nordquist N, et al: Development of depression: sex and the interaction between environment and a promoter polymorphism of the serotonin transporter gene. Int J Neuropsychopharmacol 9:443–449, 2006

Sklar P, Gabriel SB, McInnis MG, et al: Family-based association study of 76 candidate genes in bipolar disorder: BDNF is a potential risk locus. Brain-derived neutrophic factor. Mol Psychiatry 7:579–593, 2002

Sklar P, Pato MT, Kirby A, et al: Genome-wide scan in Portuguese Island families identifies 5q31–5q35 as a susceptibility locus for schizophrenia and psychosis. Mol Psychiatry 9:213–218, 2004

Smoller JW, Finn CT: Family, twin, and adoption studies of bipolar disorder. Am J Med Genet C Semin Med Genet 123:48–58, 2003

Smoller JW, Perlis RH: Family and genetic studies of depression, in Handbook of Chronic Depression. Edited by Alpert JE, Fava M. New York, Marcel Dekker, 2004, pp 97–138

Smoller J, Tsuang M: Panic and phobic anxiety: defining phenotypes for genetic studies. Am J Psychiatry 155:1152–1162, 1998

Smoller JW, Acierno JS Jr, Rosenbaum JF, et al: Targeted genome screen of panic disorder and anxiety disorder proneness using homology to murine QTL regions. Am J Med Genet 105:195–206, 2001

Smoller JW, Yamaki LH, Fagerness JA, et al: The corticotropin-releasing hormone gene and behavioral inhibition in children at risk for panic disorder. Biol Psychiatry 57:1485–1492, 2005

Somanath CP, Jain S, Reddy YC: A family study of early onset bipolar I disorder. J Affect Disord 70:91–94, 2002

Spencer TJ, Biederman J, Wozniak J, et al: Parsing pediatric bipolar disorder from its associated comorbidity with the disruptive behavior disorders. Biol Psychiatry 49:1062–1070, 2001

Stein MB, Chartier MJ, Hazen AL, et al: A direct-interview family study of generalized social phobia. Am J Psychiatry 155: 90–7, 1998

Stein MB, Jang KL, Taylor S, et al: Genetic and environmental influences on trauma exposure and posttraumatic stress disorder symptoms: a twin study. Am J Psychiatry 159:1675–1681, 2002

Strauss J, Barr CL, George CJ, et al: Association study of brain-derived neurotrophic factor in adults with a history of childhood onset mood disorder. Am J Med Genet B Neuropsychiatr Genet 131:16–19, 2004

Strauss J, Barr CL, George CJ, et al: Brain-derived neurotrophic factor variants are associated with childhood-onset mood disorder: confirmation in a Hungarian sample. Mol Psychiatry 10:861–867, 2005

Strober M, Morrell W, Burroughs J, et al: A family study of bipolar I disorder in adolescence: early onset of symptoms linked to increased familial loading and lithium resistance. J Affect Disord 15:255–268, 1988

Sullivan PF, Neale MC, Kendler KS: Genetic epidemiology of major depression: review and meta-analysis. Am J Psychiatry 157:1552–1562, 2000

Surtees PG, Wainwright NW, Willis-Owen SA, et al: Social adversity, the serotonin transporter (5-HTTLPR) polymorphism and major depressive disorder. Biol Psychiatry 59:224–229, 2006

Tadic A, Rujescu D, Szegedi A, et al: Association of a MAOA gene variant with generalized anxiety disorder, but not with panic disorder or major depression. Am J Med Genet B Neuropsychiatr Genet 117:1–6, 2003

Taylor M, Abrams R: Early- and late-onset bipolar illness. Arch Gen Psychiatry 38:58–61, 1981

Taylor MA, Berenbaum SA, Jampala VC, et al: Are schizophrenia and affective disorder related? Preliminary data from a family study. Am J Psychiatry 150:278–285, 1993

Taylor SE, Way BM, Welch WT, et al: Early family environment, current adversity, the serotonin transporter promoter polymorphism, and depressive symptomatology. Biol Psychiatry 60:671–676, 2006

Thorgeirsson TE, Oskarsson H, Desnica N, et al: Anxiety with panic disorder linked to chromosome 9q in Iceland. Am J Hum Genet 72:1221–1230, 2003

Todd RD: Genetics of early onset bipolar affective disorder: are we making progress? Curr Psychiatry Rep 4:141–145, 2002

Trippitelli CL, Jamison KR, Folstein MF, et al: Pilot study on patients' and spouses' attitudes toward potential genetic testing for bipolar disorder. Am J Psychiatry 155:899–904, 1998

True WR, Rice J, Eisen SA, et al: A twin study of genetic and environmental contributions to liability for posttraumatic stress symptoms [see comments]. Arch Gen Psychiatry 50:257–264, 1993

Tsuang M, Faraone S: The Genetics of Mood Disorders. Baltimore, MD, Johns Hopkins University Press, 1990

Tsuang MT, Winokur G, Crowe RR: Morbidity risks of schizophrenia and affective disorders among first degree relatives of patients with schizophrenia, mania, depression and surgical conditions. Br J Psychiatry 137:497–504, 1980

Uhl GR, Grow RW: The burden of complex genetics in brain disorders. Arch Gen Psychiatry 61:223–229, 2004

Ustun TB, Ayuso-Mateos JL, Chatterji S, et al: Global burden of depressive disorders in the year 2000. Br J Psychiatry 184:386–392, 2004

Valles V, Van Os J, Guillamat R, et al: Increased morbid risk for schizophrenia in families of in-patients with bipolar illness. Schizophr Res 42:83–90, 2000

Van Den Bogaert A, Sleegers K, De Zutter S, et al: Association of brain-specific tryptophan hydroxylase, TPH2, with unipolar and bipolar disorder in a Northern Swedish, isolated population. Arch Gen Psychiatry 63:1103–1110, 2006

Wada K, Sasaki T, Jitsuiki H, et al: Manic/hypomanic switch during acute antidepressant treatment for unipolar depression. J Clin Psychopharmacol 26:512–515, 2006

Wang Z, Valdes J, Noyes R, et al: Possible association of a cholecystokinin promotor polymorphism (CCK_{36CT}) with panic disorder. Am J Med Genet (Neuropsychiatric Genetics) 81:228–234, 1998

Warner V, Mufson L, Weissman MM: Offspring at high and low risk for depression and anxiety: mechanisms of psychiatric disorder. J Am Acad Child Adolesc Psychiatry 34:786–797, 1995

Weissman MM, Gershon ES, Kidd KK, et al: Psychiatric disorders in the relatives of probands with affective disorders: the Yale University–National Institute of Mental Health Collaborative Study. Arch Gen Psychiatry 41:13–21, 1984a

Weissman MM, Leckman JF, Merikangas KR, et al: Depression and anxiety disorders in parents and children: results from the Yale Family Study. Arch Gen Psychiatry 41:845–852, 1984b

Weissman MM, Wickramaratne P, Merikangas KR, et al: Onset of major depression in early adulthood: increased familial loading and specificity. Arch Gen Psychiatry 41:1136–1143, 1984c

Weissman MM, Merikangas KR, Wickramaratne P, et al: Understanding the clinical heterogeneity of major depression using family data. Arch Gen Psychiatry 43:430–434, 1986

Weissman MM, Wickramaratne P, Adams PB, et al: The relationship between panic disorder and major depression: a new family study. Arch Gen Psychiatry 50:767–780, 1993

Weissman MM, Bland RC, Canino GJ, et al: Cross-national epidemiology of major depression and bipolar disorder. JAMA 276:293–299, 1996

Weissman MM, Fyer AJ, Haghighi F, et al: Potential panic disorder syndrome: clinical and genetic linkage evidence. Am J Med Genet 96:24–35, 2000

Weissman MM, Wickramaratne P, Nomura Y, et al: Families at high and low risk for depression: a 3-generation study. Arch Gen Psychiatry 62:29–36, 2005

Weissman MM, Wickramaratne P, Nomura Y, et al: Offspring of depressed parents: 20 years later. Am J Psychiatry 163:1001–1008, 2006

Wellcome Trust Case Control Consortium: Genome-wide association study of 14,000 cases of seven common diseases and 3,000 shared controls. Nature 447:661–678, 2007

Wender PH, Kety SS, Rosenthal D, et al: Psychiatric disorders in the biological and adoptive families of adopted individuals with affective disorders. Arch Gen Psychiatry 43:923–929, 1986

Wilhelm K, Mitchell PB, Niven H, et al: Life events, first depression onset and the serotonin transporter gene. Br J Psychiatry 188:210–215, 2006

Winokur G, Coryell W: Familial subtypes of unipolar depression: a prospective study of familial pure depressive disease compared to depression spectrum disease. Biol Psychiatry 32:1012–1018, 1992

Wittchen H-U, Reed V, Kessler R: The relationship of agoraphobia and panic in a community sample of adolescents and young adults. Arch Gen Psychiatry 55:1017–1024, 1998

Woo JM, Yoon KS, Yu BH: Catechol-O-methyltransferase genetic polymorphism in panic disorder. Am J Psychiatry 159:1785–1787, 2002

Woo JM, Yoon KS, Choi YH, et al: The association between panic disorder and the L/L genotype of catechol-O-methyltransferase. J Psychiatr Res 38:365–370, 2004

Xian H, Chantarujikapong SI, Scherrer JF, et al: Genetic and environmental influences on posttraumatic stress disorder, alcohol and drug dependence in twin pairs. Drug Alcohol Depend 61:95–102, 2000

You JS, Hu SY, Chen B, et al: Serotonin transporter and tryptophan hydroxylase gene polymorphisms in Chinese patients with generalized anxiety disorder. Psychiatr Genet 15:7–11, 2005

Zalsman G, Huang YY, Oquendo MA, et al: Association of a triallelic serotonin transporter gene promoter region (5-HTTLPR) polymorphism with stressful life events and severity of depression. Am J Psychiatry 163:1588–1593, 2006

Zhang X, Gainetdinov RR, Beaulieu JM, et al: Loss-of-function mutation in tryptophan hydroxylase-2 identified in unipolar major depression. Neuron 45:11–16, 2005

Zill P, Baghai TC, Zwanzger P, et al: SNP and haplotype analysis of a novel tryptophan hydroxylase isoform (TPH2) gene provide evidence for association with major depression. Mol Psychiatry 9:1030–1036, 2004

Zubenko GS, Hughes HB 3rd, Maher BS, et al: Genetic linkage of region containing the CREB1 gene to depressive disorders in women from families with recurrent, early onset, major depression. Am J Med Genet 114:980–987, 2002a

Zubenko GS, Hughes HB, Stiffler JS, et al: Genome survey for susceptibility loci for recurrent, early onset major depression: results at 10cM resolution. Am J Med Genet 114:413–422, 2002b

Zubenko GS, Hughes IH, Stiffler JS, et al: D2S2944 identifies a likely susceptibility locus for recurrent, early onset, major depression in women. Mol Psychiatry 7:460–467, 2002c

Zubenko GS, Maher B, Hughes HB 3rd, et al: Genome-wide linkage survey for genetic loci that influence the development of depressive disorders in families with recurrent, early-onset, major depression. Am J Med Genet B Neuropsychiatr Genet 123:1–18, 2003

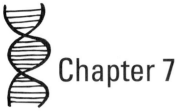

Chapter 7

Genetics of Alzheimer's Disease

Matthew B. McQueen, Sc.D.
Deborah Blacker, M.D., Sc.D.

Clinical Phenotype

Dementia is defined as an acquired loss of cognitive function in two or more domains occurring in a clear sensorium. The differential diagnosis is based on the pattern of deficits and concomitant physical findings and/or tests. Dementing disorders include Alzheimer's disease, vascular or multi-infarct dementia, dementia with Lewy bodies, frontotemporal lobe dementia, and Parkinson's dementia. In addition, a wide variety of medical and neurological conditions can produce dementia.

Alzheimer's disease is the most common and best-studied form of dementia and will be the focus of this chapter. It is estimated to represent from 50% to 90% of all dementias (Kukull and Ganguli 2000). Alzheimer's disease is a late-life dementia with insidious onset and gradual decline. Age at onset of Alzheimer's disease varies widely, from the 30s to the 90s, but the disease is rare before age 60 years. In recognition of differences in family history and genetics described later in this chapter, an onset age of 60 years is often used to separate *early-onset* from *late-onset* Alzheimer's disease, but this division is arbitrary and has little utility in clinical settings.

Alzheimer's disease is diagnosed on the basis of a characteristic pattern of deficits with progressive functional loss. The early stages of Alzheimer's disease are marked by prominent short-term memory loss and difficulty with complex tasks. Depression is also common in the early phase of the illness. Moderate to severe Alzheimer's disease is marked by increasing difficulties with memory, including long-term memory, and growing difficulties in other cognitive domains such as language and spatial reasoning. Patients also begin to have difficulty with basic activities of daily living such as

177

grooming and self-care. Behavioral symptoms such as paranoia, agitation, and wandering are also common in this phase. The profound to terminal phase of Alzheimer's disease is marked by total dependency, with incontinence, immobility, and swallowing dysfunction. For patients who live through the entire course, death generally occurs within 10–20 years of onset. However, because of the late onset, many patients succumb to other illnesses first.

More recently, a prodromal phase of Alzheimer's disease, marked by mild memory loss with little or no impact on function, is being recognized. It is most commonly known as *mild cognitive impairment* (Petersen et al. 1999), although a wide variety of other terms is seen in the research literature, including *cognitively impaired, not demented* and *age-associated memory impairment*. Mild cognitive impairment is a major focus of research to facilitate early intervention while functional status is preserved.

The clinical diagnosis of Alzheimer's disease is based on characteristic symptoms and exclusion of other causes. Two commonly used sets of diagnostic criteria, the National Institute of Neurological and Communicative Disorders and Stroke/Alzheimer's Disease and Related Disorders Association (NINCDS/ADRDA) criteria (McKhann et al. 1984) and the DSM-IV criteria (American Psychiatric Association 1994, 2000), are in common use and are quite similar. In the NINCDS/ADRDA criteria, two levels of certainty are offered, *probable Alzheimer's disease*, in which there is no evidence of other possible sources of dementia, and *possible Alzheimer's disease*, in which other potential contributing factors are present but judged insufficient to cause the patient's symptoms. A *definite Alzheimer's disease* diagnosis at autopsy is based on the density of neuritic plaques and neurofibrillary tangles, the characteristic lesions of Alzheimer's disease, in specific brain regions (Consensus Report of the Working Group on: "Molecular and Biochemical Markers of Alzheimer's Disease" 1998). The positive predictive value of a clinical diagnosis of probable Alzheimer's disease in an academic center is 80%–90% but is much lower in community settings. The ability to hone clinical diagnosis against a neuropathological gold standard, along with the biological insight gained from the neuropathological lesions themselves, is likely to be partly responsible for the more rapid progress in understanding Alzheimer's disease genetics, compared with other psychiatric disorders.

Phenotype definition for studies of Alzheimer's disease genetics includes a variety of strategies to minimize errors. In some studies, the proband or all affected family members are required to meet criteria for probable Alzheimer's disease, and in other studies, at least one autopsy-confirmed case is required. Careful screening of unaffected participants and longitudinal follow-up also improve the accuracy of phenotypic data. In addition, a variety of alternative phenotypes have been proposed, including quantitative traits such as age at onset, age-adjusted memory function, and plasma A-beta levels. Subtypes based on onset age, psychotic features, and Parkinsonian features have also been proposed.

Epidemiology

The prevalence and incidence of dementia overall and Alzheimer's disease specifically increase substantially with age. The overall prevalence of dementia is generally estimated at between 5% and 10% of older adults from a variety of diverse populations (Canadian Study of Health and Aging Working Group 1994; Evans et al. 1989), with variation likely attributable to variations in assessment procedures and age structure of the population. The prevalence of dementia is fairly low among people in their early 60s, but doubles for every 5-year increase in age, reaching as high as 25% to 40% between ages 90 and 95 (Breitner et al. 1999; Jorm and Jolley 1998).

Reliable estimates of incidence rates in the general population are more difficult to obtain, as the types of studies necessary to garner such estimates require long follow-up periods and large sample sizes. The studies available consistently show a steep rise in the incidence of Alzheimer's disease at least into the age range of 90–99 years, where incidence may finally taper off. Incidence has been estimated at 0.1% to 0.5% per year for subjects ages 65–69 years and from 5% to 10% for subjects age 85 years or older (Bachman et al. 1993; Hebert et al. 1995; Canadian Study of Health and Aging Working Group 2000; Launer et al. 1999; Miech et al. 2002). Much of the variation in incidence rates can be attributed to methodological issues such as baseline screening methods and diagnostic thresholds at follow-up.

A wide variety of demographic and environmental risk factors have been investigated for a potential role in Alzheimer's disease (Kukull and Ganguli 2000). The best-established risk factors are longevity, family history, and female gender. There is also convincing evidence that educational attainment offers some protection against the development of Alzheimer's disease. In addition, an increasing amount of evidence suggests that a wide variety of cardiovascular risk factors, including atherosclerosis, diabetes, hypertension, and elevated cholesterol levels, also increase the risk of Alzheimer's disease (Kamboh 2004). Epidemiological evidence has suggested that postmenopausal estrogen supplementation and antioxidant vitamins may be protective against the development of Alzheimer's disease, but these finding have not held up in randomized controlled trials (Petersen et al. 2005; Shumaker et al. 2004). There is also some evidence that nonsteroidal anti-inflammatory agents and statins may also be protective (Kamboh 2004; Kukull and Ganguli 2000).

Genetic Epidemiology

Alzheimer's disease is a genetically complex and heterogeneous disorder. Particularly for genetic studies, Alzheimer's disease is often categorized according to age at onset, with age 60 years as the cutoff for "early-onset" versus "late-onset" Alzheimer's disease. This division makes sense because age at onset is correlated in families (Farrer et al. 1990) and also carries important clinical and public health significance. Early-onset Alzheimer's disease is much less common and is more likely to be familial and to follow an autosomal dominant inheritance pattern.

In contrast, late-onset Alzheimer's disease follows no discernible inheritance pattern and therefore is thought to arise from more complex etiology, with likely contributions from both genes and environment. Studies consistently show that first-degree relatives of Alzheimer's disease patients have a two- to threefold higher risk of developing Alzheimer's disease than the general population (Farrer et al. 1989; Green et al. 2002; Payami et al. 1997), and this increase in risk persists into advanced ages (Lautenschlager et al. 1996; Silverman et al. 1994). It is noteworthy that family history remains a risk factor for Alzheimer's disease, even in analyses controlling for the known Alzheimer's disease gene apolipoprotein E4 (*APOE4*) (see the section on *APOE* later in this chapter) (Payami et al. 1997).

Family history is necessary but not sufficient to suggest genetic etiology, as many environmental risk factors also cluster in families. Adoption studies, which unlink genes and environment, or twin studies, which hold environment relatively constant while varying the degree of genetic relationship, are used to establish a role for genes. Adoption studies are generally not feasible for Alzheimer's disease because of the long delay between adoption and disease onset, but a number of small twin studies have been completed and are consistent with a substantial genetic contribution to disease risk (Bergem et al. 1997; Breitner et al. 1995; Raiha et al. 1997). Monozygotic twin concordance rates are well below 100%, confirming a role for environmental factors, and even in concordant pairs, age at onset can vary widely. As with results in family studies, twin concordance differences remain even after *APOE* genotype is accounted for (Bergem et al. 1997).

Segregation analysis provides another approach to assessing the role of genes. Because of the late onset of Alzheimer's disease, this approach is limited, as parental information is retrospective—if available at all—and tends to be of poor quality, reflecting substantial changes in diagnostic practices and criteria over the past decades. Available segregation analyses are consistent with genetic etiology (Daw et al. 2000; Farrer et al. 1990). The results of the analysis by Daw et al. (2000), which used age at onset as the phenotype, point to the existence of four to five additional Alzheimer's disease risk genes.

Molecular Genetics

Four genes that are involved in the etiology of Alzheimer's disease have been identified. Defects in three genes are known to cause early-onset Alzheimer's disease: the genes for amyloid-β protein precursor (*APP*) on chromosome 21 (Goate et al. 1991; Tanzi et al. 1987), presenilin 1 (*PSEN1*) on chromosome 14 (Schellenberg et al. 1992; Sherrington et al. 1995), and presenilin 2 (*PSEN2*) on chromosome 1 (Levy-Lehad et al. 1995; Rogaev et al. 1995). A variant of one gene, the apolipoprotein E gene (*APOE*) on chromosome 19, is associated primarily with late-onset Alzheimer's disease (Saunders et al. 1993; Strittmatter et al. 1993) and acts as a risk factor and modifier of age at onset. An overview of the established genes involved in Alzheimer's disease can be found in Table 7–1.

TABLE 7–1. Overview of the established Alzheimer's disease genes

Gene	Chromo-some	Mode of inheritance	Number of mutations	Mean familial onset age, years (range)
APP	21	Autosomal dominant	20	51.5 (35–60)
PSEN1	14	Autosomal dominant	144	44.1 (24–60)
PSEN2	1	Autosomal dominant	10	57.1 (46–71)
APOE	19	Complex	N/A	Onset-age modifier

Note. N/A=not available.
Source. Adapted from Bertram L, Tanzi RE: "The Current Status of Alzheimer's Disease Genetics: What Do We Tell the Patients?" *Pharmacological Research* 50:385–396, 2004. Used with permission.
Numbers of mutations updated from Alzheimer Disease and Frontotemporal Dementia Database 2005.

Early-Onset Alzheimer's Disease

Initial efforts to understand the role of genetics in Alzheimer's disease in the early 1980s focused on extremely rare, large multigenerational families with early-onset Alzheimer's disease occurring in multiple members in each generation, suggesting autosomal dominant inheritance with complete penetrance. An example of such an Alzheimer's disease pedigree, in this case a family carrying a mutation in *PSEN1*, is shown in Figure 7–1. Even this seemingly simple form of the disease is remarkably complex, involving multiple mutations in three known genes and others yet to be identified. Most of these mutations have been found in only one family or one individual and are thus genetically "private." Furthermore, it has become increasingly apparent that mutations in the *APP* and presenilin genes do not account for all cases of early-onset Alzheimer's disease (Tanzi et al. 1996).

Amyloid-Beta Protein Precursor Gene

The first gene associated with early-onset Alzheimer's disease was *APP* (Goate et al. 1991; Tanzi et al. 1987). Twenty different pathogenetic mutations have been identified in this gene in a total of 60 unrelated families; together these account for a very small proportion (~5%) of reported Alzheimer's disease pedigrees and a still smaller proportion of reported cases of early-onset Alzheimer's disease (Alzheimer Disease and Frontotemporal Dementia Mutation Database 2005). The age at onset of Alzheimer's disease reported for individuals harboring pathogenic mutations in *APP* ranges from the late 30s through the late 60s, with some variation according to the specific mutation that is present. All mutations appear to be fully penetrant, although some lead to other neurological syndromes instead of or in addition to dementia. It is noteworthy that in families harboring a pathogenic *APP* mutation, family members who carry one or especially two *APOE4* alleles experience an earlier age at onset (Sorbi et al. 1993).

Presenilin Genes

Mutations in the presenilin genes *PSEN1* and *PSEN2* (primarily *PSEN1*) account for Alzheimer's disease in roughly 50% of early-onset Alzheimer's disease pedigrees (Levy-Lehad et al. 1995; Sherrington et al. 1995; Tanzi et al. 1996). To date, 144 different Alzheimer's disease mutations have been identified in *PSEN1* in 289 unrelated families and in sporadic cases of Alzheimer's disease, but only 10 *PSEN2* Alzheimer's disease mutations have been reported in 18 families (Alzheimer Disease and Frontotemporal Dementia Database 2005). Virtually all of the Alzheimer's disease mutations identified in *PSEN1* are best characterized as autosomal dominant fully penetrant gene defects. The mean age at onset of Alzheimer's disease in *PSEN1*-linked

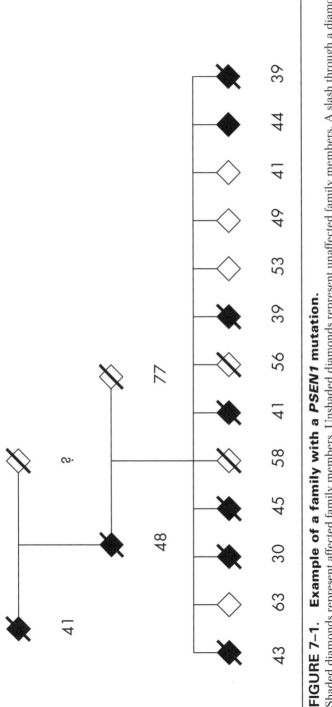

FIGURE 7–1.   Example of a family with a *PSEN1* mutation.

Shaded diamonds represent affected family members. Unshaded diamonds represent unaffected family members. A slash through a diamond indicates a deceased family member. Age at onset (for affected family members) or age at examination/age at death (for unaffected family members) is shown below the diamonds.

Source.   Adapted from Schellenberg GD, Bird TD, Wijsman EM, et al.: "Genetic Linkage Evidence for a Familial Alzheimer's Disease Locus on Chromosome 14. *Science* 258:668–671, 1992. Used with permission.

Alzheimer's disease families is approximately 45 years, with a range from the early 30s to the late 50s. Differences in mean age at onset have been associated with specific mutations and even with groups of mutations in the same gene segment (Tanzi et al. 1996). The mean age at onset in families with the most common mutation in *PSEN2*–called the Volga German mutation because it was first identified in a group of ethnic Germans who had settled in Russia (Schellenberg, 1995)–is 52 years, and individual age at onset varies widely from 40 to 85 years (Tanzi et al. 1996). In families harboring *PSEN2* mutations, individuals with one or especially two copies of the *APOE4* allele appear to have earlier age at onset of Alzheimer's disease (Wijsman et al. 2005), although in families with *PSEN1* mutations, the *APOE4* allele has no effect on age at onset (Van Broeckhoven et al. 1994).

Late-Onset Alzheimer's Disease

Given the complexity of genetics for early-onset Alzheimer's disease, which represents only a small fraction of cases of the disorder, it is likely that the far more common late-onset form of the disease has still more complex genetics. Several additional factors contribute to the difficulty of studying genes involved in late-onset Alzheimer's disease. First, the prevalence of the disorder is high and rises steeply with age, so some clustering in families may be due to chance alone, and multiple sources of disease may co-occur in a single family. Second, late-onset Alzheimer's disease occurs very near the end of the life span, so that many individuals do not survive the age of risk. Because of this characteristic, it is difficult to assess the mode of inheritance or even to derive an accurate estimate of the increase in risk for relatives of Alzheimer's disease cases. In addition, no one can be said to be past the age of risk, so unaffected family members contribute less to linkage analysis. Third, elderly patients are at increased risk for other causes of cognitive decline, elevating the rate of diagnostic errors and hence phenocopies (individuals who appear to have the disease but do not carry any disease-causing genes).

Despite these obstacles, investigators were able to identify, in 1993, a powerful risk factor gene: *APOE4*. A number of other putative late-onset Alzheimer's disease genes have been reported in the scientific literature (Alzheimer Research Forum 2005), but none of these can be considered an established risk factor for late-onset Alzheimer's disease.

Apolipoprotein E Gene

The apolipoprotein E gene (*APOE*) has three alleles, designated 2 (allele frequency ~0.08), 3 (allele frequency ~0.80), and 4 (allele frequency ~0.12) (Myers et al. 1996). The E4 allele is associated with increased risk of Alzheimer's disease *and* cardiovascular disease and with decreased longevity, and the E2 allele is associated with decreased risk of Alzheimer's disease *and* cardiovascular disease and with increased longevity. Investigators first noted that that the E4 allele was overrepresented in early- and late-onset familial and sporadic cases (Saunders et al. 1993; Strittmatter et al. 1993), and these findings have been subsequently confirmed in a meta-analysis (Farrer et al. 1997) and numerous population-based studies (e.g., Breitner et al. 1999; Myers et al. 1996). Similarly, the *APOE2* effect was first noted in familial and sporadic cases (Corder et al. 1994) but has been confirmed in a large meta-analysis (Farrer et al. 1997).

However, instead of acting deterministically, *APOE4* acts as a risk factor and *APOE2* as a protective factor for the disease. *APOE4* is clearly not necessary for the development of the disease at any age: in fact, some 35%–60% of Alzheimer's disease case patients do not carry the E4 allele, and only 12%–15% have two copies ("Apolipoprotein E Genotyping in Alzheimer's Disease" 1996; Schellenberg 1995; "Statement on Use of Apolipoprotein E Testing for Alzheimer's Disease" 1995). Based on figures such as these, some researchers have estimated that the *APOE4* allele accounts for susceptibility to Alzheimer's disease in no more than 50% of cases (Saunders et al. 1993; Schellenberg 1995). However, such estimates must be interpreted with caution because the E4 allele is present in 20%–30% of the general population, so its presence in an Alzheimer's disease subject does not necessarily mean it is responsible for the disease. More critically, even two copies of *APOE4* are not sufficient to cause the disease. For instance, in a study of 310 families with at least two living members affected with Alzheimer's disease, there were 15 cognitively normal individuals with two copies of *APOE4* who were older than their two affected siblings, often by as much as 10 years (Blacker et al. 1997).

The primary role of *APOE4* may be as a modifier of age at onset (Meyer et al. 1998), as it has already been documented to act with both *APP* and *PSEN2*. Its effect on age at onset is dose-dependent, with homozygotes experiencing onset much earlier than heterozygotes, whose onset is only modestly earlier than in individuals who do not carry the E4 allele (Corder et al. 1993; Farrer et al. 1997; Myers et al. 1996). In addition, the *APOE4* effect appears to be age-dependent, with the gene's peak effect on Alzheimer's disease risk occurring in individuals who experience onset of the disease in their 60s (Blacker et al. 1997; Farrer et al. 1997).

Beyond *APOE*

Despite the strong effect of *APOE4* on the risk of Alzheimer's disease, the majority of genetic culprits effectively remain "at large." Several lines of evidence suggest the presence of additional Alzheimer's disease genes. For example, the effect of family history (Payami et al. 1997) or monozygotic twin status (Bergem et al. 1997) remains after *APOE4* is controlled for. In addition, a segregation analysis points to the existence of several additional late-onset Alzheimer's disease genes (Daw et al. 2000), and the peak age at onset is in the 60s (Farrer et al. 1997), while the disease incidence continues to rise steeply for decades.

Linkage analysis has provided several clues to where such Alzheimer's disease genes may reside (reviewed in Bertram and Tanzi 2004; Kamboh 2004). Other than the *APOE* region on chromosome 19, the most consistent linkage signals have been observed on chromosomes 9, 10, and 12 (Blacker et al 2003; Myers et al. 2002). Follow-up in these regions has been extensive, particularly with candidate gene studies using the case-control study design. More than 200 genes have been tested for association with Alzheimer's disease, with discouraging results (Alzheimer Research Forum 2005; Kamboh 2004). Initial reports of association between Alzheimer's disease and a particular gene have generally not been replicated, and thus the field has yet to produce even a second established Alzheimer's disease risk factor gene.

Chromosome 9 holds two distinct linkage regions—on 9p21 and 9q22 (Blacker et al. 2003; Myers et al. 2002). For the 9p peak, perhaps the most interesting candidate is the gene encoding the very low-density lipoprotein receptor (*VLDLR*) (Okuizumi et al. 1995). However, consistent with other genes, replication has been less than convincing (reviewed in Alzheimer Research Forum 2005; Bertram and Tanzi 2004). For the 9q peak, the finding of association to the gene encoding ubiquilin (*UBQLN*) in two independent samples (Bertram et al. 2005) is promising, but preliminary efforts at replication are mixed (Alzheimer Research Forum 2005).

The chromosome 10 peak has received the greatest amount of attention (Bertram et al. 2000; Ertekin-Taner et al. 2000; Myers et al. 2000). Perhaps the most attractive candidate gene in this large region is the gene encoding insulin-degrading enzyme (*IDE*) (Abraham et al. 2001), and a large number of association studies have been published (for review, see Alzheimer Research Forum 2005). Other promising candidates include the genes encoding glutathione *S*-transferase omega 1 and 2 (*GSTO1* and *GSTO2*) (Li et al. 2004) and plasminogen activator urokinase (*PLAU*), but results have been equally disappointing (Alzheimer Research Forum 2005).

Evidence for linkage on chromosome 12 has been reported by multiple groups (Myers et al. 2002; Pericak-Vance et al. 1997; Rogaeva et al. 1998). A variety of candidate genes have been tested in this region, including the genes encoding alpha$_2$-macroglobulin (*A2M*) (Saunders et al. 2003) and the low-density lipoprotein receptor–related protein 1 (*LRP1*) (Kang et al. 1997).

Of these genes, *LRP1* may be the most promising (see Alzheimer Research Forum 2005); *A2M* has been controversial, with many null reports across a large number of case-control studies (for a meta-analysis, see Bertram et al. 2007) and modest confirmation in the majority of family-based studies (Saunders et al. 2003).

Clinical and Public Health Implications of Alzheimer's Disease Genetics

The potential benefits of greater understanding in Alzheimer's disease genetics are many. The discovery of *APP*, *PSEN1*, and *PSEN2* has already contributed enormously to the understanding of Alzheimer's disease pathophysiology, and at least 20 drugs already in development are based in genetics research. *APOE* and any subsequently discovered late-onset Alzheimer's disease genes may play a role in early detection, early intervention, and prevention, and may also show specific pharmacogenomic effects. In addition, knowledge gained in genetic research can be used to provide genetic counseling and, in some cases, genetic testing for those with a family history of Alzheimer's disease. What can be offered depends on the specific family history.

Where there is a history of autosomal dominant, early-onset Alzheimer's disease, a referral to a specialized center for formal genetic counseling and possibly genetic testing may be in order. Genetic testing for *PSEN1* is commercially available and is generally targeted to families with onset ages before age 50 years. Testing is sometimes offered for confirmation of diagnosis, although testing adds little to diagnostic certainty in this context. It can also be used to predict disease onset in unaffected individuals with an autosomal dominant family history of Alzheimer's disease with onset at or before age 50 years. However, because of the marked allelic heterogeneity, testing requires sequencing the gene, ideally done by testing a known affected family member. Because the illness is untreatable, the current standard is to offer pre- and posttest counseling following a Huntington's disease model (Bird 1999; Liddell et al. 2001; Williamson and LaRusse 2004). Testing for the other two early-onset Alzheimer's disease genes is not commercially available but is sometimes feasible in a research setting (Lannfelt et al. 1995; Steinbart et al. 2001). As with Huntington's disease, there has been limited interest in predictive testing for Alzheimer's disease among family members at risk for early-onset autosomal dominant Alzheimer's disease (Karlinsky et al. 1996; Steinbart et al. 2001).

For more typical Alzheimer's disease, genetic counseling typically provides risk estimates based on λ, the risk in relatives compared with the general population. In typical families (i.e., those with non-Mendelian inheritance), there is only modest increase in risk, on the order of two- to three-fold. Because Alzheimer's disease is a common disease, *relative* risk may be more palatable than *absolute* risk. It is critical to reassure patients that genetic risk is not deterministic, and it is often helpful to point out that age at onset tends to be correlated in families (Farrer et al. 1990). Genetic testing for *APOE* is currently available as an adjunct to diagnosis, although it offers only marginal improvement in diagnostic accuracy and does not obviate need for a careful workup (Mayeux et al. 1998). Multiple formal panels have recommended against the use of testing to predict future risk (e.g., "Apolipoprotein E Genotyping in Alzheimer's Disease" 1996; McConnell et al. 1998; "Statement on Use of Apolipoprotein E Testing for Alzheimer's Disease" 1995) because the predictive value is insufficient for this purpose. However, it is possible that *APOE* testing will have a future role in targeting prevention or therapy, and a randomized controlled trial of *APOE* testing in clinical practice is ongoing (Roberts et al. 2004).

Overall, Alzheimer's disease genetics is likely to become one of the test cases for the introduction of genetic knowledge into clinical practice, of particular interest to persons who are preparing for the possibility of genetic testing for psychiatric disorders. In addition to the potential benefits of genetic findings in developing and targeting treatments, these findings may carry potential costs. For example, although *APOE* testing lacks sufficient predictive value to be clinically useful at the individual level, it is highly predictive at the group level, and insurance companies are quite aware of its potential actuarial value (Zick et al. 2005). Careful attention to these issues, along with better education about genetics and probabilistic reasoning for physicians and their patients, will be critical as genetic risk concepts are introduced into clinical settings.

In the meantime, clinicians should adopt a long-term perspective and suggest that Alzheimer's disease patients and their families do the same. A great deal remains to be done, including the identification of more genes involved in early-onset and especially late-onset Alzheimer's disease and the development of a fuller understanding of how these genes might act alone and/or in concert with other genes and environmental factors to produce the disease. Drug development based on genetic findings, while very exciting, is in its early stages, and preventive treatments are not yet on the horizon. Of course, modestly effective treatments, developed on the basis of other lines of research, are already available. In addition, effective and underutilized treatments are available for associated symptoms such as psychosis, depression, and sleep disturbances (American Psychiatric Association 1997). Although Alzheimer's disease genetic findings offer little at present in the way of improved therapy or risk assessment (other than for those from rare autosomal dominant families), they hold considerable promise for treating or even preventing Alzheimer's disease in generations to come. In the meantime, investigators, clinicians, patients, and families must be cautious not to overinterpret–or overvalue–genetic research.

References

Abraham R, Myers A, Wavrant-DeVrieze F, et al: Substantial linkage disequilibrium across the insulin-degrading enzyme locus but no association with late-onset Alzheimer's disease. Hum Genet 109:646–652, 2001

Alzheimer Disease and Frontotemporal Dementia Mutation Database. Available at: http://www.molgen.ua.ac.be/ADMutations/default.cfm?MT=1andML=3 andPage=MutByPublication. Accessed November 14, 2005.

Alzheimer Research Forum. AlzGene–Published AD Candidate Genes [AlzGene database]. Available at: http://www.alzgene.org. Accessed November 14, 2005.

American Psychiatric Association: Diagnostic and Statistical Manual of Mental Disorders, 4th Edition. Washington, DC, American Psychiatric Association, 1994

American Psychiatric Association: Diagnostic and Statistical Manual of Mental Disorders, 4th Edition, Text Revision. Washington, DC, American Psychiatric Association, 2000

American Psychiatric Association: Practice guideline for the treatment of patients with Alzheimer's disease and other dementias of late life. Am J Psychiatry 154 (suppl):1–39, 1997

Apolipoprotein E genotyping in Alzheimer's disease. National Institute on Aging/ Alzheimer's Association Working Group. Lancet 347:1091–95, 1996

Bachman DL, Wolf PA, Linn RT, et al: Incidence of dementia and probable Alzheimer's disease in a general population: the Framingham Study. Neurology 43:515–519, 1993

Bergem AL, Engedal K, Kringlen EL: The role of heredity in late-onset Alzheimer disease and vascular dementia: a twin study. Arch Gen Psychiatry 54:264–270, 1997

Bertram L, Tanzi RE: The current status of Alzheimer's disease genetics: what do we tell the patients? Pharmacol Res 50:385–396, 2004

Bertram L, Blacker D, Mullin K, et al: Evidence for genetic linkage of Alzheimer's disease to chromosome 10q. Science 290:2302–2303, 2000

Bertram L, Hiltunen M, Parkinson M, et al: Family-based association of Alzheimer's disease and UBQLN1 on chromosome 9q22, New Engl J Med 352:884–894, 2005

Bertram L, McQueen MB, Mullin K, et al: Systematic meta-analysis of Alzheimer's disease genetic association studies: the AlzGene database. Nat Genet 39:17–23, 2007

Bird TD: Risks and benefits of DNA testing for neurogenetic disorders. Semin Neurol 19:253–259, 1999

Blacker D, Haines JL, Rodes L, et al: *APOE*-4 and age-at-onset of Alzheimer's disease: the NIMH Genetics Initiative. Neurology 48:139–147, 1997

Blacker D, Bertram L, Saunders AJ, et al: Results of a high-resolution genome screen of 437 Alzheimer's disease families. Hum Mol Genet 12:23–32, 2003

Breitner JCS, Welsh KA, Gau BA, et al: Alzheimer's disease in the National Academy of Sciences–National Research Council Registry of Aging Twin Veterans: III: detection of cases, longitudinal results, and observations on twin concordance. Arch Neurol 52:763–771, 1995

Breitner JCS, Wyse BW, Anthony JC: APOE-e4 count predicts age when prevalence of AD increases, then declines: the Cache County Study. Neurology 53:321–331, 1999

Canadian Study of Health and Aging Working Group: Study methods and prevalence of dementia. Canad Med Assoc J 150:899–913, 1994

Canadian Study of Health and Aging Working Group: The incidence of dementia in Canada. Neurology 55:66–73, 2000

Consensus Report of the Working Group on: "Molecular and Biochemical Markers of Alzheimer's Disease." The Ronald and Nancy Reagan Research Institute of the Alzheimer's Association and the National Institute on Aging Working Group. Neurobiol Aging 19:109–116, 1998

Corder EH, Saunders AM, Strittmatter WJ, et al: Gene dose of apolipoprotein E type 4 allele and the risk of Alzheimer's disease in late onset families. Science 261:921–923, 1993

Corder EH, Saunders AM, Risch NJ, et al: Protective effect of apolipoprotein E type 2 allele for late onset Alzheimer disease. Nat Genet 7:180–184, 1994

Daw EW, Payami H, Nemens EJ, et al: The number of trait loci in late-onset Alzheimer's disease. Am J Hum Genet 66:196–204, 2000

Ertekin-Taner N, Graff-Radford N, Younkin LH, et al: Linkage of plasma Abeta42 to a quantitative locus on chromosome 10 in late-onset Alzheimer's disease pedigrees. Science 290:2303–2304, 2000

Evans DA, Funkenstein HH, Albert MS, et al: Prevalence of Alzheimer's disease in a community population of older persons higher than previously reported. JAMA 262:2661–2556, 1989

Farrer LA, O'Sullivan D, Cupples LA, et al: Assessment of genetic risk for Alzheimer's disease among first-degree relatives. Ann Neurol 25:485–493, 1989

Farrer LA, Myers RH, Cupples LA, et al: Transmission and age-at-onset patterns in familial Alzheimer's disease: evidence for heterogeneity. Neurology 38:395–403, 1990

Farrer LA, Cupples LA, Haines JL, et al: Effects of age, sex, and ethnicity on the association between apolipoprotein E genotype and Alzheimer disease: a meta-analysis. APOE and Alzheimer Disease Meta-Analysis Consortium. JAMA 278:1349–1356, 1997

Goate AM, Chartier-Harlin MC, Mullan MC, et al: Segregation of a missense mutation in the amyloid precursor protein gene with familial Alzheimer's disease. Nature 349:704–706, 1991

Green RC, Cupples LA, Go R, et al: Risk of dementia among white and African-American relatives of patients with Alzheimer's disease. JAMA 287:329–336, 2002

Hebert LE, Scherr PA, Beckett LA, et al: Age-specific incidence of Alzheimer's disease in a community population. JAMA 273:1354–1359, 1995

Jorm AF, Jolley D: The incidence of dementia: a meta-analysis. Neurology 51:728–733, 1998

Kamboh MI: Molecular genetics of late-onset Alzheimer's disease. Ann Hum Genet 68:381–404, 2004

Kang DE, Saitoh T, Chen X, et al: Genetic association of the low-density lipoprotein receptor-related protein gene (LRP), an apolipoprotein E receptor, with late-onset Alzheimer's disease. Neurology 49:56–61, 1997

Karlinsky H, Geiger O, MacDougall A, et al: A pilot experience in genetic counseling for Alzheimer's disease. Ann New York Acad Sci 802:120–127, 1996

Kukull WA, Ganguli M: Epidemiology of dementia: concepts and overview. Neurol Clin 18:923–949, 2000

Lannfelt L, Axelman K, Lilius L, et al: Genetic counseling in a Swedish Alzheimer family with amyloid precursor protein mutation. Am J Hum Genet 56:332–335, 1995

Launer LJ, Andersen K, Dewey ME, et al: Rates and risk factors for dementia and Alzheimer's disease: results from EURODEM pooled analyses. EURODEM Incidence Research Group and Work Groups. European Studies of Dementia. Neurology 52:78–84, 1999

Lautenschlager NT, Cupples LA, Rao VS, et al: Risk of dementia among relatives of Alzheimer's disease patients in the MIRAGE study: what is in store for the oldest old? Neurology 46:641–650, 1996

Levy-Lehad E, Wasco W, Poorkaj P, et al: Candidate gene for the chromosome 1 familial Alzheimer's disease locus. Science 269:973–977, 1995

Li YJ, Oliveira SA, Xu P, et al: Glutathione S-transferase omega-1 modifies age-at-onset of Alzheimer disease and Parkinson disease. Hum Mol Genet 12:3259–3267, 2004

Liddell MB, Lovestone S, Owen MJ: Genetic risk of Alzheimer's disease: advising relatives. Br J Psychiatry 178:62–66, 2001

Mayeux R, Saunders AM, Shea S, et al: Utility of the apolipoprotein E genotype in the diagnosis of Alzheimer's disease. Alzheimer's Disease Centers Consortium on Apolipoprotein E and Alzheimer's Disease. New Engl J Med 338:506–511, 1998

McConnell LM, Koenig LM, Greely HT, et al: Genetic testing and Alzheimer disease: has the time come? Nature Med 4:757–759, 1998

McKhann G, Drachman D, Folstein M, et al: Clinical diagnosis of Alzheimer's disease: report of the NINCDS-ADRDA Work Group under the auspices of Department of Health and Human Services Task Force on Alzheimer's Disease. Neurology 34:939–944, 1984

Meyer MR, Tschanz JT, Norton MC, et al: APOE genotype predicts when—not whether—one is predisposed to develop Alzheimer disease. Nat Genet 19:321–322, 1998

Miech RA, Breitner JC, Zandi PP, et al: Incidence of AD may decline in the early 90s for men, later for women: the Cache County study. Neurology 58:209–218, 2002

Myers A, Holmans P, Marshall H, et al: Susceptibility locus for Alzheimer's disease on chromosome 10. Science 290:2304–2305, 2000

Myers A, Wavrant De-Vrieze F, Holmans P, et al: Full genome screen for Alzheimer disease: stage II analysis. Am J Med Genet 114:235–244, 2002

Myers RH, Schaefer EJ, Wilson PWF, et al: Apolipoprotein E4 associated with dementia in a population-based study: the Framingham Study. Neurology 45:673–677, 1996

Okuizumi K, Onodera O, Namba Y, et al: Genetic association of the very low density lipoprotein (VLDL) receptor gene with sporadic Alzheimer's disease. Nat Genet 11:207–209, 1995

Payami H, Grimslid H, Oken B, et al: A prospective study of cognitive health in the elderly (Oregon Brain Aging Study): effects of family history and apolipoprotein E genotype. Am J Hum Genet 60:948–956, 1997

Pericak-Vance MA, Bass MP, Yamaoka LH, et al: Complete genomic screen in late-onset familial Alzheimer disease: evidence for a new locus on chromosome 12. JAMA 278:1237–1241, 1997

Petersen RC, Smith GE, Waring SC, et al: Mild cognitive impairment: clinical characterization and outcome. Arch Neurol 56:303–308, 1999

Petersen RC, Thomas RG, Grundman M, et al: Vitamin E and donepezil for the treatment of mild cognitive impairment. N Engl J Med 352:2379–2388, 2005

Raiha I, Kaprio J, Kosenvuo M, et al: Alzheimer's disease in twins. Biomed Pharmacother 51:101–04, 1997

Roberts JS, Barber M, Brown T, et al: Who seeks genetic susceptibility testing for Alzheimer's disease? Findings from a multi-site, randomized clinical trial. Genet Med 6:197–203, 2004

Rogaev EI, Sherrington R, Rogaeva EA, et al: Familial Alzheimer's disease in kindreds with missense mutation in a gene on chromosome 1 related to the Alzheimer's disease type 3 gene. Nature 376:775–778, 1995

Rogaeva E, Premkumar S, Song Y, et al: Evidence for an Alzheimer disease susceptibility locus on chromosome 12 and for further locus heterogeneity. JAMA 280:614–618, 1998

Saunders AJ, Bertram L, Mullin K, et al: Genetic association of Alzheimer's disease with multiple polymorphisms in alpha-2-macroglobulin. Hum Mol Genet 12:2765–2776, 2003

Saunders AM, Strittmatter WJ, Schmechel D, et al: Association of apolipoprotein E allele ε4 with late-onset familial and sporadic Alzheimer's disease. Neurology 43:1467–1472, 1993

Schellenberg GD: Genetic dissection of Alzheimer disease, a heterogeneous disorder. Proc Natl Acad Sci U S A 92:8552–8559, 1995

Schellenberg GD, Bird TD, Wijsman EM, et al: Genetic linkage evidence for a familial Alzheimer's disease locus on chromosome 14. Science 258:668–671, 1992

Sherrington R, Rogaev EI, Liang Y, et al: Cloning of a novel gene bearing missense mutations in early familial Alzheimer disease. Nature 375:754–760, 1995

Shumaker SA, Legault C, Kuller L, et al: Conjugated equine estrogens and incidence of probable dementia and mild cognitive impairment in postmenopausal women: the Women's Health Initiative Memory Study. JAMA 291:2947–2958, 2004

Silverman JM, Li G, Zaccario ML, et al: Patterns of risk in first-degree relatives of patients with Alzheimer's disease. Arch Gen Psych 51:577–586, 1994

Sorbi S, Nacmias B, Forleo P, et al: Epistatic effect of *APP717* mutation and apolipoprotein E genotype in familial Alzheimer's disease. Ann Neurol 38:124–127, 1993

Statement on use of apolipoprotein E testing for Alzheimer's disease. American College of Medical Genetics/American Society of Human Genetics Working Group on ApoE and Alzheimer Disease. JAMA 274:1627–1629, 1995

Steinbart EJ, Smith CO, Pookaj P, et al: Impact of DNA testing for early onset familiar Alzheimer disease and frontotemporal dementia. Arch Neurol 58:1828–1831, 2001

Strittmatter WJ, Saunders AM, Schmechel D, et al: Apolipoprotein E: high avidity binding to b-amyloid and increased frequency of type 4 allele in late-onset familial Alzheimer disease. Proc. Natl Acad Sci U S A 90:1977–1981, 1993

Tanzi R, Gusella JF, Watkins PC, et al: The amyloid beta protein gene: cDNA cloning, mRNA distribution, and genetic linkage near the Alzheimer locus. Science 235:880ñ884, 1987

Tanzi RE, Kovacs DM, Kim T-W: The gene defects responsible for familial Alzheimer's disease. Neurobiol Dis 3:159–168, 1996

Van Broeckhoven C, Backhovens H, Cruts M, et al: APOE genotype does not modulate age of onset in families with chromosome 14 encoded Alzheimer's disease. Neurosci Lett 169:179–180, 1994

Wijsman EM, Daw EW, Yu X, et al: APOE and other loci affect age-at-onset in Alzheimer's disease families with PS2 mutation. Am J Med Genet B Neuropsychiatr Genet 132:14–20, 2005

Williamson J, LaRusse S: Genetics and genetic counseling: recommendations for Alzheimer's disease, frontotemporal dementia, and Creutzfeldt-Jakob disease. Curr Neurol Neurosci Rep 4:351–357, 2004

Zick CD, Mathews CJ, Roberts JS, et al: Genetic testing for Alzheimer's disease and its impact on insurance purchasing behavior. Health Aff (Millwood) 24:483–490, 2005

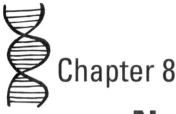

Chapter 8

Neuropsychiatric Aspects of Genetic Disorders

Christine T. Finn, M.D.

Compared with major psychiatric disorders, genetic conditions that are accompanied by psychiatric or behavioral symptoms are quite rare. However, in some populations, including individuals with psychiatric symptoms, occurrence of genetic syndromes may be significantly elevated compared with general population rates. For example, the genetic condition velocardiofacial syndrome, which occurs in approximately 1 in 3,000 individuals in the general population, is estimated to occur in 2% of the adult schizophrenia population; that number rises to 6% when patients with childhood-onset psychosis are considered, representing a 200-fold increased risk for the syndrome in these children (Bassett and Chow 1999; Sporn et al. 2004). The potential for this increased risk makes it essential to rule out the presence of a genetic syndrome or inborn error of metabolism in the diagnostic workup of selected psychiatric patients, because the presence of a disorder may affect long-term prognosis, direct treatment options, highlight the potential for associated medical conditions, increase eligibility for support services, or influence recurrence risks for other family members.

This chapter consists of an overview of genetic principles and selected genetic conditions that are transmitted in a Mendelian fashion and that should be considered in the differential diagnosis of patients with psychiatric and behavioral symptoms accompanied by associated medical conditions or with a personal or family history suggestive of such disorders.

Brief Overview of Mendelian Genetics

Humans are thought to have an estimated 25,000–30,000 genes, distributed unequally among 23 pairs of chromosomes. For each pair, one chromosome is normally inherited from each parent. Mendelian disorders have defined genetic etiologies (e.g., chromosomal abnormalities or single-gene mutations) that dictate mode of transmission in families and result in the patterns of inheritance described in the next section. The recognition that symptoms among family members appear to follow a classic pattern of inheritance may be the first suggestion of an underlying genetic syndrome or metabolic disorder in a patient. Visual depiction of a family history as a pedigree may aid pattern identification. Patterns of inheritance are determined by gene location, depending on whether the pattern is autosomal (chromosomes 1–22) or sex-linked (chromosome X or Y) and whether the gene is dominantly or recessively expressed. This chapter will first review selected genetics topics that may be applicable to a variety of conditions. More information on these subjects as well as information on a variety of genetic disorders can be found in the general genetics references provided (Cassidy and Allanson 2001; Estrov et al. 2000; Finn et al. 2003; Golomb 2002; Korf 2000; MacIntyre et al. 2003; Moldavsky et al. 2001; Nussbaum et al. 2004).

Patterns of Inheritance

Autosomal Recessive

An autosomal recessive pattern of inheritance is the mechanism of inheritance for the majority of metabolic syndromes. An autosomal recessive disorder will occur in an individual who inherits two nonfunctional copies of a gene (and is therefore said to be homozygous for a mutated allele). Individuals who have one functional allele and one nonfunctional allele are heterozygous at this location and are called carriers. Carriers of an autosomal recessive disorder are usually asymptomatic, although for some disorders, symptoms may also manifest in the carrier state. When two carriers reproduce, in each pregnancy there is a 25% chance for the offspring to inherit two gene mutations and be affected, a 50% chance of being a carrier, and a 25% chance of being neither affected nor a carrier. Both males and females have equal chances of being affected.

Most often, individuals with an autosomal recessive disorder have two unaffected carrier parents, although new mutations can occur during gametogenesis in a parent's egg or sperm. Increased carrier rates are reported for some disorders based on specific population features (e.g., increased rates of cystic fibrosis in Caucasians, increased risk of Tay-Sachs disease among

Ashkenazi Jews). Pedigrees of autosomal recessive disorders may show small numbers of affected individuals in the same generation among siblings and no affected individuals among more distantly related family members. Most often, individuals with autosomal recessive disorders have no previous family history of the disorder.

Autosomal Dominant

In a typical autosomal dominant disorder, each affected person will have one copy of a mutated allele, either from an affected parent or as the result of a new mutation. Unlike in autosomal recessive disorders, the presence of one functional copy of a gene cannot compensate for the malfunctioning copy in autosomal dominant disorders. Because of the rarity of these disorders in the general population, individuals with autosomal dominant disorders usually have unaffected partners. Therefore, the risk for each offspring of a parent affected with an autosomal dominant condition to inherit the disease-causing mutation is 50%. Again, males and females are equally likely to be affected and may transmit the disorder to offspring of either sex. Pedigrees of autosomal dominant conditions typically show multiple generations affected with the disorder.

In addition to single-gene disorders, several disorders known as microdeletion syndromes (e.g., velocardiofacial syndrome, Williams syndrome) are also transmitted in an autosomal dominant manner. Microdeletion syndromes are characterized by deletions ranging from hundreds to thousands of kilobases in length and result in an affected person having only one copy of multiple contiguous genes on the chromosome without the deletion. For some disorders, the deletion of a single gene in the chromosomal region may mediate at least some features of disease, while for others, the loss of multiple genes may be important in producing the disease state. These deletions can sometimes be seen on high- resolution karyotype analysis, or other techniques may be required that allow a closer examination of chromosomes (see section "Laboratory Work-Up for Genetic Syndromes and Inborn Errors of Metabolism" later in this chapter).

X-Linked

Genes that are found on the X chromosome are designated as X-linked. Females have two copies of the X chromosome (one copy of which is randomly turned off by the process of X inactivation). Males have one X chromosome and one Y chromosome and are designated as "hemizygous" for X-linked loci. X-linked disorders may be either recessive or dominant. X-linked recessive disorders are more common, are seen almost exclusively in males, and are inherited from an unaffected carrier mother approximately two-thirds of the time. Symptoms of variable severity are sometimes seen in carrier females because of unequal X inactivation. An X-linked recessive disorder is never passed from father to son. X-linked dominant disorders are seen in females heterozygous for the mutation and may be passed from mother to daughters and sons equally (similar to an autosomal dominant pedigree) and from fathers to all daughters and no sons. Many X-linked dominant disorders are lethal in males, which may obfuscate the inheritance pattern. Y-linked inheritance can also occur, and mutations are passed from affected fathers to all sons.

Mitochondrial Inheritance

In humans, a small number of genes are found on the mitochondrial chromosome, located in the cytoplasm of cells. Each mitochondrion has many copies of its own chromosome, and each cell has many mitochondria; the presence of symptoms related to mutations in mitochondrial DNA is thus largely dependent on the ratio of normal to mutated copies. Mitochondrial DNA is inherited from the mother, as it is present in the egg at conception, and all cells contain mitochondria derived from the original maternal mitochondria. For this reason, a mother may pass on mutations in mitochondrial DNA to both sons and daughters. An affected male, however, will not pass on mutations to any of his offspring. Women who pass on the mutated DNA may be asymptomatic themselves, again because of ratio of normal to abnormal mitochondrial DNA in each cell.

Additional Issues to Consider With Genetic Inheritance

Genetic inheritance may be complicated by several additional factors. Some disorders may exhibit decreased *penetrance,* meaning that the disorder may not show clinical symptoms in all individuals who carry the mutated gene(s). Penetrance is an all-or-none phenomenon in an individual (i.e., symptoms are either present or absent). In a population, however, symptoms of a disorder described as "80% penetrant" would be exhibited by 80% of individuals with the gene mutation. Penetrance may also be affected by age (e.g., Alzheimer's dementia) or be sex-limited, which may complicate determination of the inheritance pattern in a family. Expressivity, or how genes manifest themselves in affected individuals, may also be variable from person to person, differing in severity or in the specific symptoms associated with the genetic defects. For example, individuals with Marfan syndrome may have involvement of the skeletal and cardiovascular systems, as well as eye findings. However, one person with the syndrome may be tall, with minimal aortic involvement and a dislocated lens of the eye, and a second person could present with an aortic dissection and a history of joint instability. Overall, each person may show all symptoms of a disorder or a selected few.

Additional genetic mechanisms may produce atypical patterns of inheritance, including imprinting. *Imprinting* is a process where genes are turned off and on based on the parent of origin of the chromosome where the gene is located. Imprinting is a reversible form of gene inactivation, does not affect the sequence of underlying DNA, and takes place in the germline during gametogenesis prior to fertilization. Imprinted genes are not expressed. For imprinted genes, the development of a medical disorder depends on the parent of origin of a genetic mutation in the imprinted region. Imprinting plays a role in the development of several genetic disorders, including Prader-Willi syndrome (see Table 8–1).

Another mechanism that influences genetic inheritance is that of *anticipation,* which is the phenomenon of earlier onset of illness, or more severe illness, occurring in successive generations. Anticipation occurs with triplet repeat disorders, such as Huntington's disease, in which stretches of repetitive DNA may undergo expansion when being passed from parent to child. For some disorders (e.g., Huntington's disease), greatest expansion may occur when the mutation is passed from father to child, although for others (e.g., fragile X syndrome), maternal origin of mutation leads to risk of expansion to a disease-causing length.

Clues to the Presence of Genetic Syndromes and Inborn Errors of Metabolism

Ruling out the contribution of an underlying organic etiology to observed psychiatric symptoms is part of the general assessment of all psychiatric patients and may routinely include checking thyroid function studies in a patient with depression or screening for drugs of abuse in a patient with new-onset psychosis. For a subset of patients, however, inclusion of an expanded set of conditions may be indicated when formulating a differential diagnosis. A psychiatrist would not be expected to be able to diagnose all the genetic and metabolic syndromes reviewed in this chapter (Tables 8–1 and 8–2) but hopefully will begin to develop a sense of which psychiatric patients would benefit from referral to genetics colleagues for additional assessment regarding the etiology of their psychiatric symptoms. Suspicion regarding the likelihood of a genetic or metabolic syndrome may be derived from a review of the medical or family history, physical examination, or routine laboratory studies.

TABLE 8–1. Selected genetic syndromes with psychiatric and behavioral symptoms

Syndrome and incidence	Etiology	Inheritance	Diagnostic clues and other behavioral symptoms	Psychosis	Mood symptoms	Obsessions/compulsions	ADHD	Delirium	PDD spectrum	Dementia	References
Fragile X syndrome 1 in 4,000 (males)	Dysfunction of *FMR1* at Xq27.3	XL	Males: large testes, connective tissue disease (loose joints), low muscle tone, and characteristic facial appearance (large head with prominent forehead and jaw, long face with large ears) Mental retardation in the moderate to severe range Carrier females with full mutation may be symptomatic Oppositional defiant disorder, avoidant personality disorder and traits Premutation female carriers may show increased rates of depression and social phobia		●		●		●		Backes et al. 2000; Franke et al. 1996, 1998; Goldson and Hagerman 1992; Hagerman et al. 2004; Hundscheid et al. 2003; Jacquemont et al. 2003, 2004

TABLE 8–1. Selected genetic syndromes with psychiatric and behavioral symptoms *(continued)*

Syndrome and incidence	Etiology	Inheritance	Diagnostic clues and other behavioral symptoms	Psychosis	Mood symptoms	Obsessions/ compulsions	ADHD	Delirium	PDD spectrum	Dementia	References
Huntington's disease 1 in 20,000	Mutation in *HD* on 4p16	AD	Dysarthria, clumsiness, chorea Characteristic atrophy of the caudate and putamen may be apparent on magnetic resonance imaging or computed tomography scan of the brain Changes in personality, apathy	•	•					•	Kirkwood et al. 2001, 2002; Paulsen et al. 2001
Inv dup(15) 1 in 4,000 risk of marker, 50% of those with marker have inv dup(15)	Marker chromosome or other cytogenetic arrangement, often involving 15q11–q14	—[a]	Seizures (especially infantile spasms and hypsarrythmia) ataxia, hypotonia, genitourinary malformations Mental retardation and developmental delay of variable severity Symptoms of Prader-Willi and Angelman's syndromes possible depending on size of involved region and parent of origin						•		Battaglia 2005; Borgatti et al. 2001

TABLE 8–1. Selected genetic syndromes with psychiatric and behavioral symptoms *(continued)*

Syndrome and incidence	Etiology	Inheritance	Diagnostic clues and other behavioral symptoms	Psychosis	Mood symptoms	Obsessions/compulsions	ADHD	Delirium	PDD spectrum	Dementia	References
Klinefelter's syndrome 1 in 600 (boys)	47, XXY (addition of one X chromosome)		Males, typically tall, may have small penis and testes, gynecomastia, low testosterone level and associated physical findings IQ usually normal, some learning disabilities Social immaturity		•		•		•		Boone et al. 2001; Cassidy et al. 2001; Mandoki et al. 1991
Neurofibromatosis 1 in 3000	Mutation in *NF1* on 17q11	AD	Skin findings of café au lait macules, axillary/inguinal freckling, neurofibromas, Lisch nodules on iris, osseous lesions, optic glioma Learning disabilities				•		•		Kayl and Moore 2000

TABLE 8–1. Selected genetic syndromes with psychiatric and behavioral symptoms *(continued)*

Syndrome and incidence	Etiology	Inheritance	Diagnostic clues and other behavioral symptoms	Psychosis	Mood symptoms	Obsessions/ compulsions	ADHD	Delirium	PDD spectrum	Dementia	References
Prader-Willi syndrome 1 in 10,000–22,000	Most due to deletion at 15q11–q13	—[a]	Obesity, short stature, small hands and feet, small external genitalia, fair skin and hair coloring, characteristic facial appearance Decreased IQ and specific learning problems, although areas of strength (visual-spatial) Hyperphagia, skin picking, and temper tantrums	•	•	•	•		•		Boer et al. 2002; Clarke et al. 2002; Descheemaeker et al. 2002; Dykens and Shah 2003; Dykens et al. 1992, 1996; State and Dykens 2000
Rett syndrome 1 in 10,000–20,000 (girls)	Mutations in *MECP2* at Xq28		Initially normal with progressive loss of developmental skills associated with acquired microcephaly, loss of purposeful hand movements, gait abnormalities, seizures, and bruxism						•		Amir and Zoghbi 2000; Clayton-Smith et al. 2000

TABLE 8–1. Selected genetic syndromes with psychiatric and behavioral symptoms *(continued)*

Syndrome and incidence	Etiology	Inheritance	Diagnostic clues and other behavioral symptoms	Psychosis	Mood symptoms	Obsessions/ compulsions	ADHD	Delirium	PDD spectrum	Dementia	References
Smith-Magenis syndrome 1 in 25,000	Microdeletion at 17p11.2 Mutations in *RAI1* also implicated	AD	Prominent sleep disturbances, abnormal lipid profiles, characteristic facial appearance, "self hug" when happy. IQ range borderline intelligence to moderate mental retardation. Tantrums, impulsivity self-injurious behaviors (onychotillomania, polyembolokoilamania, skin picking)		•		•				Bi et al. 2004; Finucane et al. 1994; Shelley and Robertson 2005; Smith et al. 1998a, 1998b
Tuberous sclerosis 1 in 6,000	Mutations in *TSC1* on 9q23 or *TSC2* on 16p13.3	AD	Seizures, skin findings (ash leaf spots, shagreen patches, angiofibromas), dental pits, tumors in multiple organ systems (central nervous system tubers, retinal hamartomas, cardiac rhabdomyomas, and renal angiomyolipomas)				•		•		Hunt and Dennis 1987

TABLE 8–1. Selected genetic syndromes with psychiatric and behavioral symptoms *(continued)*

Syndrome and incidence	Etiology	Inheritance	Diagnostic clues and other behavioral symptoms	Psychosis	Mood symptoms	Obsessions/ compulsions	ADHD	Delirium	PDD spectrum	Dementia	References
Turner's syndrome 1 in 3,000 (girls)	45, X (absence of one X chromosome)		Females, with physical characteristics of short stature, webbed neck, and a flat, broad chest; failure to achieve secondary sexual development; infertility IQ usually normal, some learning disabilities Anxiety, problems with social skills		•		•				Lesniak-Karpiak et al. 2003; Ross et al. 2000
Velocardiofacial syndrome 1 in 2,500	Microdeletion at 22q11	AD	Cleft palate, congenital heart defect, immune problems, low calcium levels, characteristic appearance Learning disabilities (nonverbal learning disorders) Oppositional defiant disorder	•	•	•	•		•		Bassett and Chow 1999; Bassett et al. 1998; Gothelf et al. 2004; Karayiorgou et al. 1995; McDonald-McGinn et al. 1997; Papolos et al. 1996; Pulver et al. 1994; Sporn et al. 2004; Usiskin et al. 1999

TABLE 8–1. Selected genetic syndromes with psychiatric and behavioral symptoms *(continued)*

Syndrome and incidence	Etiology	Inheritance	Diagnostic clues and other behavioral symptoms	Psychosis	Mood symptoms	Obsessions/ compulsions	ADHD	Delirium	PDD spectrum	Dementia	References
Williams syndrome 1 in 7,500	Microdeletion at 7q11.23	AD	Congenital heart defect (supravalvular aortic or pulmonic stenosis), short stature, microcephaly, "elfin" facial appearance IQ range mild to severe mental retardation Anxiety, circumscribed interests, may be somatically focused, socially disinhibited and overly friendly		●	●	●		●		Davies et al. 1998; Gosch and Pankau 1997

Note. AD=autosomal dominant; ADHD=attention-deficit/hyperactivity disorder; PDD=pervasive developmental disorder; XL=X-linked.
[a]Inheritance may vary depending on underlying genetic etiology.

TABLE 8–2. Selected inborn errors of metabolism with psychiatric and behavioral symptoms

Syndrome and incidence	Etiology	Inheritance	Diagnostic clues	Psychosis	Mood symptoms	Obsessions/ compulsions	ADHD	Delirium	PDD spectrum	Dementia	References
Acute intermittent porphyria 1 in 10,000–50,000	Mutations in *HMBS* on 11q23.3	AD	Acute "neurovisceral attacks" (recurrent abdominal pain, vomiting, generalized body pain, weakness) Anxiety, "histrionic" personality Episodic nature of symptoms Psychiatric medications which upregulate P450 system may exacerbate symptoms	●	●			●			Crimlisk 1997; Santosh and Malhotra 1994; Tishler et al. 1985
Adrenoleuko-dystrophy, X-linked 1 in 20,000–50,000	Mutations in *ABCD1* on Xq28	XL	In males, early difficulty with gait, handwriting, or speech; progressive loss of motor skills, vision, and hearing; elevation of ACTH, and other findings associated with adrenal dysfunction Female carriers may also be symptomatic	●	●		●			●	Cohen-Cole and Kitchin 1985; Garside et al. 1999; Kitchin et al. 1987; Rosebush et al. 1999

TABLE 8–2. Selected inborn errors of metabolism with psychiatric and behavioral symptoms *(continued)*

Syndrome and incidence	Etiology	Inheritance	Diagnostic clues	Psychosis	Mood symptoms	Obsessions/ compulsions	ADHD	Delirium	PDD spectrum	Dementia	References
Homocystinuria 1 in 200,000–350,000	Mutations in *CBS* on 21q22.3	AR	"Marfanoid" body habitus, connective tissue disease (pectus excavatum, lens dislocation, scoliosis, high-arched palate), restricted joint mobility, thrombotic events		●	●					Abbott et al. 1987; Bracken and Coll 1985; Levine et al. 2002; Picker and Coyle 2005
Lesch-Nyhan syndrome 1 in 200,000	Mutations in *HPRT1* on Xq26–27.2	XL	Mental retardation, spastic cerebral palsy, choreo-athetosis, uric acid urinary stones Self-injurious and self-mutilatory behaviors (head banging, biting lips and fingers), aggression								Schretlen et al. 2005

TABLE 8–2. Selected inborn errors of metabolism with psychiatric and behavioral symptoms *(continued)*

Syndrome and incidence	Etiology	Inheritance	Diagnostic clues	Psychosis	Mood symptoms	Obsessions/ compulsions	ADHD	Delirium	PDD spectrum	Dementia	References
Metachromatic leukodystrophy 1 in 40,000	Mutations in *ARSA* on 22q13.31	AR	Ataxia and walking difficulties, dysarthria, dysphagia, pyramidal signs, vision loss Magnetic resonance imaging of the brain may show periventricular changes with progression to white matter atrophy due to loss of myelin Personality changes Late-onset forms	•						•	Finelli 1985; Hyde et al. 1992; Waltz et al. 1987
Mitochondrial disease Unknown incidence	Various	—[a]	Multiple medical problems, often affecting different organ systems, especially those with high energy demands (i.e., brain, cardiac and skeletal muscle)	•	•		•	•	•	•	Spellberg et al. 2001

TABLE 8–2. Selected inborn errors of metabolism with psychiatric and behavioral symptoms *(continued)*

Syndrome and incidence	Etiology	Inheritance	Diagnostic clues	Psychosis	Mood symptoms	Obsessions/ compulsions	ADHD	Delirium	PDD spectrum	Dementia	References
Niemann-Pick disease, type C 1 in 150,000	Mutations in *NPC1* on 18q11–q12	AR	Ataxia, coordination problems, dysarthria; Vertical supranuclear palsy is the hallmark of the disorder; Seizures and hepatosplenomegaly may be present	•						•	Campo et al. 1998; Turpin et al. 1991
Ornithine trans-carbamylase (OTC) deficiency (carriers)	Mutations in *OTC* on Xp21.1	XL	Males: usual presentations of neonatal hyperammonemia Female carriers: symptoms may range from none to mild to severe intermittent hyper-ammonemia, depending on random X inactivation and protein load Episodic nature of symptoms may be seen in association with high protein load (from food intake or endogenous breakdown with illness and fasting)					•			Largilliere 1995; Legras et al. 2002

TABLE 8–2. Selected inborn errors of metabolism with psychiatric and behavioral symptoms *(continued)*

Syndrome and incidence	Etiology	Inheritance	Diagnostic clues	Psychosis	Mood symptoms	Obsessions/ compulsions	ADHD	Delirium	PDD spectrum	Dementia	References
Tay-Sachs disease (late onset) Rare	Mutations in *HEXA* on 15q23–q24	AR	Ataxia, coordination problems, dysarthria, dystonia, spasticity, and seizures Macular cherry red spots, the hallmark of the early-onset form, are not present in the later-onset form Catatonia	•	•						• MacQueen et al. 1998; Navon et al. 1986; Rosebush et al. 1995; Streifler et al. 1989

TABLE 8–2. Selected inborn errors of metabolism with psychiatric and behavioral symptoms *(continued)*

Syndrome and incidence	Etiology	Inheritance	Diagnostic clues	Psychosis	Mood symptoms	Obsessions/ compulsions	ADHD	Delirium	PDD spectrum	Dementia	References
Wilson's disease 1 in 30,000	Mutations in *ATP7B* on 13q14–21	AR	Signs and symptoms of liver dysfunction with abnormal liver function tests, tremor, dysarthria, muscular rigidity, parkinsonism, dyskinesia, dystonia, chorea, Kayser-Fleischer rings; copper deposits may be seen with magnetic resonance imaging of the brain or in the liver via a liver biopsy. Personality changes, pseudo-bulbar palsy, cognitive decline	•	•					•	Akil and Brewer 1995; Dening and Berrios 1989, 1990

Note. ACTH=adrenocorticotropic hormone; AD=autosomal dominant; ADHD=attention-deficit/hyperactivity disorder; AR=autosomal recessive; PDD=pervasive developmental disorder; XL=X-linked.
[a]Inheritance may vary depending on underlying genetic etiology.

Medical History and Review of Systems

A comprehensive review of the medical history begins with questions regarding the prenatal period. Many genetic and metabolic syndromes may be associated with abnormalities seen on ultrasound or may affect maternal health during pregnancy. Asking about a history of medical issues or surgeries in the newborn period or whether neonatal intensive care was required may uncover a resolved (and sometimes forgotten) medical problem such as a congenital heart defect that has undergone surgical repair. Specific inquiry regarding birth defects or other congenital anomalies may provide important information to guide additional genetic evaluation. Obtaining a history of exposure to medications, drugs, alcohol, toxins, or radiation may reveal a teratogenic origin of related medical and behavioral symptoms, as is seen in fetal alcohol syndrome.

Developmental history is also an important area of investigation when thinking about genetic and metabolic syndromes, because developmental delays or cognitive deficits are frequently associated with these conditions but are not typical for the average psychiatric patient. Questions regarding a history of verbal or motor delays, the need for treatment of developmental deficits (physical, occupational, or speech therapy) as part of early intervention or school programs, and a history of special education classes or other academic supports should be explored. Uncovering a history of developmental regression or decline in school performance may be especially important for metabolic disorders of later onset that involve accumulation of toxic by-products in the brain (e.g., lysosomal storage disorders).

Additional questions should be included with the standard medical review of systems to alert the clinician to the need to consider the presence of an underlying inborn error of metabolism. These questions include inquiry about a history of poor feeding and growth, history of food intolerance or unusual food preferences, history of decompensation with viral illness, or the presence of neurological symptoms, including those that occur on an episodic basis.

Family History

When the clinician is taking a family history, it is often helpful to gather information on a person-by-person basis and to visually depict the gathered history in the form of a pedigree to help with recognition of patterns of inheritance (Bennett et al. 1995). It is important to include historical information on both sides of the family and, when possible, to review both psychiatric and medical history for all first- and second-degree family members. Information regarding unexplained infertility, frequent miscarriages, stillbirths, infant or childhood deaths, or children requiring surgery at a young age should also be included, as they may represent individuals with medical conditions or anomalies that require further investigation. Specific inquiries regarding comorbid neurological symptoms may also be helpful. In addition, questions regarding ethnicity and race and the presence of consanguinity may help to pinpoint increased risks for certain genetic and metabolic syndromes that occur at increased rates in selected populations. Asking a general question such as, "Is there anyone in the family with special needs?" may also elicit important history regarding associated medical and developmental conditions.

Physical Examination Findings

It is likely that most psychiatrists do not frequently complete physical examinations of patients in their outpatient practices, but they may do so on the inpatient setting or as part of an emergency department or consultation-liaison psychiatric evaluation. However, careful notice of facial features, with attention to dysmorphic or asymmetric features, is easily accomplished in all settings. Persons with certain genetic and metabolic disorders have characteristic facial appearances, so attention to dysmorphic craniofacial findings may prove critical. Reviewing records from the patient's primary care physician or neurologist may supplement information that can be obtained by direct observation.

Results of Routine Laboratory Studies

The results of routine laboratory studies obtained for psychiatric patients will rarely confirm the presence of an underlying genetic or metabolic syndrome, but the findings may help guide additional laboratory workup of patients. Certain genetic syndromes may have associated abnormalities (e.g., low calcium levels in velocardiofacial syndrome), which are reviewed in the next section. Metabolic derangements such as acidosis, an elevated anion gap, abnormal liver function tests, and elevated ammonia, lactate, or pyruvate levels may all be associated with a variety of metabolic syndromes. Table 8–3 reviews laboratory findings associated with selected metabolic conditions.

Laboratory Workup for Genetic Syndromes and Inborn Errors of Metabolism

Once suspicion has been raised regarding the possibility of an underlying genetic or metabolic condition, patients should be referred to a genetics or metabolic specialist for further evaluation. These clinicians are likely to be

TABLE 8–3. Laboratory findings and associated metabolic conditions

Laboratory abnormality	Associated disorders
Acidosis/abnormal anion gap	Associated with many metabolic disorders; use blood gas results and electrolyte panel results to determine
Liver dysfunction (⇑ transaminases)	Storage disorders with deposition of abnormal substances in liver
Ammonia ⇑	Primary elevation in urea cycle disorders
	Secondary elevation in organic acidemias, disorders of fatty acid oxidation
Lactate ⇑	Disorders of energy metabolism
Pyruvate ⇑	Disorders of energy metabolism
Amino acids (abnormal pattern in plasma or cerebrospinal fluid)	Amino acid disorders (e.g., urea cycle defects, homocystinuria)
Organic acids (abnormal pattern in urine)	Organic acidemias, fatty acid oxidation disorders
Acylcarnitine profile (abnormal pattern)	Disorders of fatty acid oxidation, organic acidemias
Very long chain fatty acids ⇑	Peroxisomal disorders
Urine mucopolysaccharides or urine oligosaccharides ⇑	Lysosomal storage disorders

aware of available testing options for genetic and metabolic conditions and are able to proceed in a stepwise fashion to evaluate psychiatric patients. A variety of testing methods are reviewed here to inform the psychiatric clinician about a few common options for genetic testing. Generally, it may be less helpful for psychiatrists to attempt to direct this workup on their own, as the interpretation of test results for genetic and metabolic conditions can be challenging. Furthermore, a negative test result does not rule out the presence of all genetic conditions, and genetics colleagues may also consider other genetic syndromes that are beyond the scope of knowledge of most psychiatrists.

Testing for Structural Abnormalities of Chromosomes

Most physicians are likely familiar with a karyotype analysis of chromosomes. A karyotype is a microscopic view of the total number of chromosomes, usually from the metaphase stage of mitosis, when each chromosome is condensed and has duplicated itself, as seen by pairs of sister chromatids that consist of the shorter "p" arms and longer "q" arms joined at the constricted area known as the centromere. Chromosomes are organized in homologous pairs, from larger to smaller, except for the sex chromosomes, X and Y, which are depicted last (and chromosome 21, which is actually smaller than chromosome 22). A normal human female karyotype is designated as 46, XX, indicating a total of 46 chromosomes including two X chromosomes, and a normal male karyotype is designated as 46, XY (Figure 8–1). A variety of staining techniques is available to visualize chromosomal bands and to look for the addition or loss of entire chromosomes, smaller areas of deletions, duplications, or translocations (i.e., the transfer of material between or among chromosomes).

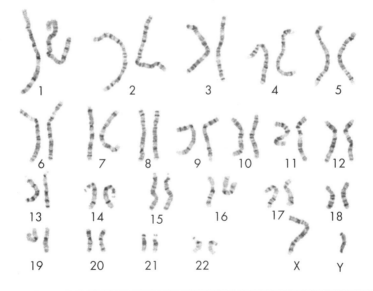

FIGURE 8–1. Normal human male karyotype 46, XY.
Source. Provided by Azra H. Ligon, Ph.D and Joana Carvalho Da Costa, Cytogenetics Laboratory, Brigham and Women's Hospital, Boston, MA. Used with permission.

Karyotype analysis is limited by the degree of resolution of the chromosomes and cannot be used to detect smaller structural abnormalities, including microdeletion syndromes, which are often evaluated by a technique called *fluorescence in situ hybridization* (FISH). This technique involves the denaturation of DNA on slides (i.e., "in situ"), thus exposing the DNA strands and allowing binding of sequence-specific fluorescent probes to regions of interest. When the slides are viewed under fluorescent light, a probe signal indicates the presence of the chromosomal area of interest (Figure 8–2). Fluorescence in situ hybridization may be used to look at a single location on a chromosome (e.g., to investigate a specific microdeletion syndrome) or may be employed as a panel of probes to look at multiple regions in a sample, as when the subtelomeric regions of chromosomes (areas prone to deletion and associated with mental retardation) are examined (Knight et al. 1999; Sogaard et al. 2005; Walter et al. 2004).

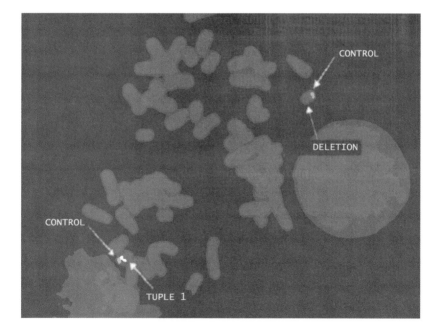

FIGURE 8–2. Fluorescence in situ hybridization (FISH) showing deletion at 22q11.2 using TUPLE 1 probe.

A related technology currently being quickly adopted for the clinical evaluation of patients is *comparative genomic hybridization,* which allows the simultaneous comparison of submicroscopic regions of chromosomes between a patient and a reference sample to investigate various loci throughout the genome (Figure 8–3). Comparative genomic hybridization has the advantage of allowing analysis of selected loci across the entire genome in a single experiment. Each sample is painted with a different color probe, and after the samples are combined, ratios of the two colors are analyzed to determine relative gains (amplification or duplications) or losses (deletions) in DNA. Depending on how the test is designed, probes may be specific for known genetic disorders or may be chosen to provide spaced coverage across the genome. Regions identified as abnormal may require further investigation or confirmation by other techniques. If a specific disorder is suspected that involves a single gene, a variety of techniques are available to look at genetic changes.

Selected Genetic Syndromes With Psychiatric and Behavioral Symptoms

Genetic syndromes are combinations of medical findings that occur together in organized patterns and are secondary to a single underlying etiology. Many genetic syndromes may have psychiatric or behavioral symptoms as part of their presentation. In fact, these symptoms may sometimes help to identify an underlying syndrome, as they may be quite characteristic of it. A short description of selected genetic syndromes and a listing of associated medical and psychiatric symptoms are summarized in Table 8–1. For the interested clinician, two clinical genetics resources that may be helpful are GeneTests, sponsored by the University of Washington (http://www.geneclinics.org) and the Online Mendelian Inheritance in Man (OMIM) website, accessed through the National Center for Biotechnology Information (http://www.ncbi.nlm.nih.gov/). Additional information on genetic conditions, as well as photographs of facial features, can also often be found on disorder-specific websites.

Selected Inborn Errors of Metabolism With Psychiatric and Behavioral Symptoms

Metabolic disorders result from deficiencies of enzymes or their cofactors, and symptoms may be secondary to problems with biosynthesis, transport, or degradation of metabolic pathway by-products. Many metabolic disor-

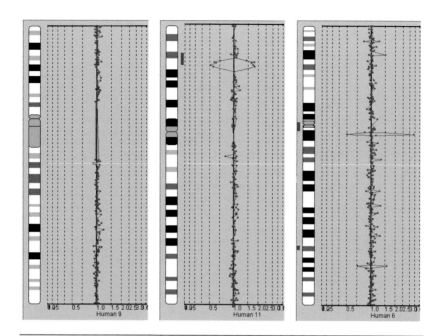

FIGURE 8–3. Comparative genomic hybridization micro-array analysis of chromosome regions.

The middle panel shows a comparative genomic hybridization analysis for a patient with an interstitial chromosome 11 duplication. The left panel shows a chromosome 9–specific profile from the same patient showing normal results. The right panel shows a chromosome 6–specific profile in which copy number variations are present.

Source. Provided by Charles Lee, Ph.D., F.A.C.M.G. Used with permission.

ders affect the brain and have associated psychiatric symptoms. Clues to the presence of an underlying inborn error of metabolism may come from review of the medical or family history and physical examination findings, as well as the results of common and specialized laboratory testing. Some metabolic disorders are tested for by state newborn screening programs, but these programs vary greatly from state to state and change over time. In addition to websites listed in the previous section, an excellent resource for information about metabolic disorders is Metabolic and Molecular Bases of Inherited Disease Online (OMMBID; http://genetics. accessmedicine. com). Selected inborn errors of metabolism and their psychiatric and behavioral findings are presented in Table 8–2.

Conclusions

For most individuals, the occurrence of a psychiatric disorder is secondary to a complex interplay of genetic and environmental factors that are as yet undefined. However, for a subset of patients with psychiatric and behavioral symptoms, accompanying physical and historical features may hint at the presence of a specific genetic or metabolic syndrome that is inherited in a Mendelian manner. On an individual basis, a parsimonious explanation for psychiatric and medical symptoms in the form of a genetic syndrome can be of great benefit to the affected patient and the patient's family members, as it may direct medical management, affect pharmacological or other treatment options, and identify other family members who may be at risk for developing the disorder. A healthy suspicion of alternative explanations for psychiatric symptoms and a willingness to refer to genetics colleagues can improve the clinical care of patients. In addition, the psychiatric research community can benefit from the progress already made in understanding these disorders with more simple patterns of inheritance. Uncovering the genetic basis for psychiatric symptoms in disorders with defined genetic etiologies may provide insight into the cause of psychiatric disorders in the general population and serve to inform further research studies. Continued interest in Mendelian disorders is essential to increased understanding of psychiatric and behavioral symptoms.

References

Abbott MH, Folstein SE, Abbey H, et al: Psychiatric manifestations of homocystinuria due to cystathionine beta-synthase deficiency: prevalence, natural history, and relationship to neurologic impairment and vitamin B6-responsiveness. Am J Med Genet 26:959–969, 1987

Akil M, Brewer GJ: Psychiatric and behavioral abnormalities in Wilson's disease. Adv Neurol 65:171–178, 1995

Amir RE, Zoghbi HY: Rett syndrome: methyl-CpG-binding protein 2 mutations and phenotype-genotype correlations. Am J Med Genet 97:147–152, 2000

Backes M, Genc B, Schreck J, et al: Cognitive and behavioral profile of fragile X boys: correlations to molecular data. Am J Med Genet 95:150–156, 2000

Bassett AS, Chow EW: 22q11 deletion syndrome: a genetic subtype of schizophrenia. Biol Psychiatry 46: 882–891, 1999

Bassett AS, Hodgkinson K, Chow EW, et al: 22q11 deletion syndrome in adults with schizophrenia. Am J Med Genet 81:328–337, 1998

Battaglia A: The inv dup(15) or idic(15) syndrome: a clinically recognisable neurogenetic disorder. Brain Dev 27:365–369, 2005

Bennett RL, Steinhaus KA, Uhrich SB, et al: Recommendations for standardized human pedigree nomenclature. Pedigree Standardization Task Force of the National Society of Genetic Counselors. Am J Hum Genet 56:745–752, 1995

Bi W, Saifi GM, Shaw CJ, et al: Mutations of RAI1, a PHD-containing protein, in nondeletion patients with Smith-Magenis syndrome. Hum Genet 115:515–524, 2004

Boer H, Holland A, Whittington J, et al: Psychotic illness in people with Prader Willi syndrome due to chromosome 15 maternal uniparental disomy. Lancet 359:135–136, 2002

Boone KB, Swerdloff RS, Miller BL, et al: Neuropsychological profiles of adults with Klinefelter syndrome. J Int Neuropsychol Soc 7:446–456, 2001

Borgatti R, Piccinelli P, Passoni D, et al: Relationship between clinical and genetic features in "inverted duplicated chromosome 15" patients. Pediatr Neurol 24: 111–116, 2001

Bracken P, Coll P: Homocystinuria and schizophrenia: literature review and case report. J Nerv Ment Dis 173:51–55, 1985

Campo JV, Stowe R, Slomka G, et al: Psychosis as a presentation of physical disease in adolescence: a case of Niemann-Pick disease, type C. Dev Med Child Neurol 40:126–129, 1998

Cassidy SB, Allanson JE: Management of Genetic Syndromes. New York, Wiley-Liss, 2001

Clarke DJ, Boer H, Whittington J, et al: Prader-Willi syndrome, compulsive and ritualistic behaviours: the first population-based survey. Br J Psychiatry 180:358–362, 2002

Clayton-Smith J, Watson P, Ramsden S, et al: Somatic mutation in MECP2 as a non-fatal neurodevelopmental disorder in males. Lancet 356: 830–832, 2000

Cohen-Cole S, Kitchin W: Adrenoleukodystrophy and psychiatric disorder. Am J Psychiatry 142:1224–1225, 1985

Crimlisk HL: The little imitator—porphyria: a neuropsychiatric disorder. J Neurol Neurosurg Psychiatry 62:319–328, 1997

Davies M, Udwin O, Howlin P: Adults with Williams syndrome: preliminary study of social, emotional and behavioural difficulties. Br J Psychiatry 172:273–276, 1998

Dening TR, Berrios GE: Wilson's disease: psychiatric symptoms in 195 cases. Arch Gen Psychiatry 46:1126–1134, 1989

Dening TR, Berrios GE: Wilson's disease: a longitudinal study of psychiatric symptoms. Biol Psychiatry 28:255–265, 1990

Descheemaeker MJ, Vogels A, Govers V, et al: Prader-Willi syndrome: new insights in the behavioural and psychiatric spectrum. J Intellect Disabil Res 46:41–50, 2002

Dykens E, Shah B: Psychiatric disorders in Prader-Willi syndrome: epidemiology and management. CNS Drugs 17:167–178, 2003

Dykens EM, Hodapp RM, Walsh K, et al: Adaptive and maladaptive behavior in Prader-Willi syndrome. J Am Acad Child Adolesc Psychiatry 31:1131–1136, 1992

Dykens EM, Leckman JF, Cassidy SB: Obsessions and compulsions in Prader-Willi syndrome. J Child Psychol Psychiatry 37:995–1002, 1996

Estrov Y, Scaglia F, Bodamer OA: Psychiatric symptoms of inherited metabolic disease. J Inherit Metab Dis 23:2–6, 2000

Finelli PF: Metachromatic leukodystrophy manifesting as a schizophrenic disorder: computed tomographic correlation. Ann Neurol 18:94–95, 1985

Finn CT, Stoler JM, Smoller JW: Genetics and genetic disorders, in Massachusetts General Hospital Handbook of General Hospital Psychiatry. Edited by Cassem NH, Stern TA, Rosenbaum JR, et al. St. Louis, MO, Mosby, 2003

Finucane BM, Konar D, Haas-Givler B, et al: The spasmodic upper-body squeeze: a characteristic behavior in Smith-Magenis syndrome. Dev Med Child Neurol 36:78–83, 1994

Franke P, Maier W, Hautzinger M, et al: Fragile-X carrier females: evidence for a distinct psychopathological phenotype? Am J Med Genet 64:334–339, 1996

Franke P, Leboyer M, Gansicke M, et al: Genotype-phenotype relationship in female carriers of the premutation and full mutation of FMR-1. Psychiatry Res 80:113–127, 1998

Garside S, Rosebush PI, Levinson AJ, et al: Late-onset adrenoleukodystrophy associated with long-standing psychiatric symptoms. J Clin Psychiatry 60:460–468, 1999

Goldson E, Hagerman RJ: The fragile X syndrome. Dev Med Child Neurol 34:826–832, 1992

Golomb M: Psychiatric symptoms in metabolic and other genetic disorders: is our "organic" workup complete? Harv Rev Psychiatry 10:242–248, 2002

Gosch A, Pankau R: Personality characteristics and behaviour problems in individuals of different ages with Williams syndrome. Dev Med Child Neurol 39:527–533, 1997

Gothelf D, Presburger G, Zohar AH, et al: Obsessive-compulsive disorder in patients with velocardiofacial (22q11 deletion) syndrome. Am J Med Genet B Neuropsychiatr Genet 126:99–105, 2004

Hagerman RJ, Leavitt BR, Farzin F, et al: Fragile-X-associated tremor/ataxia syndrome (FXTAS) in females with the FMR1 premutation. Am J Hum Genet 74:1051–1056, 2004

Hundscheid RD, Smits AP, Thomas CM, et al: Female carriers of fragile X premutations have no increased risk for additional diseases other than premature ovarian failure. Am J Med Genet A 117:6–9, 2003

Hunt A, Dennis J: Psychiatric disorder among children with tuberous sclerosis. Dev Med Child Neurol 29:190–198, 1987

Hyde TM, Ziegler JC, Weinberger DR: Psychiatric disturbances in metachromatic leukodystrophy: insights into the neurobiology of psychosis. Arch Neurol 49:401–406, 1992

Jacquemont S, Hagerman, RJ Leehey M, et al: Fragile X premutation tremor/ataxia syndrome: molecular, clinical, and neuroimaging correlates. Am J Hum Genet 72:869–878, 2003

Jacquemont S, Hagerman RJ, Leehey MA, et al: Penetrance of the fragile X-associated tremor/ataxia syndrome in a premutation carrier population. JAMA 291:460–469, 2004

Karayiorgou M, Morris MA, Morrow B, et al: Schizophrenia susceptibility associated with interstitial deletions of chromosome 22q11. Proc Natl Acad Sci U S A 92:7612–7616, 1995

Kayl AK, Moore BD: Behavioral phenotypes of neurofibromatosis, type 1. Ment Retard Dev Disabil Res Rev 6:117–124, 2000

Kirkwood SC, Su JL, Conneally P, et al: Progression of symptoms in the early and middle stages of Huntington disease. Arch Neurol 58:273–278, 2001

Kirkwood SC, Siemers E, Viken R, et al: Longitudinal personality changes among presymptomatic Huntington disease gene carriers. Neuropsychiatry Neuropsychol Behav Neurol 15:192–197, 2002

Kitchin W, Cohen-Cole SA, Mickel SF: Adrenoleukodystrophy: frequency of presentation as a psychiatric disorder. Biol Psychiatry 22:1375–1387, 1987

Knight SJ, Regan R, Nicod A, et al: Subtle chromosomal rearrangements in children with unexplained mental retardation. Lancet 354:1676–1681, 1999

Korf BR: Human Genetics: A Problem-Based Approach. Malden, MA, Blackwell Science, 2000

Largilliere C: Psychiatric manifestations in a girl with ornithine transcarbamylase deficiency. Lancet 345(8957):1113, 1995

Legras A, Labarthe F, Maillot F, et al: Late diagnosis of ornithine transcarbamylase defect in three related female patients: polymorphic presentations. Crit Care Med 30:214–244, 2002

Lesniak-Karpiak K, Mazzocco MM, Ross JL: Behavioral assessment of social anxiety in females with Turner or fragile X syndrome. J Autism Dev Disord 33:55–67, 2003

Levine J, Stahl Z, Sela BA, et al: Elevated homocysteine levels in young male patients with schizophrenia. Am J Psychiatry 159:1790–1792, 2002

MacIntyre DJ, Blackwood DH, Porteous DJ, et al: Chromosomal abnormalities and mental illness. Mol Psychiatry 8:275–287, 2003

MacQueen GM, Rosebush PI, Mazurek MF: Neuropsychiatric aspects of the adult variant of Tay-Sachs disease. J Neuropsychiatry Clin Neurosci 10:10–19, 1998

Mandoki MW, Sumner GS, Hoffman RP, et al: A review of Klinefelter's syndrome in children and adolescents. J Am Acad Child Adolesc Psychiatry 30:167–172, 1991

McDonald-McGinn DM, LaRossa D, Goldmuntz E, et al: The 22q11.2 deletion: screening, diagnostic workup, and outcome of results; report on 181 patients. Genet Test 1:99–108, 1997

Moldavsky M, Lev D, Lerman-Sagie T: Behavioral phenotypes of genetic syndromes: a reference guide for psychiatrists. J Am Acad Child Adolesc Psychiatry 40:749–761, 2001

Navon R, Argov Z, Frisch A: Hexosaminidase A deficiency in adults. Am J Med Genet 24:179–196, 1986

Nussbaum RL, McInnes RR, Willard HF, et al: Thompson and Thompson Genetics in Medicine. Philadelphia, PA, WB Saunders, 2004

Papolos DF, Faedda GL, Veit S, et al: Bipolar spectrum disorders in patients diagnosed with velo-cardio-facial syndrome: does a hemizygous deletion of chromosome 22q11 result in bipolar affective disorder? Am J Psychiatry 153:1541–1547, 1996

Paulsen JS, Ready RE, Hamilton JM, et al: Neuropsychiatric aspects of Huntington's disease. J Neurol Neurosurg Psychiatry 71:310–314, 2001

Picker JD, Coyle JT: Do maternal folate and homocysteine levels play a role in neurodevelopmental processes that increase risk for schizophrenia? Harv Rev Psychiatry 13:197–205, 2005

Pulver AE, Nestadt G, Goldberg R, et al: Psychotic illness in patients diagnosed with velo-cardio-facial syndrome and their relatives. J Nerv Ment Dis 182:476–478, 1994

Rosebush PI, MacQueen GM, Clarke JT, et al: Late-onset Tay-Sachs disease presenting as catatonic schizophrenia: diagnostic and treatment issues. J Clin Psychiatry 56:347–353, 1995

Rosebush PI, Garside S, Levinson AJ, et al: The neuropsychiatry of adult-onset adrenoleukodystrophy. J Neuropsychiatry Clin Neurosci 11:315–327, 1999

Ross J, Zinn A, McCauley E: Neurodevelopmental and psychosocial aspects of Turner syndrome. Ment Retard Dev Disabil Res Rev 6:135–141, 2000

Santosh PJ, Malhotra S: Varied psychiatric manifestations of acute intermittent porphyria. Biol Psychiatry 36:744–747, 1994

Schretlen DJ, Ward J, Meyer SM, et al: Behavioral aspects of Lesch-Nyhan disease and its variants. Dev Med Child Neurol 47:673–677, 2005

Shelley BP, Robertson MM: The neuropsychiatry and multisystem features of the Smith-Magenis syndrome: a review. J Neuropsychiatry Clin Neurosci 17:91–97, 2005

Smith AC, Dykens E, Greenberg F: Behavioral phenotype of Smith-Magenis syndrome (del 17p11.2). Am J Med Genet 81:179–185, 1998a

Smith, AC Dykens E, Greenberg F: Sleep disturbance in Smith-Magenis syndrome (del 17 p11.2). Am J Med Genet 81:186–191, 1998b

Sogaard M, Tumer Z, Hjalgrim H, et al: Subtelomeric study of 132 patients with mental retardation reveals 9 chromosomal anomalies and contributes to the delineation of submicroscopic deletions of 1pter, 2qter, 4pter, 5qter and 9qter. BMC Med Genet 6:21, 2005

Spellberg B, Carroll RM, Robinson E, et al: mtDNA disease in the primary care setting. Arch Intern Med 161:2497–2500, 2001

Sporn A, Addington A, Reiss AL, et al: 22q11 deletion syndrome in childhood onset schizophrenia: an update. Mol Psychiatry 9: 225–6, 2004

State MW, Dykens EM: Genetics of childhood disorders: XV. Prader-Willi syndrome: genes, brain, and behavior. J Am Acad Child Adolesc Psychiatry 39:797–800, 2000

Streifler J, Golomb M, Gadoth N: Psychiatric features of adult GM2 gangliosidosis. Br J Psychiatry 155:410–413, 1989

Tishler PV, Woodward B, O'Connor J, et al: High prevalence of intermittent acute porphyria in a psychiatric patient population. Am J Psychiatry 142:1430–1436, 1985

Turpin JC, Masson M, Baumann N: Clinical aspects of Niemann-Pick type C disease in the adult. Dev Neurosci 13:304–306, 1991

Usiskin SI, Nicolson R, Krasnewich DM, et al: Velocardiofacial syndrome in childhood-onset schizophrenia. J Am Acad Child Adolesc Psychiatry 38:1536–1543, 1999

Walter S, Sandig K, Hinkel GK, et al: Subtelomere FISH in 50 children with mental retardation and minor anomalies, identified by a checklist, detects 10 rearrangements including a de novo balanced translocation of chromosomes 17p13.3 and 20q13.33. Am J Med Genet A 128:364–373, 2004

Waltz G, Harik SI, Kaufman B: Adult metachromatic leukodystrophy: value of computed tomographic scanning and magnetic resonance imaging of the brain. Arch Neurol 44:225–227, 1987

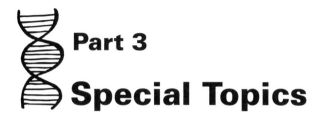

Part 3

Special Topics

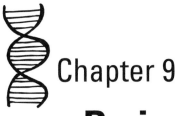

Chapter 9

Perinatal Psychiatry and Teratogenicity

Alexia Koukopoulos, M.D.
Adele C. Viguera, M.D.
Ruta Nonacs, M.D.
Laura F. Petrillo, M.D.
Lee S. Cohen, M.D.

Although the postpartum period has been identified as a time of increased vulnerability to mood and anxiety disorders, pregnancy has often been considered a time of emotional well-being (Zajicek 1981). A growing literature, however, suggests that relapse of an existing mood or anxiety disorder or the emergence of a new disorder is often seen during pregnancy (Cohen et al. 2006; Northcott and Stein 1994; O'Hara et al. 1986; Viguera et al. 2000). Mood and anxiety disorders are highly prevalent among women of childbearing age (Eaton et al. 1994; Kessler et al. 1994) as is psychopharmacological treatment of these disorders (Einarson et al. 2001; Marcus et al. 2005; Wisner et al. 2000). Despite increasing evidence for significant morbidity associated with mood disorders during pregnancy, issues around family planning for women with psychiatric illness have not been examined adequately (Packer 1992; Viguera et al. 2002b, 2007). Currently, most pregnant women with mood or anxiety disorders are either untreated or undertreated (Flynn et al. 2006). Moreover, clinical practice appears to favor discontinuation of maintenance pharmacotherapy during pregnancy in order to avoid potential adverse developmental effects on the fetus and consequent liability risks (Einarson et al. 2001; Viguera et al. 2002a).

Although evidence-based guidelines for the clinical care of pregnant women with mood and anxiety disorders remain sparse, substantial progress has been made in several areas including accumulating information on the reproductive safety of psychotropic drugs, improved understanding of the course of these disorders during pregnancy, and quantification of risk of recurrence during pregnancy and the postpartum period (Wisner et al. 2000; Yonkers et al. 2004). Increasingly, women with mood and anxiety disorders who wish to conceive are seeking preconception consultation to better understand the risks and benefits of the various treatment options available (Bonari et al. 2005; Einarson et al. 2001; Viguera et al. 2002b). In this chapter , we consider the course of mood and anxiety disorders during pregnancy, review the reproductive safety data for the major categories of psychotropic medications, and discuss the risk-benefit assessment process for the treatment of psychiatric illness in pregnant women.

Family Planning Decisions Among Women With a History of Mood or Anxiety Disorder

Typically, women with psychiatric illness encounter significant obstacles from the professional community with respect to pregnancy; they are often counseled to avoid becoming pregnant or to terminate an established pregnancy in order to prevent fetal exposure to potentially teratogenic medications or risk of recurrent illness (Bonari et al. 2005; Cohen et al. 1994a, Einarson et al. 2001; Viguera et al. 2002b). Women who decide to pursue pregnancy, even those with a history of highly recurrent psychiatric illness, are likely to discontinue treatment during attempts to conceive or after conception, because most perceive psychotropic drugs as more dangerous to the fetus than other, nonpsychotropic medications during pregnancy (Bonari et al. 2005; Cohen et al. 2006; Einarson et al. 2001).

In a study of family planning decisions made by women with a history of bipolar disorder, investigators observed that the majority of women, regardless of educational and socioeconomic status, were ill-informed about the perinatal course of their illness and treatment (Viguera et al. 2002b). Nearly 50% of the respondents had been advised against pregnancy by a mental health professional, primary care physician, obstetrician, or family member. Despite this initial advice, all of the respondents sought out a specialized perinatal psychiatric consultation to gather information on the course of mood disorders during pregnancy and reproductive safety data for mood-stabilizing medications. After consultation, just over 60% of the women surveyed attempted to conceive. However, approximately 40% of the patients chose not to pursue pregnancy, even when presented with the same risk-benefit information at consultation. These findings are consistent with those of another study in which the efficacy of evidence-based counseling was examined among pregnant women who were deciding whether to continue or discontinue antidepressant medications (Bonari et al. 2005). The investigators found that personal feelings, intuition, values, and beliefs were powerful determinants of risk perception, and a patient's perceived risk did not always match risk communicated by a professional. However, in both studies, evidence-based consultation appeared to reduce patients' fear and positively influence an informed and thoughtful decision-making process (Bonari et al. 2005; Viguera et al. 2002b).

Genetics of Perinatal Mood Disorders

Although major depression and anxiety disorders have been shown to be familial, it remains unclear whether genetic factors influence vulnerability to these disorders during or after pregnancy (Forty et al. 2006; Jones and Craddock 2001; Jones et al. 2000, 2001; Murphy-Eberenz et al. 2006; Robertson et al. 2005). Postpartum depression and postpartum psychosis, in particular, may represent homogeneous subtypes of complex genetic disorders. In molecular genetic studies, the existence of these subtypes has allowed investigators to evaluate a hierarchy of hypotheses concerning the involvement of neurosteroid pathways in the pathophysiology of the disorders (Jones et al. 2001). Thus far, the available evidence from clinical, outcome, and genetic studies supports the hypothesis that genes are involved in susceptibility to a mood disorder diathesis and a puerperal trigger (Forty et al. 2006; Jones and Craddock 2001; Jones et al. 2000, 2001; Murphy-Eberenz et al. 2006; Robertson et al. 2005).

With respect to postpartum depression, results from recent family studies have suggested that episodes of depression cluster in families (Forty et al. 2006; Murphy-Eberenz et al. 2006). In one study, postpartum depression (within a narrowly defined time period of 4 weeks after childbirth) was found to cluster in families, but no significant evidence of familial clustering was found for more broadly defined postpartum depression (onset within 6 months). Among women with a family history of narrowly defined postpartum episodes, 42% experienced depression after their first delivery, whereas only 15% of women with no such family history experienced depression after their first delivery (Forty et al. 2006). The investigators concluded that a narrowly defined postnatal onset of depression within 6–8 weeks of delivery may be optimal in genetic studies of puerperal triggering of mood episodes.

Similarly, postpartum psychosis may provide a more homogeneous subtype for the genetic studies of bipolar disorder (Jones et al. 2001; Robertson et al. 2005). Postpartum psychosis, defined as an episode of mania or an abrupt onset of severe psychosis precipitated by childbirth, occurs shortly after childbirth in approximately 1–2 of 1,000 deliveries. The available evidence supports the hypothesis that the majority of puerperal psychotic episodes are manifestations of bipolar disorder with a puerperal trigger (Jones and Craddock 2001; Jones et al. 2000, 2001; Robertson et al. 2005). Family studies of puerperal psychosis have consistently demonstrated familial aggregation of bipolar disorder and have also suggested a major overlap in the familial factors predisposing to puerperal psychosis, bipolar disorder, and a puerperal trigger (Jones and Craddock 2001; Jones et al. 2000, 2001; Robertson et al. 2005). Efforts have been made to identify candidate genes involved in the triggering mechanism. In one study, the "short" allele of the serotonin transporter gene promoter polymorphism was associated with a fourfold increase in risk for developing postpartum psychosis (Coyle et al. 2000).

Course of Mood and Anxiety Disorders During Pregnancy

While the genetic vulnerability for mood and anxiety disorders during pregnancy remains uncertain, recent data suggest that pregnancy does not have a salutary effect on mood but rather may act as an independent physiological stressor, predisposing vulnerable women (i.e., those with a prior history of mood and anxiety disorders) to illness during pregnancy (Cohen et al. 2006; Viguera et al. 2000, 2007). Findings in a recent landmark prospective study indicate that the risk for depression is particularly high among women with a history of major depression (Cohen et al. 2006). In a sample of 201 women followed prospectively, 43% experienced a relapse of major depression during pregnancy. Of the women who maintained antidepressant treatment throughout pregnancy, 26% relapsed ($n=82$), compared with 68% of women who discontinued medication. Risk of illness was greatest among women with a history of severe illness, such as a history of four or more depressive episodes or duration of illness of greater than 5 years.

A similar high risk of recurrence has been found among women with a prior history of bipolar disorder (Viguera et al. 2000). In one retrospective study, rates of recurrence among pregnant women with bipolar disorder were greater than 50% after discontinuation of maintenance pharmacotherapy. A recent prospective study found even higher rates of recurrence, with risk nearly three times greater among women who discontinued treatment (85%) versus those who maintained treatment (37%) (Viguera et al. 2007). Risk was greatest during the first trimester and with rapid discontinuation of mood-stabilizing treatment.

Anxiety disorders are common among women, but little is known about the prevalence of anxiety disorders during pregnancy and the postpartum period (Ross and McLean 2006). For women with anxiety disorders, including panic disorder and obsessive-compulsive disorder, the perinatal course may be variable. Pregnancy may ameliorate symptoms of panic in some patients, but in other studies persistence or worsening of panic symptoms during pregnancy have been noted (Cohen et al. 1994b; Klein 1994; Northcott and Stein 1994). For example, in patients with preexisting obsessive-compulsive disorder, symptoms appear to worsen during pregnancy and the postpartum period (Buttolph and Holland 1990; Sichel et al. 1993). Given the limited information available, further study with prospective assessments is needed to better quantify the risk for recurrence of anxiety disorders during and after pregnancy.

In general, women with a history of mood or anxiety disorder should be informed of their high risk of relapse during pregnancy, especially if they are contemplating discontinuation of their maintenance pharmacotherapy. Given the evolving information on the risk for relapse after discontinuation of medication, it may be prudent for women with more recurrent or severe depressive illness to choose to maintain pharmacotherapy during attempts to conceive and during pregnancy in order to limit their risk.

Treatment of Mood and Anxiety Disorders During Pregnancy: A Risk-Benefit Assessment

Women of childbearing age who have a history of mood or anxiety disorder should be counseled appropriately about family planning. Patients should be made aware of the attendant risks of psychotropic medications and should be encouraged to continue using contraception unless they are willing to accept such risks. Planning for pregnancy while the patient has been well and clinically stable for a prolonged period of time provides for thoughtful treatment choices and avoids precipitous changes in treatment decisions in response to an unplanned pregnancy (Cohen et al. 2006; Viguera et al. 2002a; Wisner et al. 2000).

All decisions regarding the continuation or initiation of treatment during pregnancy must follow an assessment of the following factors: 1) the currently available reproductive safety data for the medications; 2) the substantial risks of untreated psychiatric illness in the mother to the patient, fetus, and family; and 3) the typically high risk of relapse associated with discontinuation of maintenance treatment, particularly when discontinuation is abrupt. Each of these risks should be discussed frankly with the patient and her partner, ideally on more than one occasion before and after conception and in conjunction with ongoing communication with the patient's obstetrician. All of these discussions should be documented in the patient's medical record.

Patients and their clinicians must face the difficult realities that no decision is risk-free and that no decision is perfect. The role of the psychiatrist who manages women with mood or anxiety disorders during pregnancy is to share the spectrum of risks associated with continuing or discontinuing available treatment. Our own research and clinical experience suggest that patients presented with the same information, including women with similar clinical illness histories, will make very different decisions about psychotropic medication use during pregnancy (Cohen et al. 2006; Viguera et al. 2002b). Thus, decisions about what constitutes "reasonable risk during pregnancy" ultimately rests with the informed patient.

Risks Associated With Untreated Maternal Mood and Anxiety Disorders During Pregnancy

Clinicians have focused primarily on the effect of psychotropic medications on the developing fetus, with the result that the potential impact of untreated psychiatric illness on the well-being of the fetus and on the mother has often been overlooked and underestimated (Newport et al. 2002; Weissman et al. 2006). Current research findings suggest that maternal depression itself may adversely affect the developing fetus. Associations have been found between maternal depressive symptoms and preterm birth, lower birth weight, smaller head circumference, and lower Apgar scores (Orr and Miller 1995; Steer et al. 1992; Zuckerman et al. 1990).

The physiological mechanisms by which symptoms of depression might affect neonatal outcome are not clear. Increased serum cortisol and catecholamine levels, which are typically observed in patients with depression, may affect placental function by altering uterine blood flow and inducing uterine irritability (Glover 1997; Teixeira et al. 1999). Dysregulation of the hypothalamic-pituitary-adrenal (HPA) axis, which is associated with depression, may also have a direct effect on fetal development. Findings from animal studies suggest that stress during pregnancy is associated with neuronal death and abnormal development of neural structures in the fetal brain as well as with sustained dysfunction of the HPA axis in the offspring (Alves et al. 1997; Newport et al. 2002; Uno et al. 1990).

Psychiatric illness during pregnancy is also associated with significant morbidity in the mother and may contribute to poor self-care and inattention to prenatal care (Zuckerman et al. 1990). Women with depression often have decreased appetite and consequently lower-than-expected weight gain in pregnancy. These factors have been associated with negative pregnancy outcomes (Zuckerman et al. 1989). In addition, pregnant women with depression or anxiety are more likely to smoke and to use either alcohol or illicit drugs (Meshberg-Cohen and Svikis 2007; Zuckerman et al. 1989), which further increases the risk of negative outcomes for the fetus. Depression in the mother also has an adverse effect on the family unit. Depression is typically associated with interpersonal difficulties, including disruptions in mother-child interactions and attachment, which may have a profound impact on infant development (Murray and Cooper 1997; Weinberg and Tronick 1998). In a recent study, children of depressed mothers and fathers were three times more likely than children of nondepressed parents to be at risk for anxiety disorders, major depression, and substance dependence (Weissman et al. 2006). In addition, these children were also at greater risk for social impairment, medical problems, and untimely death, compared with the control group.

Risk of Recurrence Associated With Discontinuation of Maintenance Treatments

Although the potential for teratogenesis is of serious concern, so too is the high risk for morbidity and mortality associated with discontinuation of maintenance psychotropic medication. A growing body of literature in nongravid populations indicates that the discontinuation of maintenance pharmacological treatment is associated with high rates of relapse (Baldessarini et al. 1996, 1999; Suppes et al. 1991; Viguera et al. 1998, 2000). For example, among patients with bipolar disorder, approximately 50% experience recurrence within 6 months of lithium discontinuation (Baldessarini et al. 1996, 1999; Suppes et al. 1991). This risk appears to be particularly high in the setting of abrupt rather than a slowly tapered discontinuation of mood-stabilizing medication (Baldessarini et al. 1996; Faedda et al. 1993). In addition, studies have shown that the discontinuation of maintenance lithium in patients with bipolar disorder was followed by a dramatic increase in suicide risk (Baldessarini et al. 1999). Similar findings have also been noted in patients with unipolar depression and anxiety disorders (Kupfer et al. 1992; Pollack and Smoller 1995; Viguera et al. 1997, 1998). Given these findings, cessation of pharmacotherapy during pregnancy must be viewed as potentially dangerous. As such, the decision to discontinue maintenance treatment should be made only after careful consideration.

Potential Risks of Pharmacotherapy

All medications diffuse readily across the placenta, and no psychotropic drug has yet been approved by the U.S. Food and Drug Administration

(FDA) for use during pregnancy. When considering the use of a psychiatric medication during pregnancy, the clinician must factor in three types of risk to the developing fetus: 1) risk of organ malformation or teratogenesis, 2) risk of neonatal toxicity or withdrawal syndromes during the acute neonatal period, and 3) risk of long-term neurobehavioral sequelae (Cohen and Altshuler 1997).

Risk of Teratogenesis

The baseline incidence of major congenital malformations in newborns born in the United States is estimated to be approximately 2%–4% (Fabro 1987). During the earliest stages of pregnancy, formation of major organ systems is complete within the first 12 weeks of gestation. A teratogen is defined as an agent that interferes with this process and causes some type of organ malformation or dysfunction. Exposure to a toxic agent before 2 weeks of gestation does not typically result in congenital malformations but is more likely to result in a nonviable or blighted ovum. During development of each organ or organ system, there exists a critical period of particular susceptibility to the effects of teratogens. For example, neural tube folding and closure, by which the brain and spinal cord are formed, occur within the first 4 weeks of gestation. Formation of the heart and great vessels takes place from 4–9 weeks after conception.

Risk of Neonatal Symptoms or Syndromes

Perinatal syndromes, neonatal toxicity, or *poor neonatal adaptation* refer to a spectrum of physical and behavioral symptoms observed in the acute neonatal period that can be attributed to drug exposure at or near the time of delivery. Recently, attention has focused on a range of transient neonatal distress syndromes associated with exposure to or withdrawal from, antidepressants in utero; however, it is unclear how often these syndromes occur (Laine et al. 2003; Oberlander et al. 2004). Anecdotal reports that attribute these syndromes to drug exposure must be interpreted with caution and larger samples must be studied in order to establish a causal link between exposure to a particular medication and a perinatal syndrome.

Risk of Long-Term Neurobehavioral Effects

Although the data suggest that some medications may be used safely during pregnancy, our knowledge regarding the long-term effects of prenatal exposure to psychotropic medications is incomplete. Because neuronal migration and differentiation occur throughout pregnancy and into the early years of life, the central nervous system remains particularly vulnerable to toxic agents throughout pregnancy. Although insults that occur early in pregnancy may result in gross abnormalities, exposures that occur after neural tube closure at 32 days of gestation may produce more subtle changes in behavior and functioning.

Behavioral teratogenesis refers to the potential of a psychotropic drug administered during pregnancy to have long-term neurobehavioral effects. For example, children who have been exposed to an antidepressant in utero may be at risk for cognitive or behavioral problems at a later point during their development. To date, few studies have systematically investigated the impact of exposure to psychotropic medications in utero on development and behavior in humans (Nulman and Koren 1996; Nulman et al. 1997, 2002).

Antidepressant Use During Pregnancy

To date, studies have not demonstrated a statistically increased risk of congenital malformations associated with prenatal exposure to antidepressants (Alwan et al. 2007; Green 2007; Louik et al. 2007) . Two meta-analyses combining studies with exposures to tricyclic antidepressants (TCAs) and selective serotonin reuptake inhibitors (SSRIs) did not demonstrate an increase in risk of congenital malformation (Addis and Koren 2000; Altshuler et al. 1996). Data supporting the reproductive safety of fluoxetine (Chambers et al. 1996; Cohen et al. 2000; Goldstein 1995; Goldstein et al. 1991, 1997; Loebstein and Koren 1997; McElhatton et al. 1996; Nulman and Koren 1996) and citalopram (Ericson et al. 1999) are particularly robust.

However, several studies and reports have raised concerns regarding the use of paroxetine during pregnancy (Alwan et al. 2005; GlaxoSmithKline 2005; Wogelius et al. 2005). A report from the Swedish Medical Birth Registry demonstrated a 1.8-fold increase in risk of cardiovascular malformations in paroxetine-exposed children (N=822) (Hallberg and Sjoblom 2005); however, infants exposed to other SSRIs did not have an increased risk of cardiac or other defects (Hallberg and Sjoblom 2005).

Paroxetine has also been associated with an increased risk for omphalocele, an abnormality in which the intestines or other abdominal organs protrude from the abdomen. This abnormality occurs in approximately 1 of 4,000 births. In a case-control study, investigators from the University of British Columbia, Vancouver, analyzed data from the National Birth Defects Prevention Study (Alwan et al. 2005) and found a strong association between exposure to paroxetine during the first trimester and a threefold increase in risk for omphalocele.

Given these recent reports, the FDA issued a public health advisory about paroxetine in December 2005. The report released by the FDA also included preliminary results from two unpublished studies that indicated that paroxetine exposure in the first trimester may increase the risk of congenital malformations, particularly cardiac malformations. At the FDA's request, the manufacturer GlaxoSmithKline changed the pregnancy category label for paroxetine from C to D. In addition, the American College of Obstetricians and Gynecologists recently issued a Committee Opinion on the use of SSRIs (American College of Obstetricians and Gynecologists 2006). The report recommended that paroxetine use among pregnant women or women planning to become pregnant be avoided if possible. The report also included the caution that the potential risk of SSRI use throughout pregnancy must be considered in the context of the risk of relapse of depression if maintenance treatment is discontinued. However, the committee recommended that decisions about treatment with SSRIs or selective norepinephrine reuptake inhibitors during pregnancy should be individualized.

Although these recent reports do raise concerns about paroxetine, it is important to note that they are inconsistent with older studies (Ericson et al. 1999; Kulin et al. 1998). A more recent meta-analysis of seven prospective studies that included a total of 1,774 infants exposed to antidepressants in utero found no association between SSRI exposure and increased risk of major malformations (Einarson and Einarson 2005).

More recently, the teratogenic effect of SSRI use during the first trimester of pregnancy was examined in two large case-control studies from multisite surveillance programs (Alwan et al. 2007; Louik et al. 2007). In the National Birth Defects Prevention Study, no significant associations were found between SSRI use overall and congenital heart defects (Alwan et al. 2007). However, an association was found between paroxetine during early pregnancy and anencephaly, craniosynostosis, and omphalocele, but the absolute risk associated with SSRI use remained small. In the Slone Epidemiology Center Birth Defects Study, no increased risk of craniosynostosis, omphalocele, or heart defects associated with SSRI use overall during early pregnancy was found (Louik et al. 2007). An association was seen between paroxetine and right ventricular outflow defects as well as between sertraline and omphalocele and atrial/ventricular septum defects. However, both studies are limited by the small number of exposed infants for each individual malformation and by the fact that the authors conducted multiple comparisons for their main hypothesis.

The current data on SSRI exposure during early pregnancy provide conflicting data on the risk for specific malformations. However, these recent reports taken together may signal an increase in risk of malformations in children exposed to paroxetine, although it is important to put this risk in perspective. Absolute risk is of far greater clinical value than relative risk and should be taken into consideration before patients are counseled to discontinue antidepressants during pregnancy. Even if we assume the associations from the newer case-control study are true, a 6.4-fold increase in risk for omphalocele translates into an absolute risk of only 0.16% (approximately 2 of 1,200 births). Patients who are planning to conceive and are at significant risk for depressive relapse associated with antidepressant discontinuation may benefit from switching to an antidepressant for which there exists substantial data supporting reproductive safety. These antidepressants include fluoxetine, citalopram, and escitalopram, as well as the older tricyclics. However, for women who are already pregnant and are using SSRIs, including paroxetine, discontinuation should not be pursued arbitrarily, because of the potential associated threats to maternal affective well-being.

Risk of Neonatal Symptoms

Several studies have suggested that exposure to SSRIs at the time of delivery may be associated with poor perinatal outcomes (Casper et al. 2003; Laine et al. 2003; Simon et al. 2002; Zeskind and Stephens 2004). These findings have prompted the FDA to include warnings in the package inserts regarding the use of certain antidepressants, including the SSRIs and venlafaxine, during pregnancy. The most commonly reported symptoms in neonates exposed to the drugs include tremor, restlessness, increased muscle tone, and increased crying. Although the investigators suggest that these symptoms represent a withdrawal phenomenon, others have hypothesized that they reflect serotonergic hyperstimulation (Laine et al. 2003).

A recent report suggests that infants exposed to SSRI antidepressants, such as fluoxetine, sertraline, citalopram, and paroxetine, may be at risk for developing withdrawal symptoms after delivery (Levinson-Castiel et al. 2006). In this study, the most commonly observed symptoms were tremor, increased muscle tone, sleep disruption, gastrointestinal disturbances, and high-pitched crying. In the infants who exhibited severe symptoms, the symptoms were most severe within 2 days after birth. No infants with symptoms required any specific medical treatment. The symptoms usually disappeared within 48 hours and did not require medical intervention.

It is reassuring that the reported adverse events appear to be relatively mild and short-lived and rarely require any type of medical intervention. Further research is essential; pending more study appropriate vigilance of exposed newborns after delivery is good clinical practice. It is unclear at this point whether discontinuing or decreasing the dose of the antidepressant shortly before delivery will reduce the risk of neonatal toxicity; however, it is clear that this type of intervention may significantly increase the risk of depressive relapse in the mother. Given the adverse effects of maternal depression on the child, maintaining mood stability in the mother should remain the highest priority.

Risk of Long-Term Neurobehavioral Effects

To date only a few studies with human subjects have systematically investigated the effects of exposure to antidepressants in utero on development and behavior. The first of these landmark studies followed a cohort of 135 children who had been exposed to either TCAs or fluoxetine during pregnancy, most commonly during the first trimester, and compared these subjects with a cohort of nonexposed control subjects (Nulman et al. 1997). The results indicated no significant differences in IQ, temperament, behavior, reactivity, mood, distractibility, or activity level between exposed and nonexposed children. A more recent report from the same group followed a cohort of children exposed to fluoxetine ($n=40$) or TCAs ($n=47$) for the entire duration of the pregnancy. This study yielded similar results (Nulman et al. 2002). The authors concluded that their findings support the hypothesis that fluoxetine and TCAs are not behavioral teratogens and do not have a significant effect on cognitive development, language, or behavior. In contrast, they observed that depression in the mother is associated with lower cognitive and language achievement in offspring.

A study by Casper and colleagues (2003) assessed children ages 6–40 months and compared 13 children of women who were depressed but had not taken antidepressant medication during pregnancy with 31 children who had been exposed to an SSRI prenatally. The investigators found no differences in global cognition, but they did observe lower psychomotor scores for the SSRI-exposed group. In another study, Oberlander and colleagues (2004) evaluated SSRI-exposed children and controls at ages 2 and 8 months and reported no differences between the two groups with respect to cognitive or motor development. Although these data are reassuring, it is important to note that the findings are preliminary. Further investigation into the long-term neurobehavioral effects of prenatal exposure to antidepressants, as well as other psychotropic medications, is clearly warranted.

Mood Stabilizer Use During Pregnancy

Lithium

Since the early 1970s, there has been concern about an association between prenatal exposure to lithium and risk for major congenital anomalies. Reports from an early International Register of Lithium Babies based on a voluntary physician-reporting system described an excess of cardiovascular malformations, particularly Ebstein's anomaly, in lithium-exposed newborns (Schou 1990; Schou et al. 1973). This anomaly is characterized by right ventricular hypoplasia and downward displacement of the tricuspid valve, often with varying septal defects. The risk for this malformation in infants with lithium exposure in the first trimester was initially determined to be 400 times higher than the background baseline rate of about 1 of 20,000 live births found in the general population (Cohen et al. 1994a; Schou et al. 1973). Despite the fact that the reliability of this initial estimate was highly suspect in view of almost certain selective reporting of adverse outcomes to such registers, this risk estimate influenced clinical practice for the next two decades.

More recent controlled epidemiological studies have suggested a real but more modest teratogenic risk for Ebstein's anomaly following lithium exposure in the first trimester (Cohen et al. 1994a). On the basis of a pooled analysis of the data, Cohen et al. (1994a) and others estimated the risk for Ebstein's anomaly following first-trimester exposure to be between 1 in 1,000 (0.1%) and 1 in 2,000 (0.05%) of all births. Rates of other congenital cardiovascular defects among lithium-exposed infants based on relatively well-designed studies have varied from 0.9% to 12% (Cohen et al. 1994a). Although the estimated risk of Ebstein's anomaly in lithium-exposed infants is 10–20 times higher than in the general population, the absolute risk is small (0.05%–0.1%), and lithium arguably remains the safest mood stabilizer for use during pregnancy. Nevertheless, the FDA pregnancy category label for lithium is D. Prenatal screening with a high-resolution ultrasound and fetal echocardiography is recommended at 16–18 weeks gestation to screen for cardiac anomalies (Cohen et al. 1994a; Yonkers et al. 2004).

Risk of Neonatal Symptoms

Although reintroduction of lithium after the first trimester is not associated with increased risk for major malformations, additional risks arise from exposure later in pregnancy. Neonatal toxicity in offspring exposed to lithium during labor and delivery has been reported. These reports include several cases of muscular hypotonia with impaired breathing and cyanosis, often referred to as "floppy baby" syndrome (Newport et al. 2005; Schou et al. 1973). Isolated cases of neonatal hypothyroidism, nephrogenic diabetes insipidus, and polyhydramnios also have been described (Newport et al. 2005).

On the basis of a number of case reports of toxicity in infants born to mothers treated with lithium, some authors have recommended discontinuation of lithium several days or weeks prior to delivery to minimize the risk of neonatal toxicity (Ananth 1976; Woody et al. 1971). However, given the low incidence of neonatal toxicity with lithium exposure, this practice carries significant risk. because it withdraws treatment from patients precisely as they are about to enter the postpartum period, a time of greatest risk for recurrent illness. A naturalistic survey found no direct evidence of neonatal toxicity in newborns whose mothers received lithium either during pregnancy or during labor and delivery (Cohen et al. 1995).

Risk of Long-Term Neurobehavioral Effects

Limited information is available regarding behavioral outcomes of children exposed to lithium in utero, but one 5-year follow-up study of 60 children exposed to lithium during the second and third trimesters of pregnancy showed no evidence of significant behavioral problems (Schou 1976). In a preliminary report on children of women with bipolar disorder, no significant differences in neurobehavioral outcome were found between a group of 32 children (average age=3.5 years) who had been exposed to lithium in utero and a group of 24 children (average age=3.3 years) who had not been exposed to medication in utero (Viguera et al. 2005). This study used blinded and well-validated neurocognitive assessments. However, the small sample size precludes conclusions about lithium exposure and childhood neurocognitive development.

Anticonvulsant Medications

Anticonvulsants are being used with increasing regularity for the treatment of women with bipolar disorder (Yonkers et al. 2004). All commonly used older anticonvulsants have been associated with teratogenicity, and the risk for major birth defects in infants born to women receiving anticonvulsants is two to three times greater than that in the general population (Holmes et al. 2002). Although most information on the reproductive safety of anticonvulsants is derived from patients with epilepsy rather than patients with bipolar disorder, more recent findings suggest that exposure to certain anticonvulsants, rather than the presence of a seizure disorder, is the relevant variable (Holmes et al. 2002; Viguera et al. 2007).

Risk of Neonatal Symptoms

Fetal exposure to anticonvulsants has been associated not only with relatively high rates of neural tube defects such as spina bifida but also with multiple anomalies, including midface hypoplasia (also known as the "anticonvulsant face"), congenital heart disease, cleft lip and/or palate, growth retardation, and microcephaly (Holmes et al. 2002; Morrell 1996). Factors that may increase the risk for teratogenesis include high maternal anticonvulsant serum levels and exposure to more than one anticonvulsant medication (Holmes et al. 2002). When anticonvulsants are used during pregnancy, the lowest effective dose should be used, anticonvulsant serum levels should be monitored closely, and the dosage should be adjusted appropriately (Morrell 1992). High peak serum levels of anticonvulsants have been associated with adverse effects and should be avoided by administering the drug in frequent divided doses over the course of the day (Crawford 2005). Prenatal screening for congenital malformations, including cardiac anomalies, with fetal ultrasound at 18–22 weeks of gestation is recommended. The possibility of fetal neural tube defects should be evaluated with maternal serum alpha fetoprotein and ultrasonography. In addition, folic acid 4 mg/day before conception and in the first trimester is recommended for women who take anticonvulsants. Whether supplemental folic acid can attenuate the risk of neural tube defects in the setting of anticonvulsant exposure has not been examined.

First-trimester exposure to carbamazepine is associated with a risk of neural tube defects estimated to be about 1.0% (Rosa 1991). Infants with prenatal exposure to carbamazepine are also at increased risk for craniofacial abnormalities, microcephaly, and growth retardation. It is not known whether the new derivative medication, oxcarbazepine, is associated with similar fetal risks (Devinsky and Cramer 2000). Among the anticonvulsants used to treat bipolar disorder, valproic acid and its various derivatives and preparations, including divalproex, may be even more serious teratogens, having been recently associated with rates of around 10% for overall malformations, including craniofacial abnormalities, cardiovascular malformations, limb defects, and genital anomalies (Wyszynski et al. 2005).

Data regarding the reproductive safety of many of the newer anticonvulsants, such as gabapentin, oxcarbazepine, topiramate, tiagabine, levetiracetam, and zonisamide, are limited. Over the last decade, however, pregnancy registries have emerged as a new method for collecting data on fetal risks associated with exposure to anticonvulsants. These registries include the International Registry of Antiepileptic Drugs and Pregnancy (EURAP), the North American Antiepileptic Drug Pregnancy Registry, the International Lamotrigine Pregnancy Registry, the United Kingdom Epilepsy and Pregnancy Register, and the Australian Pregnancy Registry. A main advantage of a pregnancy registry is that it allows accumulation of enough data with the necessary sample size to make a definitive interpretation. The methodology among registries varies, but most registries are largely prospective in design.

Until fairly recently, data on the reproductive safety of lamotrigine suggested that rates of malformation in lamotrigine-exposed infants are similar to those observed in the general population (Cunnington and Tennis 2005; Tennis and Eldridge 2002). Data from the North American Antiepileptic Drug Pregnancy Registry, however, recently presented at the Annual Meeting of the Teratology Society demonstrated an increase in the frequency of oral clefts among infants exposed to lamotrigine. The investigators reported that the overall prevalence of major malformation in a total of 564 children exposed to lamotrigine monotherapy was 2.7%; however, five infants had oral clefts, indicating a prevalence rate of 8.9 per 1,000 births (Holmes et al. 2006). In a comparison group of 221,746 unexposed infants, the prevalence of oral clefts was 0.37 per 1,000, indicating a 24-fold increase in risk of oral cleft in infants exposed to lamotrigine. The other established registries, however, have not demonstrated such a significant increase in risk for oral clefts. In fact, among a total of 1,623 lamotrigine-exposed infants surveyed in the other anticonvulsant registries, only four infants with oral clefts were identified, indicating a frequency of 1:405 or 2.5 per 1,000. While these preliminary data suggest an increased risk of oral clefts with lamotrigine exposure, the absolute risk overall remains small. More data are essential to better evaluate the reproductive safety of lamotrigine. Important questions regarding the safety of lamotrigine and other anticonvulsants may be best addressed by collaboration between multiple registries, including EURAP and the North American Antiepileptic Drug Pregnancy Registry.

Risk of Long-Term Neurobehavioral Effects

Neurobehavioral teratogenesis is another important risk to consider when prescribing anticonvulsants. Although there is no evidence to suggest increased risk for mental retardation after antenatal exposure to anticonvulsants, negative cognitive effects have been suggested (Adab et al. 2001). Researchers in the United Kingdom surveyed 721 women in a regional epilepsy clinic about the schooling of their children (Adab et al. 2001). They found that the use of special education supports was highly correlated with maternal use of specific anticonvulsants. Children exposed to valproate in utero had a threefold increased risk of developmental difficulties requiring additional resources, compared with children who were not exposed to valproate. Children exposed in utero to carbamazepine and other medications as monotherapy had no greater risk of developmental difficulties than children not exposed to any drug. These findings are consistent with two other studies that also noted lower mean IQ among children exposed to valproic acid in utero, compared with control subjects (Adab et al. 2004; Gaily et al. 2004).

Currently, a prospective study known as the Neurodevelopmental Effects of Antiepileptic Drugs (NEAD) Study, supported by the National Institute of Mental Health, is under way to study neurodevelopmental effects of in utero exposure to several anticonvulsants, including carbamazepine, lamotrigine, phenytoin, and valproic acid monotherapy (Meador 2005). This study involves more than 25 sites in the United States and the United Kingdom. Preliminary data to date are consistent with other studies that suggest that children exposed to valproic acid have an increased risk for developmental delay, compared with children exposed to other anticonvulsants such as phenytoin, lamotrigine, or carbamazepine monotherapy.

Antipsychotic Medications

The reproductive safety of the older typical antipsychotic medications or first-generation neuroleptics, such as haloperidol, is supported by extensive data accumulated since the 1950s (Altshuler et al. 1996; Einarson and Einarson 2005). In clinical practice, high-potency neuroleptic agents such fluphenazine, haloperidol, perphenazine, and trifluoperazine may be preferable to low-potency agents or the newer atypical antipsychotics for use in pregnancy, on the basis of a commonsense attempt to limit fetal exposure to potentially toxic molecules-per-time (Altshuler et al. 1996).

Far less reproductive safety data exist for the newer "atypical" class of antipsychotics, including olanzapine, risperidone, quetiapine, aripiprazole, ziprasidone, and clozapine. The atypical neuroleptics are used widely to treat a spectrum of psychiatric disorders, including major depression, bipolar disorder, and anxiety disorders. Thus far, most of the data on the reproductive safety of these agents have been limited to manufacturers' accumulated case series and spontaneous reports that may be inherently biased toward overreporting of poor outcomes. Overall, the available evidence tentatively does not suggest an increased risk for malformations, nor does it indicate any specific pattern of abnormalities among drug-exposed infants. At this point, however, we can make only limited conclusions from this information while noting the fact that it has not suggested any particular concerns regarding the use of atypical antipsychotic drugs in pregnancy.

The first prospective study of the reproductive safety of atypical neuroleptics in the literature was published in 2005, and it provides reassuring data regarding the risk of malformations in children exposed to these medications, albeit in a relatively small sample of 151 patients (McKenna et al. 2005). Investigators from the Motherisk Program in Toronto prospectively followed women who took olanzapine, risperidone, quetiapine, or clozapine during pregnancy. All of the women had taken one of these agents during the first trimester, and 48 women took medication throughout pregnancy. A control group of 151 pregnant women who had taken a nonteratogenic drug was also followed. The rates of malformations were not statistically different between the two groups; in the atypical-exposed group, one infant was born with a major malformation (0.9%), compared with two infants (1.5%) in the control group.

Given the limited data regarding the reproductive safety of the atypical agents, patients taking an antipsychotic drug may choose to discontinue their medication or replace treatment with a better-characterized conventional antipsychotic agent such as perphenazine or haloperidol. However, many women do not respond well to the typical agents or have such severe illness that changes to their regimen may place them at significant risk. Although the Motherisk data are not a guarantee of safety, they do provide information that, in combination with the manufacturers' data, is moderately reassuring. On the basis of these data, women and their clinicians may choose to use atypical agents during pregnancy in order to sustain well-being, while acknowledging that information regarding their reproductive safety remains incomplete.

Risk of Neonatal Symptoms

Several case reports have documented symptoms of poor neonatal adaptation in neonates exposed to neuroleptics in utero. These symptoms, which include motor restlessness, tremor, hypertonicity, dystonia, and parkinsonism (Auerbach et al. 1992; Levy and Wisniewski 1974), have typically been of short duration and are followed by apparently normal motor development (Desmond et al. 1967). Risks of potential neurobehavioral or cognitive effects associated with prenatal exposure to older neuroleptics have also been considered, but the available data remain limited and inconclusive. A longitudinal study that evaluated general intelligence and behavior of children exposed to low-potency neuroleptics in utero found no evidence of dysfunction or developmental delays up to age 5 years (Slone et al. 1977).

Anxiolytic Medications

Benzodiazepines are used commonly as adjunctive medications for mood stabilization or for anxiety, agitation, and insomnia. The most commonly prescribed benzodiazepines during pregnancy are lorazepam and clonazepam (Yonkers et al. 2004). Despite the fact that benzodiazepines have been marketed for almost 50 years, their safety during pregnancy remains controversial (Altshuler et al. 1996; Dolovich et al. 1998; Einarson and Einarson 2005). Although initial reports suggested that there might be an increased risk of cleft lip and cleft palate in infants exposed to these medications in utero, more recent reports have shown no association between exposure to benzodiazepines and risk for cleft lip or palate (Aarskog 1975; Heinonen et al. 1999; McElhatton 1994). A meta-analysis of 23 studies found an association between oral cleft and benzodiazepine use only among case-control studies (odds ratio $=1.79$) and not in cohort studies. Although this risk is significantly increased above the baseline risk for oral clefts in the general population (11 per 10,000 births vs. 6 per 10,000 births), the absolute risk remains small at less than 1% (Dolovich et al. 1998).

Poor neonatal adaptation among infants exposed to benzodiazepines at delivery has also been described. Case reports have described cases of sedation, hypotonia, poor suck, apnea, and cyanosis. However, these effects appear to be self-limited (Koren et al. 1998). In one small study ($N=39$) of a series of infants whose mothers had taken clonazepam (0.5–3.5 mg/day) for treatment of panic disorder during pregnancy, neonatal toxicity was not found (Weinstock et al. 1996).

Systematically derived data on the long-term neurobehavioral effects of benzodiazepines exposure are sparse. Some investigators have noted motor and developmental delays associated with drug exposure while others have not (Bergman et al. 1992; Laegreid et al. 1992).

Currently, no systematic data are available on the reproductive safety of nonbenzodiazepine anxiolytic agents such as buspirone and hypnotic agents such as zolpidem and zaleplon. Therefore, these medications are not recommended for use in pregnancy.

Guidelines for Treatment of Psychiatric Illness During Pregnancy

General Guidelines for the Treatment of Mood and Anxiety Disorders During Pregnancy

Management of the pregnant woman with mood or other psychiatric illness is particularly difficult given that clinical decisions regarding care of this population are not derived from abundant evidence-based data. Rather, treatment decisions are based on a series of partially quantified risks. The most important factor influencing clinical treatment planning during pregnancy is the nature of the patient's illness. Factors such as severity of illness and impairment, duration of euthymia both while taking medication and while not taking medication, prodromal symptoms of relapse, time to relapse following medication discontinuation, and time to recovery with reintroduction must be factored into the treatment plan.

Patients with a history of a single past episode of illness with sustained affective well-being may be able to taper and even discontinue pharmacotherapy before attempting to conceive. Given the recent data that indicate discontinuation of maintenance pharmacological treatment is associated with high rates of relapse when done abruptly, the taper should be done gradually. The clinical maxim "slower is better" applies in this case, because no standard definition of "gradual" exists, other than a minimum taper period of 2 weeks or greater. A pregravid trial of a medication taper allows the clinician and patient to assess clinical status during the taper and when the patient is untreated. Any signs of early relapse may then be followed with reintroduction of the medication. Any plan for discontinuation of medication during pregnancy should then be reevaluated in light of the pregravid trial results.

Women with a history of recurrent illness present a greater challenge. Some patients may choose to gradually discontinue their maintenance antidepressant or mood stabilizer prior to conception. If the patient becomes symptomatic during the taper, the maintenance medication may be easily resumed and the feasibility of trying to conceive without medication should be reassessed. Alternatively, psychotropic discontinuation could await early documentation of pregnancy. This strategy minimizes exposure and affords relapse prophylaxis for the longest period of time while conception is attempted. Maintenance of pharmacotherapy until early documentation of pregnancy may be particularly prudent for older patients, because the time required for conception may be longer than for younger patients.

For women who are able to discontinue medications successfully, the decision to restart medication after the first trimester remains controversial. With sparse data informing a particular treatment path, some women may elect the "wait and see" approach and may reintroduce medication only with early signs of illness relapse. Others may opt to reintroduce medications as a prophylactic approach to reduce the risk of a potential relapse. If the patient's illness history includes episodes of self-harm, protracted recovery time, or evidence that the support system cannot tolerate another episode, empiric treatment may reduce overall risk to both the mother and fetus.

For women with the most severe forms of illness, maintenance of treatment before and during pregnancy is advisable. Accepting the relatively small absolute increase in teratogenic risk with exposure to lithium in the first trimester seems particularly justified since these patients are at highest risk for clinical deterioration in the absence of treatment. Relapse of mood disorders during pregnancy is potentially dangerous to mother and fetus and may require aggressive treatment, including hospitalization and introduction of multiple psychotropic medications at high doses. Thus, an informed decision to assume a small amount of quantifiable risk associated with fetal exposure to a medicine such as lithium may be preferable to the negative outcomes associated with relapse and intense pharmacological treatment to stabilize a severe affective episode. If the clinical decision is to continue medication, it is important to treat effectively with adequate dose and duration. Partial treatment of symptoms exposes the fetus to the effects of both the medication and maternal illness.

Treatment Planning During Pregnancy and the Postpartum Period

Treatment of mood and anxiety disorders during pregnancy and the postpartum period is dynamic. Each period represents a distinct time of variable risk for new onset or relapse of illness. Use of medications may have a specific set of clinical implications, depending on whether the patient is pregnant, postpartum, and/or breastfeeding. The patient should be informed that treatment recommendations and decisions might change over the course of her pregnancy and the puerperium depending on her clinical progress. For example, the treatment plan for managing a woman with affective disorder during pregnancy and the puerperium should include anticipation of the emergence of mania and/or depressive symptoms and possible introduction or reintroduction of medications. These contingencies are best addressed before pregnancy and during preconception planning when a patient is clinically well.

Nonpharmacological treatment strategies should always be explored and may be useful in either limiting or obviating the need for medication. These techniques may be used before conception to facilitate medication discontinuation or during pregnancy to either treat or prevent recurrent symptoms. In general, pharmacological treatment is pursued on the basis of the assessment that the risks associated with psychiatric illness outweigh the risks of fetal exposure to a particular medication.

When pharmacological treatment is indicated, a thorough inventory of medication trials and response to medications is critical. Such an inventory may also reveal medications that are either redundant or ineffective. For example, a nonpregnant woman may seek information on the appropriate treatment of her disorder during a future pregnancy while currently receiving treatment with a compound that is not recommended for use during pregnancy. In such a case, switching to a medication for which there are more reassuring reproductive safety data may be a reasonable option. As newer agents are introduced (e.g., newer anticonvulsants and atypical antipsychotics), the clinician should be reminded that certain older medications for which there are more reproductive safety data provide a "known" risk versus an "unknown" risk. Moreover, because exposure to one drug is better than exposure to multiple medications, streamlining the medication regimen to only the most effective agents is also encouraged. The clinician should attempt to select the safest medication regimen. Often this selection may necessitate substituting psychotropic agents with a better reproductive safety profile (e.g., an SSRI in place of a monoamine oxidase inhibitor). In certain cases, however, one may decide to use a medication for which information regarding reproductive safety is sparse. For instance, a woman with refractory depressive illness who has responded only to one antidepressant for which data on reproductive safety are limited, such as sertraline or paroxetine, may choose to continue this medication during pregnancy rather than risk illness relapse with discontinuation or introduction of a different agent.

Many women, particularly those with refractory illness, require more than one medication to maintain euthymia; while remaining mindful of that fact, every attempt should be made to simplify the medication regimen during pregnancy. This strategy is especially important for women treated with multiple anticonvulsants, because data suggest that polytherapy with anticonvulsants confers more risk to the fetus than monotherapy.

Finally, one must use the appropriate dosage of medication. Many clinicians tend to undertreat psychiatric illness during pregnancy by decreasing the medication dose in an attempt to minimize the possible risks of fetal exposure. This type of modification in treatment may place the woman at greater risk for recurrent illness. This approach exposes the patient to all the risks of adverse effects on her and the fetus without the benefits of effective pharmacological treatment.

Close clinical monitoring during pregnancy is essential because early detection of impending relapse of illness and rapid intervention may significantly reduce morbidity and improve overall prognosis. It may be helpful to conceptualize a model of care for pregnant women with mood and anxiety disorders after the standard of care for "high-risk" pregnancy in obstetrical practice. Even if all psychotropic medicines have been safely discontinued, women with mood and anxiety disorders should be monitored closely for emergence of symptoms. They are at elevated risk not only because of their past history but also because of the impending postpartum period, which is a well-established time of risk for illness.

Conclusions

Although pregnancy is typically considered a time of emotional well-being for many women, it has not been shown to be protective for women with psychiatric illness. Although nonpharmacological treatment strategies may be helpful for some women, others may require pharmacological treatment during pregnancy. Psychotropic medications may be used during pregnancy when the risk of untreated psychiatric illness in the mother outweighs the potential risks of fetal drug exposure. While concerns regarding the teratogenic effects of psychotropic medications have kindled appropriate vigilance, discontinuation of these maintenance medications may result in significant morbidity for the patient and her child. Of growing concern is the risk of untreated psychiatric illness on fetal development. When a patient asks questions regarding the use of psychotropic medications during pregnancy, all risks must be weighed carefully on a case-by-case basis to arrive at an appropriate, individualized, and optimally effective treatment plan.

References

Aarskog D: Association between maternal intake of diazepam and oral clefts (letter). Lancet 2:921, 1975

Adab N, Jacoby A, Smith D, et al: Additional educational needs in children born to mothers with epilepsy. J Neurol Neurosurg Psychiatry 70:15–21, 2001

Adab N, Kini U, Vinten J, et al: The longer term outcome of children born to mothers with epilepsy. J Neurol Neurosurg Psychiatry 75:1575–1583, 2004

Addis A, Koren G: Safety of fluoxetine during the first trimester of pregnancy: a meta-analytical review of epidemiological studies. Psychol Med 30:89–94, 2000

Altshuler LL, Cohen LS, Szuba MP, et al: Pharmacologic management of psychiatric illness in pregnancy: dilemmas and guidelines. Am J Psychiatry 153:592–606, 1996

Alves SE, Akbari HM, Anderson GM, et al: Neonatal ACTH administration elicits long-term changes in forebrain monoamine innervation: subsequent disruptions in hypothalamic-pituitary-adrenal and gonadal function. Ann NY Acad Sci 814:226–251, 1997

Alwan S, Reefhuis J, Rasmussen SA, et al: Maternal use of selective serotonin reuptake inhibitors and risk for birth defects (abstract). Birth Defects Res A Clin Mol Teratol 73:291, 2005

Alwan S, Reefhuis J, Rasmussen S, et al: Use of selective serotonin reuptake inhibitors in pregnancy and risk of birth defects. N Engl J Med 356:2684–2692, 2007

American College of Obstetricians and Gynecologists: Treatment with selective serotonin reuptake inhibitors during pregnancy. ACOG Committee Opinion No. 354. Obstet Gynecol 108:1601–1603, 2006

Ananth J: Side effects on fetus and infant of psychotropic drug use during pregnancy. Int Pharmacopsychiatry 11:246–260, 1976

Auerbach JG, Hans SL, Marcus J, et al: Maternal psychotropic medication and neonatal behavior. Neurotoxicol Teratol 14:399–406, 1992

Baldessarini RJ, Tondo L, Faedda GL, et al: Effects of rate of discontinuing lithium maintenance treatment. J Clin Psychiatry 57:441–448, 1996

Baldessarini RJ, Tondo L, Viguera AC: Discontinuing lithium maintenance treatment in bipolar disorders: risks and implications. Bipolar Disord 1:17–24, 1999

Bergman U, Rosa FW, Baum C, et al: Effects of exposure to benzodiazepine during fetal life. Lancet 340:694–696, 1992

Bonari L, Koren G, Einarson TR, et al: Use of antidepressants by pregnant women: evaluation of perception of risk, efficacy of evidence based counseling and determinants of decision making. Arch Women Ment Health 8:214–220, 2005

Buttolph ML, Holland A: Obsessive compulsive disorders in pregnancy and childbirth, in Obsessive-Compulsive Disorders: Theory and Management. Edited by Jenike M, Baer L, Minichiello WE. Chicago, IL, Year Book Medical, 1990

Casper RC, Fleisher BE, Lee-Ancajas JC, et al: Follow-up of children of depressed mothers exposed or not exposed to antidepressant drugs during pregnancy. J Pediatr 142:402–408, 2003

Chambers CD, Johnson KA, Dick LM, et al: Birth outcomes in pregnant women taking fluoxetine. N Engl J Med 335:1010–1015, 1996

Cohen L, Altshuler L: Pharmacologic management of psychiatric illness during pregnancy and the postpartum period, in Psychiatric Clinics of North America Annual of Drug Therapy. Edited by Dunner D, Rosenbaum J. Philadelphia, PA, WB Saunders, 1997, pp 21–60

Cohen LS, Friedman JM, Jefferson JW, et al: A reevaluation of risk of in utero exposure to lithium. JAMA 271:146–150, 1994a

Cohen LS, Sichel DA, Dimmock JA, et al: Impact of pregnancy on panic disorder: a case series. J Clin Psychiatry 55:284–288, 1994b

Cohen LS, Sichel DA, Robertson LM, et al: Postpartum prophylaxis for women with bipolar disorder. Am J Psychiatry 152:1641–1645, 1995

Cohen LS, Heller VL, Bailey JW, et al: Birth outcomes following prenatal exposure to fluoxetine. Biol Psychiatry 48:996–1000, 2000

Cohen LS, Altshuler LL, Harlow BL, et al: Relapse of major depression during pregnancy in women who maintain or discontinue antidepressant treatment. JAMA 295:499–507, 2006

Coyle N, Jones I, Robertson E, et al: Variation at the serotonin transporter gene influences susceptibility to bipolar affective puerperal psychosis. Lancet 356:1490–1491, 2000

Crawford P: Best practice guidelines for the management of women with epilepsy. Epilepsia 46(suppl 9):177–124, 2005

Cunnington M, Tennis P: Lamotrigine and the risk of malformations in pregnancy. International Lamotrigine Pregnancy Registry Scientific Advisory Committee. Neurology 64:955–960, 2005

Desmond MM, Rudolph AJ, Hill RM: Behavioral alterations in infants born to mothers on psychoactive medication during pregnancy, in Congenital Mental Retardation. Edited by Farrell G. Austin, TX, University of Texas Press, 1967

Devinsky O, Cramer J: Safety and efficacy of standard and new antiepileptic drugs. Neurology 55(11 Suppl 3):S5–S10, 2000

Dolovich LR, Addis A, Vaillancourt JM, et al: Benzodiazepine use in pregnancy and major malformations or oral cleft: meta-analysis of cohort and case-control studies. BMJ 317:839–843, 1998

Eaton WW, Kessler RC, Wittchen H-U, et al: Panic and panic disorder in the United States. Am J Psychiatry 151:413–420, 1994

Einarson A, Selby P, Koren G: Abrupt discontinuation of psychotropic drugs during pregnancy: fear of teratogenic risk and the impact of counseling. J Psychiatry Neurosci 26:44–48, 2001

Einarson TR, Einarson A: Newer antidepressants in pregnancy and rates of major malformations: a meta-analysis of prospective comparative studies. Pharmacoepidemiol Drug Saf 14:823–827, 2005

Ericson A, Kallen B, Wilhom B: Delivery outcome after the use of antidepressants in early pregnancy. Eur J Clin Psychopharm 55:503–508, 1999

Fabro SE: Clinical Obstetrics. New York, Wiley, 1987

Faedda GL, Tondo L, Baldessarini RJ, et al: Outcome after rapid vs gradual discontinuation of lithium treatment in bipolar mood disorders. Arch Gen Psychiatry 50:448–455, 1993

Flynn HA, Blow FC, Marcus SM: Rates and predictors of depression treatment among pregnant women in hospital affiliated obstetric practices. Gen Hosp Psychiatry 28: 289–295, 2006

Forty L, Jones L, Macgregor S, et al: Familiality of postpartum depression in unipolar disorder: results of a family study. Am J Psychiatry 163:1549–1553, 2006

Gaily E, Kantola-Sorsa E, Hiilesmaa V, et al: Normal intelligence in children with prenatal exposure to carbamazepine. Neurology 62:28–32, 2004

GlaxoSmithKline: "Dear Doctor" letter. September 2005. Available at http://www. fda.gov/medwatch/SAFETY/2005/Paxil_dearhcp_letter.pdf. Accessed January 31, 2007.

Glover V: Maternal stress or anxiety in pregnancy and emotional development of the child. Br J Psychiatry 171:105–106, 1997

Goldstein DJ: Effects of third trimester fluoxetine exposure on the newborn. J Clin Psychopharmacol 15:417–420, 1995

Goldstein DJ, Williams ML, Pearson DK: Fluoxetine-exposed pregnancies. Clin Res 39(3):768A, 1991

Goldstein DJ, Sundell KL, Corbin LA: Birth outcomes in pregnant women taking fluoxetine. N Engl J Med 336:872–873; author reply 873, 1997

Green MF: Teratogenicity of SSRIs–serious concern or much ado about little? N Engl J Med 356:2732–2733, 2007

Hallberg P, Sjoblom V: The use of selective serotonin reuptake inhibitors during pregnancy and breast- feeding: a review and clinical aspects. J Clin Psychopharmacol 25:59–73, 2005

Heinonen OP, Slone D, Shapiro S: Birth Defects and Drugs in Pregnancy. Littleton, MA, Publishing Sciences, 1999

Holmes LB, Harvey EA, Coull BA, et al: Teratogenicity of anticonvulsant drugs. N Engl J Med 334:1132–1138, 2002

Holmes LB, Wyszynski DF, Baldwin EJ, et al: Increased risk for non-syndromic cleft palate among infants exposed to lamotrigine during pregnancy. Paper presented at the 46th annual meeting of the Teratology Society, Tucson, AZ, June 2006

Jones I, Craddock N: Familiality of the puerperal trigger in bipolar disorder: results of a family study. Am J Psychiatry 158:913–7, 2001

Jones I, Middle F, McCandless F, et al: Molecular genetic studies of bipolar disorder and puerperal psychosis at two polymorphisms in the estrogen receptor alpha gene (ESR 1). Am J Med Genet 96:850–853, 2000

Jones I, Lendon C, Coyle N, et al: Molecular genetic approaches to puerperal psychosis. Prog Brain Res 133:321–331, 2001

Kessler RC, McGonagle KA, Zhao S, et al: Lifetime and 12-month prevalence of DSM-III-R psychiatric disorders in the United States: results from the National Comorbidity Study. Arch Gen Psychiatry 51:8–19, 1994

Klein DF: Pregnancy and panic disorder. J Clin Psychiatry 55:293–294, 1994

Koren G, Pastuszak A, Ito S: Drugs in pregnancy. N Engl J Med 338:1128–1137, 1998

Kulin NA, Pastuszak A, Sage S, et al: Pregnancy outcome following maternal use of the new selective serotonin reuptake inhibitors: a prospective controlled multicenter study. JAMA 279:609–610, 1998

Kupfer DJ, Frank E, Perel JM, et al: Five-year outcome for maintenance therapies in recurrent depression. Arch Gen Psychiatry 49:769–773, 1992

Laegreid L, Hagberg G, Lundberg A: The effect of benzodiazepines on the fetus and the newborn. Neuropediatrics 23:18–23, 1992

Laine K, Heikkinen T, Ekblad U, et al: Effects of exposure to selective serotonin reuptake inhibitors during pregnancy on serotonergic symptoms in newborns and cord blood monoamine and prolactin concentrations. Arch Gen Psychiatry 60:720–726, 2003

Levinson-Castiel R, Merlob P, Linder N, et al: Neonatal abstinence syndrome after in utero exposure to selective serotonin reuptake inhibitors in term infants. Arch Pediatr Adolesc Med 160:173–176, 2006

Levy W, Wisniewski K: Chlorpromazine causing extrapyramidal dysfunction in newborn infants of psychotic mothers. N Y State J Med 74:684–685, 1974

Loebstein R, Koren G: Pregnancy outcome and neurodevelopment of children exposed in utero to psychoactive drugs: the Motherisk experience. J Psychiatry Neurosci 22:192–196, 1997

Louik C, Lin AE, Werler MM, et al: First-trimester use of selective serotonin reuptake inhibitors and the risk of birth defects. N Engl J Med 356:2675–2683, 2007

Marcus SM, Flynn HA, BlowF, et al: A screening study of antidepressant treatment rates and mood symptoms in pregnancy. Arch Wom Ment Health 8:25–27, 2005

McElhatton PR: The effects of benzodiazepine use during pregnancy and lactation. Reprod Toxicol 8:461–475, 1994

McElhatton P, Garbis H, Elefant E, et al: The outcome of pregnancy in 689 women exposed to theraputic doses of antidepressants: a collaborative study of the European Network of Teratology Information Services (ENTIS). Reprod Toxicol 10:285–294, 1996

McKenna K, Koren G, Tetelbaum M, et al: Pregnancy outcome of women using atypical antipsychotic drugs: a prospective comparative study. J Clin Psychiatry 66:444–449, 2005

Meador K: Anatomical and behavioral effects of in utero exposure to antiepileptic drugs. Epilepsy Curr 5:212–216, 2005

Meshberg-Cohen S, Svikis D: Panic disorder, trait anxiety, and alcohol use in pregnant and nonpregnant women. Compr Psychiatry 48:504–510, 2007

Morrell MJ: Hormones and epilepsy through the lifetime. Epilepsia 33(suppl 4):S49–S61, 1992

Morrell MJ: The new antiepileptic drugs and women: efficacy, reproductive health, pregnancy, and fetal outcome. Epilepsia 37 (suppl 6):S34–S44, 1996

Murphy-Eberenz K, Zandi PP, March D, et al: Is perinatal depression familial? J Affect Disord 90:49–55, 2006

Murray L, Cooper P: Effects of postnatal depression on infant development. Arch Dis Child 77:99–101, 1997

Newport, DJ, Wilcox MM, Stowe ZN: Maternal depression: a child's first adverse life event. Sem Clin Neuropsychiatry 7:113–119, 2002

Newport DJ, Viguera AC, Beach AJ, et al: Lithium placental passage and obstetrical outcome: implications for clinical management during late pregnancy. Am J Psychiatry 162:2162–2170, 2005

Northcott CJ, Stein MB: Panic disorder in pregnancy. J Clin Psychiatry 55:539–542, 1994

Nulman I, Koren G: The safety of fluoxetine during pregnancy and lactation. Teratology 53:304–308, 1996

Nulman I, Rovet J, Stewart DE, et al: Neurodevelopment of children exposed in utero to antidepressant drugs. N Engl Med 336:258–262, 1997

Nulman I, Rovet J, Stewart DE, et al: Child development following exposure to tricyclic antidepressants or fluoxetine throughout fetal life: a prospective, controlled study. Am J Psychiatry 159:1889–1895, 2002

Oberlander TF, Misri S, Fitzgerald CE, et al: Pharmacologic factors associated with transient neonatal symptoms following prenatal psychotropic medication exposure. J Clin Psychiatry 65:230–237, 2004

O'Hara MW: Social support, life events, and depression during pregnancy and the pueperium. Arch Gen Psychiatry 43:569–573, 1986

Orr ST, Miller CA: Maternal depressive symptoms and the risk of poor pregnancy outcome: review of the literature and preliminary findings. Epidemiol Rev 17:165–171, 1995

Packer S: Family planning for women with bipolar disorder. Hosp Community Psychiatry 43:479–482, 1992

Pollack MH, Smoller JW: The longitudinal course and outcome of panic disorder. Psychiatr Clin North Am 18:785–801, 1995

Robertson E, Jones I, Haque S, et al: Risk of puerperal and non-puerperal recurrence of illness following bipolar affective puerperal (post-partum) psychosis. Brit J Psychiatry 186:258–259, 2005

Rosa FW: Spina bifida in infants of women treated with carbamazepine during pregnancy. N Engl J Med 324:674–676, 1991

Ross LE, McLean LM: Anxiety disorders during pregnancy and the postpartum period: a systematic review. J Clin Psychiatry 67:1285–1298, 2006

Schou M: What happened later to the lithium babies: a follow-up study of children born without malformations. Acta Psychiatr Scand 54:193–197, 1976

Schou M: Lithium treatment during pregnancy, delivery, and lactation: an update. J Clin Psychiatry 51:410–413, 1990

Schou M, Goldfield MD, Weinstein MR, et al: Lithium and pregnancy, I: report from the register of lithium babies. BMJ 2:135–136, 1973

Sichel DA, Cohen LS, Dimmock JA, et al: Postpartum obsessive-compulsive disorder: a case series. J Clin Psychiatry 54:156–159, 1993

Simon G, Cunningham M, Davis R: Outcomes of prenatal antidepressant exposure. Am J Psychiatry 159:2055–2061, 2002

Slone D, Siskind V, Heinonen OP, et al: Antenatal exposure to the phenothiazines in relation to congenital malformations, perinatal mortality rate, birth weight, and intelligence quotient score. Am J Obstet Gynecol 128:486–488, 1977

Steer RA, Scholl TO, Hediger ML, et al: Self-reported depression and negative pregnancy outcomes. J Clin Epidemiol 45:1093–1099, 1992

Suppes T, Baldessarini RJ, Faedda GL, et al: Risk of recurrence following discontinuation of lithium treatment in bipolar disorder. Arch Gen Psychiatry 48:1082–1088, 1991

Teixeira JM, Fisk NM, Glover V: Association between maternal anxiety in pregnancy and increased uterine artery resistance index: cohort-based study. BMJ 318:153–157, 1999

Tennis P, Eldridge RR, for the International Lamotrigine Pregnancy Registry Scientific Advisory Committee: Preliminary results on pregnancy outcomes in women using lamotrigine. Epilepsia 43:1161–1167, 2002

Uno H, Lohmiller L, Thieme C, et al: Brain damage induced by prenatal exposure to dexamethasone in fetal rhesus macaques. Dev Brain Res 53:157–167, 1990

Viguera AC, Baldessarini RJ, Hegarty JD: Clinical risk following abrupt and gradual withdrawal of maintenance neuroleptic treatment. Arch Gen Psychiatry 54:49–55, 1997

Viguera AC, Baldessarini RJ, Friedberg J: Discontinuing antidepressant treatment in major depression. Harv Rev Psychiatry 5:293–306, 1998

Viguera AC, Nonacs R, Cohen LS, et al: Risk of recurrence of bipolar disorder in pregnant and nonpregnant women after discontinuing lithium maintenance. Am J Psychiatry 157:179–184, 2000

Viguera AC, Cohen LS, Baldessarini RJ, et al: Managing bipolar disorder in pregnancy: weighing the risks and benefits. Can J Psychiatry 47:426–436, 2002a

Viguera AC, Cohen LS, Bouffard S, et al: Reproductive decisions by women with bipolar disorder after prepregnancy psychiatric consultation. Am J Psychiatry 159:2102–2104, 2002b

Viguera AC, Whitfield T, Sherman J, et al: Neurobehavioral outcome following lithium exposure: what happens to lithium babies. Poster presented at the annual meeting of the Society of Biological Psychiatry, Atlanta, GA, May 2005

Viguera AC, Whitfield T, Baldessarini RJ, et al: Risk of recurrence in women with bipolar disorder during pregnancy: prospective study of mood stabilizer discontinuation. Am J Psychiatry 164:1817–1824, 2007

Weinberg MK, Tronick EZ: The impact of maternal psychiatric illness on infant development. J Clin Psychiatry 59(suppl 2):53–61, 1998

Weinstock L, Cohen LS, Bailey JW, et al: Obstetrical and neonatal outcome following clonazepam use during pregnancy: a case series. Psychother Psychosom 70:158–162, 1996

Weissman MM, Wickramaratne P, Nomura Y, et al: Offspring of depressed parents: 20 years later. Am J Psychiatry 163:1001–1008, 2006

Wisner K, Zarin D, Appelbaum P, et al: Risk-benefit decision making for treatment of depression during pregnancy. Am J Psychiatry 157:1933–1940, 2000

Wogelius P, Norgaard M, Muff Munk E, et al. Maternal use of selective serotonin reuptake inhibitors and risk of adverse pregnancy outcomes (abstract). Pharmacoepidemiol Drug Saf 14:S143, 2005

Woody JN, London WL, Wilbanks G D Jr: Lithium toxicity in a newborn. Pediatrics 47:94–99, 1971

Wyszynski DF, Nambisan M, Surve T, et al: Increased rate of major malformations in offspring exposed to valproate during pregnancy. Neurology 64:961–965, 2005

Yonkers KA, Wisner KL, Stowe ZN, et al: Management of bipolar disorder during pregnancy and the postpartum period. Am J Psychiatry 161:608–620, 2004

Zajicek E: Psychiatric problems during pregnancy, in Pregnancy: A Psychological and Social Study. Edited by Wolkind S, Zajicek E. London, Academic Press, 1981, pp 57–73

Zeskind P, Stephens L: Maternal selective serotonin reuptake inhibitor use during pregnancy and newborn neurobehavior. Pediatrics 113:368–375, 2004

Zuckerman B, Amaro H, Bauchner H, et al: Depressive symptoms during pregnancy: relationship to poor health behaviors. Am J Obstet Gynecol 160:1107–1111, 1989

Zuckerman B, Bauchner H, Parker S, et al: Maternal depressive symptoms during pregnancy, and newborn irritability. J Dev Behav Pediatr 11:190–194, 1990

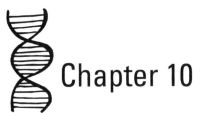

Chapter 10

Ethical, Legal, and Social Implications of Psychiatric Genetics and Genetic Counseling

Steven K. Hoge, M.D., M.B.A.
Paul S. Appelbaum, M.D.

We are in the early stages of a revolution in medicine brought about by genetic research. It is not yet clear how rapidly this scientific revolution will progress or how dramatically the new technology will affect our understanding of psychiatric disorders and treatments. Consequently, it is not possible to foresee what the full ethical, legal, and social implications will be in our field. It is apparent, however, that the new genetics promises to transform clinical practice in two fundamental ways that inevitably will raise legal and ethical questions. First, genetic information promises to provide new predictive capabilities regarding individuals' relative risk of developing mental disorders, vulnerability to environmental factors, and responsiveness to treatment. Second, genetic information has implications that extend beyond the individual from whom it was obtained. As people share genes with their biological relatives and pass them on to their children, the predictive capabilities ripple out from the individual, encompassing not only those currently alive, but also future generations. As the power of the science grows, the law and ethics of practice will need to evolve to address the concerns of the professions, patients, and society.

In this chapter we explore the legal and ethical ramifications of the new genetic capabilities. The reader should keep in mind that the problems and solutions discussed are necessarily preliminary in nature. The science itself is a rapidly moving target, as new findings are announced and published at a steady rate. Psychiatrists and other mental health clinicians have only begun the slow process of assimilating research findings and considering their implications for practice. Perhaps more importantly, the public has to be educated more deeply about the science and engaged in discussions about its appropriate use. And it should be acknowledged that academic reflections take us only so far; ultimately, ethics, policies, and law will be forged in the crucible of experience. Only when the fruits of the science are applied in a meaningful way in the lives of ordinary individuals will the dialogue truly begin.

History

Public and professional thought about the new genetic technology has been shaped by the historical specter of eugenics, which is notable for several reasons. First, eugenics-based laws and policies were often used to assert the primacy of society and race over the rights of the individual. Second, while the "science" of eugenics was ultimately discredited, during its ascendancy, political leaders exploited its apparent legitimacy in enacting broad-sweeping programs of social transformation. Third, physicians took active roles in promoting and implementing eugenic policies that often were contrary to patients' and other individuals' interests. Psychiatrists, as will be discussed, played important roles in the eugenics movement in some countries.

The eugenics (literally, "well born") movement, which flourished in the early twentieth century, focused on improving the genetic stock of the population. Eugenicists feared that modern social policies were providing support and sustenance to the "unfit," allowing them to survive and to reproduce. As a result, the thinking went, the population or "race" faced progressive degeneration if these "suicidal" policies were not counteracted. The cardinal features of the movement included the belief that scientific methods should be harnessed to improve the genetic stock of mankind. Eugenic laws and policies were implemented in many countries; these measures were designed to discourage or prevent people with "undesirable" characteristics from reproducing. Alternatively, those who were regarded as having superior genetics were encouraged to marry and reproduce. In the United States, compulsory sterilization of the mentally retarded, the mentally ill, and criminals was authorized by statute in many states, beginning in 1907. The U.S. Supreme Court upheld a Virginia statute that authorized sterilization of the mentally retarded in *Buck v. Bell* in 1927, a decision notorious for Justice Oliver Wendell Holmes's justification that "three generations of imbeciles are enough." Similar eugenic policies could be found in the United Kingdom, Canada, and other Western nations.

Eugenics reached its zenith (or nadir) in Nazi Germany. Psychiatrists were directly implicated in the application of eugenic programs under the Nazi regime (Hassenfeld 2002; Meyer 1988). Shortly after taking power, the Nazis implemented the Law for the Prevention of Offspring with Hereditary Diseases (*Das Gesetz zur Verhütung erbkranken Nachwuchses*). Under this law, more than 350,000 individuals were involuntarily sterilized; many of those persons had mental disorders, including schizophrenia, mental retardation, and alcoholism. More than 10% of the individuals involved actively resisted and were brought to the sterilization facility by police. With the beginning of World War II, the German state required that doctors report the names of children with deformities and other presumed hereditary disorders to a central registry. Medical experts were called on to determine whether the children should be killed. Reportedly, under this program, 5,000 children between the ages of 3 to 17 years were put to death.

Adult psychiatric patients were targeted under a program known as Action T4. Once again, the state created a central reporting process to aid in the identification of individuals for extermination. Psychiatric patients with a criminal history and those who had been chronically hospitalized or were unable to work were targets (Hassenfeld 2002; Meyer 1988). Action T4 included patients with schizophrenia, cyclothymia, and a wide variety of neurological and senile disorders who were put to death in gas chambers. Unlike compulsory sterilization and the "euthanasia" of children, Action T4 took place beneath a cloak of secrecy. In gas chambers disguised as showers, patients were systematically murdered. Families were deceived regarding the cause of death, and bodies were quickly cremated. Doctors involved in Action T4 were given cover names. Under this program, more than 70,000 patients were killed.

Action T4 was officially discontinued in 1941, following resistance from the Catholic Church. However, the killing did not stop. The staff and machinery of death used in T4 were employed to bring about the "Final Solution" to the existence of European Jews. Psychiatric patients continued to be killed in this phase of "Wild Euthanasia" by gunshot, starvation, and other methods, often with the intent of alleviating hospital bed shortages to accommodate war casualties (Meyer 1988). Psychiatrists were often called on to select and themselves to kill patients in mental hospitals.

Following World War II, eugenic policies were discredited on moral and scientific grounds. However, even in the United States they did not completely disappear and continued to be applied to persons with mental disorders. For example, state statutes that prohibited the marriage of "lunatics," "imbeciles," the "insane," and the "weak-minded" persisted into the 1980s (Brakel 1985). The eugenic intent of such statutes is made evident by exceptions provided for marriage applicants who have been sterilized or in marriages that involve women who have passed the childbearing years.

Over much of the period following World War II, genetic researchers and practitioners were careful to avoid the taint of eugenics. Controversy was easily avoided in the postwar era for several reasons. First, in relative terms, the flow of genetic information was a trickle. Second, as genetic information emerged and gained utility, it was applied almost exclusively in clinical settings and not for broad social purposes. Third, and perhaps most importantly, patients remained firmly in the driver's seat, deciding whether to undergo testing and determining what actions should be taken in the face of genetic results.

During this interlude between eugenics and the modern genetic revolution, a new class of medical providers—genetic counselors—emerged to assist patients in understanding the results of genetic testing. Genetic counselors adhered to a model of "nondirective" counseling, eschewing any attempts to influence individuals' decision making or to substitute professional judgments for individual ones. Concerns about eugenics were kept at bay by assiduous avoidance of interference with self-determination in the sphere of genetics and reproductive rights.

With the transgressions of eugenics as prologue, it is not surprising that the advent of new technologies for gene discovery and manipulation was met with some fear. The societal implications of modern genetic technologies have engaged governments, private foundations, and professional organizations around the world. From its inception, the leaders of the Human Genome Project have recognized the importance of addressing societal concerns about the use of the gene technologies. James Watson, the first director of the Human Genome Project, made a commitment to Congress that significant funds would be allocated to studies of the ethical, legal, and social implications of the Human Genome Project. The National Human Genome Research Institute at the National Institutes of Health has allocated 5% of the Human Genome Project research budget to funding research on the ethical, legal, and social implications. The U.S. Department of Energy, which also supported the Human Genome Project, dedicated 3% of its funding to these issues. By the end of 1999, more than $76 million had been spent on research and education related to legal and ethical implications of human genetics (ELSI Research and Evaluation Planning Group 2000). The cultural legacy of eugenics also has had an impact on the conduct of science. The National Human Genome Research Institute has involved ethicists in the design, conduct, and reporting of projects (International HapMap Consortium 2003, 2004).

The new technologies are generally recognized as promising revolutionary changes in health care. Therefore, it is not surprising that there has been a substantial outpouring of thought from various constituencies regarding how these technologies should be deployed. Within the universe of governmental commissions, foundation reports, professional statements, advocacy positions, and academic papers, there is a wide diversity of opinion. It is almost certain that views will change as technologies emerge and practical experience is gained.

Clinical Applications of Genetic Tests for Psychiatric Disorders

Testing in Adults

Adults may seek to ascertain their risk status for a mental disorder, perhaps because of concern deriving from an affected relative. Preliminary evidence suggests that there may be significant interest in such testing (Jones et al. 2002; Milner et al. 1998; Smith et al. 1996; Trippitelli et al. 1998). In one study, Trippitelli et al. (1998) asked patients with bipolar disorder and their spouses who desired testing how they might benefit from a genetic test for the disorder. Prevention—obtaining prophylactic treatment prior to the onset of "attacks"—was seen as the most important benefit by more than two-thirds of the respondents. Certainty about their genetic status was the second most-cited benefit, outranking the results' utility in guiding marital, reproductive, or financial decisions. It is reasonable to expect that once genetic testing is available, demand will soon follow, long before testing results have significance for clinical management.

Respect for patient autonomy in decision making regarding medical care is reflected in the notion of informed consent. The legal doctrine prescribes the nature and extent of information that must be provided to patients, requires that patients be competent to make decisions, and prohibits coercion in the consent process. The thrust of much ethical discourse regarding informed consent is to set a higher plane of aspiration for patient participation, beyond what is required by law. For example, there is a general consensus that professional ethics call for physicians to involve patients in the decision-making process to the greatest possible extent. Against this briefly drawn backdrop, we consider some challenges to informed consent posed by genetic testing of adults for psychiatric disorders.

In order to engage patients in the decision-making process, psychiatrists themselves will need to understand, if not master, complex information. As genetic research progresses and moves into clinical settings, the problem of professional mastery will grow. There is evidence that much work will need to be done to bring clinicians up to speed. A recent survey of psychiatrists found a low level of knowledge regarding general and psychiatric genetics (Finn et al. 2005). Less than one-quarter of psychiatrists felt competent to discuss genetic information with patients and their families. This finding, and other studies documenting deficiencies in physicians' understanding of genetic information (Hofman et al. 1993), underscores the need for psychiatric educators to dedicate more time and resources to genetic concepts.

Obtaining informed consent to genetic testing is more complex than obtaining consent for routine testing, in part, because it appears likely that the majority of cases will involve susceptibility testing. The results of such testing will be framed in probabilistic terms. Moreover, in most, if not all situations, probabilities will be influenced by family history and clinical factors, in addition to age, race, and gender. Currently recommended procedures for genetic counseling in psychiatry involve several stages of intervention that precede the patient's (or family member's) decision to undergo testing or to receive the results of testing (Faraone et al. 1999; Hodgkinson et al. 2001). This multistage scheme calls for extensive evaluation, including verification of diagnoses in all affected individuals in the family, which may require obtaining prior treatment records and/or the administration of research diagnostic instruments. At each stage, some probability of error will result from intrinsic variability in procedures, lack of cooperation from affected relatives, and other missing data. Comprehension of the uncertain and probabilistic nature of the results will require education. Faraone et al. (1999) recommended an assessment of the patient's (or family member's) understanding of probability and suggested that concepts be demonstrated (and practiced at home) with sets of coin flips. In sum, the informed consent process will require that significant attention be paid to probabilistic thinking in patients. The process leading up to testing must include education about the disorder or disorders in question, the availability of interventions, and the possible consequences of a positive test. Individuals undergoing testing must have the opportunity to consider their personal burden of knowing and weigh the relative benefits and risks of genetic information.

Informed consent to genetic testing must also take into account the "right not to know." Ethicists recognize a right *not* to know with respect to diagnosis and prognosis (Beauchamp and Childress 2001). Superficially, the right not to know appears to be at odds with informed consent; however, both are grounded in the principle of patient autonomy. As noted by Beauchamp and Childress (2001), the fundamental ethical obligation to respect patient autonomy is inconsistent with "forced" information. The notion of a "burden of knowing" and a corresponding right not to know has received widespread recognition and acceptance in ethical discourse regarding genetic testing. There is a remarkable consensus on the right not to know, which is reflected in the European Convention on Human Rights and Biomedicine (1996), the United Nations Educational, Scientific and Cultural Organization's Universal Declaration on the Human Genome and Human Rights (1997), the World Medical Association's Declaration on the Rights of the Patient (1981, amended 1995), the World Health Organization's Guidelines on Ethical Issues in Medical Genetics and the Provision of Genetic Services (1997), and the former United Kingdom Human Genetics Advisory Commission (1999) and its current incarnation, the Human Genetics Commission (2004). The influential Nuffield Council on Bioethics report *Mental Disorders and Genetics: The Ethical Context* (1998) presents the same conclusion.

The ethics community has given widespread endorsement to the right not to know based on the the burden of knowing. Simply put, many people would prefer not to assume the burden of knowing their future and would like to forgo the prognostic capabilities that flow from modern medical technology (Kass 2004). The burden of knowing may turn on the availability of clinical interventions. Marteau and Croyle (1998) found in a summary of the literature that only about 10% of those at risk for Huntington's disease, for which there is no effective intervention, choose to have predictive testing. In contrast, they found the rate of "uptake" of susceptibility testing for breast cancer, for which some possibility of prevention and treatment exists, to be about 50% and the rate for familial adenomatous polyposis, for which effective treatments exist, to be about 80%.

Direct-to-consumer marketing of genetic testing may exacerbate the problems of informed consent. Gollust et al. (2002) examined existing advertisements and found that they overstate the value of testing and exploit consumers' fears to drive demand. Moreover, advertising is likely to convey misinformation about genetics, including simplistic, deterministic notions about the relationship of genes to disease. Clinicians must be familiar with the content of consumer-oriented advertisements to provide a more realistic picture of risks and benefits to their patients.

Are there circumstances in which it is unethical to provide genetic testing at all? At present, the answer to this among many ethicists is yes. The standard ethical analysis turns on two factors: the availability of effective interventions for the disorder and the predictive accuracy of the test. For example, professional societies and some ethicists have taken the position that it is unethical to provide apolipoprotein E gene (*APOE*) testing for susceptibility to Alzheimer's disease. Because the results of *APOE* testing are only modestly predictive, it is argued, and there are no effective interventions, the potential harms outweigh the benefits of testing. The possible harms that are most concerning relate to misidentification of risk status. For example, it is argued that individuals who in fact will not go on to develop a disorder may experience psychological distress and stigma as a result of testing. Moreover, there are negative consequences in the form of the utilization of scarce medical resources by worried individuals who are not destined to become ill (Nuffield Council on Bioethics 1998).

Tests that are predictive for disorders that are not presently treatable, such as Huntington's disease, and presenilin 1 testing for Alzheimer's disease are permissible (Burke et al. 2001; Nuffield Council on Bioethics 1998). The use of *APOE* testing for Alzheimer's disease has been opposed in a statement endorsed by the American Psychiatric Association, the American College of Medical Genetics, the American Society of Human Genetics, the American Academy of Neurology, and the Ethical, Legal, and Social Implications Working Group of the National Center for Human Genome Research (American Psychiatric Association 1995). How these guidelines will stand up in clinical practice is open to question. Family members at risk for a genetic disorder may strongly desire genetic information, even if it is only probabilistic. Even in the absence of interventions, this information may allow at-risk individuals to better order their lives in preparation for illness. Ethical proscription of testing is a key threshold issue, as it is likely that susceptibility testing, rather than predictive testing, will prevail in the field of psychiatry; and it may take many years to establish definitive proof of the efficacy of interventions in preventing onset.

Already, the ingredients exist to create ethical tension in psychiatric practice. As discussed earlier, *APOE* testing is considered unethical with respect to informing patients of their risk for developing Alzheimer's disease. However, general medical practitioners increasingly obtain *APOE* genotyping, which provides valuable information about lipid abnormalities, risk for the development of atherosclerosis and cardiovascular disease, and responsiveness to statins. Should physicians who obtain *APOE* testing to determine cardiovascular risk discuss the risk of Alzheimer's disease, refer patients to a professional competent to interpret the results, or remain silent? At least one leading ethics body, the Nuffield Council on Bioethics (1998), has suggested that physicians' duty to discuss and disclose the risk of Alzheimer's disease should be based on existing professional duties regarding nongenetic testing and the discovery of risk for conditions not under investigation. Absent legal precedent directly on point, one can only speculate about the nature and contours of such a duty. The problem is not simply whether to inform unwitting patients. Savvy individuals will know that their *APOE* genotype also relates to their risk for developing dementia. Psychiatrists may find themselves facing patients who have the results of *APOE* testing from primary care physicians and who have questions about their risk status. In this context, it would be best to provide information to help patients interpret the results in light of their individual circumstances. One might then ask if psychiatrists should inform patients about the availability of *APOE* testing—and how to obtain it—while underlining the probabilistic nature of genetic profiling, the absence of effective interventions, and the ethical bar to ordering the test? After all, informed consent is designed to level the field with respect to information disparities. This ethical conundrum is not easily resolved and remains an issue that individual psychiatrists may have to struggle with.

In the wake of testing, it is important that psychiatrists ascertain patients' understanding of the information they have received. In routine practice, checking patients' understanding would be part of the process of ensuring that adequate consent has been obtained. In the context of genetic testing, patients may misunderstand results in such a way as to alter subsequent decision making. Clinicians must take care at every step to ensure that their patients understand the implications and results of genetic testing.

It is too early to predict how services will develop and how standards of care will evolve. However, it is worth considering the ethical and social implications of the structure of services and how the structure of services may alter patients' decision making. One alternative to addressing the current shortfall in psychiatrists' understanding of genetic information would be to rely more heavily on genetic counselors. (However, this strategy is also problematic. Faraone et al. [1999] cited a National Institute of Mental Health survey finding that less than 13% of genetic counselors had received formal training in psychiatric genetics.) Although genetic counselors have adhered to an ethic of nondirective counseling, at least one study (Finn et al. 2005) indicated that psychiatrists, like other physicians (Geller et al. 1993; Marteau et al. 1994), are more likely to give directive advice. Inevitably, directive advice will convey physicians' views regarding the net value of disorders and the desirability of acting on genetic risk. Given the rapid growth in genetic knowledge across medical specialties, it is probable that allocation decisions will be made by insurers, health care systems, and governmental entities that will determine whether and what kind of testing and counseling services will be available to various segments of the population. These decisions may be affected by value judgments. For example, establishing financing and infrastructure for genetic testing for some disorders but not others will enable some personal choices and constrain others.

Premarital Testing

Premarital testing for genetic disorders is fraught with potential difficulties. One of the potential partners, if found to be carrying problematic genes, may experience injury to his or her self-image. In addition, there may be adverse consequences of disseminating this information to others. These issues may be addressed during the pretesting counseling and informed consent process. However, other useful models may be considered. For example, Dor Yeshorim is a service established in the 1980s to assist Ashkenazi Jews who are at higher risk for Tay-Sachs disease and several other Mendelian recessive diseases. Unmarried individuals register with Dor Yeshorim, are tested for the recessive alleles, and are assigned a unique identification number. Tested individuals are not informed of their carrier status. When a man and a woman reach the point in their relationship when they want to determine their risk for having affected children, both submit their registry numbers to the service. Only if both are carriers for the same disease will they be told of the 25% probability that a child born to them will have the disease. Participants are free to decide whether to continue their relationship, despite the risk of having an affected child, and perhaps may use prenatal testing to determine whether to continue with a pregnancy. For Orthodox Jews for whom abortion is usually not an option, the service allows participants to determine, by mutual consent and fairly early in a relationship, whether they would prefer to seek another partner. Whether this model can be applied to disorders with more complex patterns of inheritance is an open question.

Prenatal Testing

Prenatal testing affords parents an opportunity to elect a therapeutic abortion on the basis of the genetic endowment of the fetus. At present, tests of tissue samples obtained by amniocentesis are available for chromosomal abnormalities (e.g., Down syndrome) and single-gene conditions (e.g., Huntington's disease, early-onset Alzheimer's disease). A handful of preliminary studies suggest that there may be strong interest in prenatal testing for psychiatric disorders (Jones et al. 2002; Milner et al. 1998; Smith et al. 1996; Trippitelli et al. 1998). Prenatal screening for psychiatric disorders may be problematic for two reasons.

First, susceptibility testing will provide information about the relative risk that a fetus will develop a disorder. For example, the lifetime risk of developing bipolar disorder is 0.75% in the general population. Genetic testing that indicates a doubling of risk establishes a probability of 1.5% that the fetus will develop bipolar disorder. In this example, while the relative risk based on testing is high, the absolute risk remains low. Such a test would provide little information to prospective parents and is unlikely to materially affect decision making. At what level of risk of a psychiatric disorder might a reasonable person decide to abort a pregnancy? The response to the question will be driven by personal attitudes toward abortion and risk-taking, willingness and resources to care for an affected child, experience with and attitudes toward the disorder, and other unpredictable factors. However, it is likely that a genetic test would need to indicate a risk many-fold greater than the general population risk before prenatal testing would be sought by the public or recommended by professionals.

Second, genetic tests that indicate higher risks for psychiatric disorders raise questions about the consequences for the gene pool. What are the implications of the systematic elimination of carriers of genes for psychiatric disorders? For example, consider the case of bipolar disorder. There is some evidence that a predisposition to bipolar disorder is linked to creativity (Jamison 1993). If this is so, then reduction in the predisposing genes would lead to a corresponding reduction in creativity in the arts, literature, music, and science. It is interesting to note that in the eugenics era, scientists tended to support policies that would result in a selective narrowing of the gene pool. Now, with greater understanding of gene–environment interactions and the value of diversity, the pendulum has swung in the other direction. As Brosius and Kreitman (2000) have suggested, "it makes no evolutionary sense to drive our species through a man-made bottleneck of genetic uniformity." At this time, it is not clear how potential parents' interests can be harmonized with societal interest in maintaining a diverse gene pool. However, it is safe to conclude that the public, the medical profession, and other interested groups will need to work with policy makers to establish acceptable practices.

Testing Children

Genetic testing of children may arise in several contexts. Testing that contributes to diagnosis of an existing condition is not problematic. For example, a test for fragile X syndrome may be a part of the diagnostic workup of a child with delayed developmental milestones. Screening programs to identify conditions for which interventions exist, such as phenylketonuria, are justifiable. In both instances, testing results in benefits to identified children in the form of treatment and other targeted interventions. However, testing children for predisposition to disorders that might appear later in life raises significant ethical concerns. Identification of genetic susceptibility provides no benefit to the individual child and deprives the child of the opportunity to make the testing choice later in life. In addition, in some cases, as a result of their genetic risk, children may be treated differently by their families. For example, parents may discriminate against an at-risk child in favor of siblings with respect to allocation of resources for education and other opportunities. On the other side of the ethical scale stands the parents' right to know and to make family decisions as they see fit. For example, parents may want to be sure that they have some children who are free of a particular disorder. The most thoughtful analysis of the issue suggests that parents should not make decisions about testing their children for adult-onset disorders but should defer to the children themselves when they reach adulthood (Clark 1994; Nuffield Council on Bioethics 1998). The exception to this rule would arise when effective clinical interventions are available in childhood.

The Nuffield Council resolution is a good starting point, but it is all but certain that scientific and clinical advances will introduce greater complexity. Studies of gene–environment interactions, such as those that have been found in longitudinal studies of subjects in New Zealand carrying "long" or "short" forms of the gene that produces the serotonin transporter protein, are likely to yield a growing body of knowledge that will make line-drawing more difficult (Caspi et al. 2003). In the New Zealand study, for example, researchers found that subjects with at least one "short" allele of the gene were more likely to become depressed after stressful life events than subjects with two "long" alleles. Only among subjects with a "short" allele was a history of childhood maltreatment predictive of adult depression. Arguably, it might be possible to prevent such maltreatment in childhood, perhaps even setting the threshold for legal interventions (e.g., removing an abused child from the family) on the basis of genetic factors. Is that sort of intervention sufficient to warrant genetic testing under the Nuffield formulation? And any benefits of testing would have to be weighed against the risks that a child might be labeled "stress sensitive," which might easily result in being overprotected and developing a self-image as defective or weak.

Pharmacogenetic Profiling

Pharmacogenetic profiling or, as it is sometimes known, *pharmacogenomics,* is the study of the genetic basis for variable drug response. Emerging data regarding genetic determination of enzymatic pathways for drug metabolism or variability at sites of drug action have raised hopes that, in the future, treatments may be designed and prescribed on the basis of individuals' genetic endowment. For example, a psychiatrist might be able to select a specific antidepressant for a patient on the basis of a genetic test, reducing or eliminating the risk of untoward side effects, adverse drug reactions, or nonresponsiveness to treatment. In addition, there have been proposals that children and adults be screened for genetic polymorphisms that may affect drug action, including the serotonin transporter, which is a marker for depression risk (Kaplan 2005).

At first, it might appear that the use of genetic markers to predict drug response would raise fewer concerns than other uses of genetic information. However, some markers for drug responsiveness may also convey information about disease risk. As described in the earlier section on testing of adults, general practitioners may obtain patients' *APOE* profiles because they predict responsiveness to statins. As we know, these profiles also convey important information about susceptibility to Alzheimer's disease. Moreover, genetic information obtained for what appears to be low-risk purposes later may have broader and more significant implications in the face of scientific developments (Netzer and Biller-Andorno 2004).

At this juncture, it would appear that genetic test results obtained *for any purpose* should be regarded as having a range of possible future applications. Patients should be informed that the results of the tests may reveal genetic information that may have unknown implications in the future.

Ethical concerns regarding pharmacogenomics may extend to the prescription of medication. We may arrive at a time when the prescription of a medication conveys important information about an individual's genetic makeup. In this event, a physician's prescription may convey significant genetic information to the pharmacy that fills the prescription, the insurer that provides reimbursement, the schools and hospitals that dispense medications, and possibly others (Moldrup 2002).

Screening Potential Adoptees

Higher rates of psychopathology have been noted in adoptees and may be the result of multiple factors other than genetic risk (Nickman et al. 2005). Nonetheless, prospective adoptive parents would have a strong interest in information regarding candidate children's vulnerability to psychiatric disorders. Genetic screening, however, could create a class of "genetically tainted" unadoptables.

In a joint statement, the American Society of Human Genetics and the American College of Medical Genetics (ACMG) described the organizations' position on the use of genetic testing in the adoption process ("Genetic Testing in Adoption" 2000). The two groups took the position that 1) genetic testing of children in the adoptive process should be consistent with the tests performed on other children for the purposes of diagnosis or identification of preventive interventions; 2) genetic testing should be limited to testing for conditions that manifest in childhood, or for which preventive interventions may be undertaken in childhood; and 3) children in the adoptive process should not be tested for the purpose of detecting variations or predispositions to physical, mental, or behavioral traits that fall within the normal range. In sum, the scope of genetic testing of children in the pre-adoption phase should be the same as the scope of testing for children in general. This position rests explicitly on an ethical framework that places the interests of the child paramount. An adverse test result reduces a child's chance of being adopted or, if adopted, may lead the parents to treat the child differently ("Genetic Testing in Adoption" 2000).

The ASHG/ACMG position has been criticized on the grounds that the interests of potential adoptive parents are given little weight. An earlier generation may have readily said, "We'll leave this in God's hands." However, not all adoptive parents would endorse this view. As noted by the Nuffield Council on Bioethics (1998), it is not in the child's best interests to be adopted into a home, "if there is a risk that he or she will later be rejected because the adoptive parents had an incomplete understanding of the child they were adopting." Similarly, Jansen and Ross (2001) have argued that more extensive genetic testing should be allowed in order to better match potential adoptees with adoptive parents. In some cases, a more particularized assessment, including genetic testing, may be relevant to the matching process.

In the end, the application of genetic testing in adoption is unlikely to be settled by medical ethicists or professional organizations. Adoption is highly regulated and often subject to litigation. Unhappy adoptive parents frequently have been inclined to take their complaints of "wrongful adoption" to the courts. Adoption agencies, for example, are under legal obligation to provide prospective adoptive parents with information on the birth parents' physical and mental health histories that might be material to the decision to adopt (Freundlich and Peterson 1999). To date, no court has enunciated a legal obligation to obtain pre-adoption testing. However, given the liability risks adoption agencies face, it seems likely that once good clinical predictive testing is available, it will be implemented.

Discrimination

There is considerable concern about the privacy of genetic information and its potential use for discriminatory purposes by insurance companies and employers. A commonly expressed fear is that genetic information, which holds such promise to improve health and well-being, will be used for harm. These concerns are certain to chill individuals' interest in utilizing genetic testing until appropriate and accepted policies are implemented.

Defining the use of genetic testing by the insurance industry is particularly problematic. Allowing health, disability, and life insurance decisions to be made on the basis of genetic testing may result in the creation of a class of uninsurable people, whose genetic risk for illness is deemed sufficiently high that no company is willing to provide coverage at an affordable rate. Exclusion of high-risk individuals from the insurance pool would reduce the payouts faced by insurers, which would result in either lower premiums or higher profits. However, this approach would undermine an important function of insurance: spreading risk among a large cohort of persons. The more people who are excluded, the less the risk is spread. The net result is socially undesirable, as uninsured persons will face obstacles in gaining access to care and in providing security for their families. In the end, uninsured persons will continue to have health and economic needs that must be met in some way in a just society.

An opposing point of view, however, has been articulated. Raithatha and Smith (2004) have argued that it may be unethical not to use genetic test results, because they improve the accuracy of risk estimation, which is the foundation of insurance underwriting. Private insurance, they point out, is based on the pooling of premiums that reflect individuals' risk. On the basis of actuarial methods, insurers estimate the cost of medical care in the future. Applicants for insurance are required to disclose information relevant to risk assessment, including medical and family history and lifestyle. Insurers strive to make accurate predictions in order to price their policies competitively. If genetic test results are placed off-limits to the underwriters, then a "moral hazard" problem arises: persons who know themselves to be at high risk will have a higher likelihood of seeking insurance coverage. As a result of this adverse selection process, payouts—and then premiums—will rise, and persons with lower risks of adverse outcomes will be unable or unwilling to pay for coverage. The net result would be the creation of a different class of uninsured individuals with unmet health and economic needs.

Insurance discrimination on the basis of genetic information—as opposed to genetic testing—is the norm. Family medical history, for example, is a proxy risk factor that reflects genetic loading for disease. In one study, 25% of respondents reported that they had been denied life insurance, 22% had been refused health insurance, and 13% had failed to get a job, all presumably on the basis of their family medical histories of genetically based disorders (Lapham et al. 1996). Genetic testing, it should be recognized, would indicate that some of these individuals are not at risk for diseases that run in their families and would be valuable in helping them obtain insurance. On the other hand, if testing were to be required and applied systematically, the problems of discrimination and exclusion would undoubtedly be extended to people without family histories signaling high risk.

Employers have powerful incentives to screen out employees with genetic predispositions to illness in general and especially to disorders that are likely to arise in their industry. Health insurance rates, particularly for small employers, are sensitive to the utilization of health care. High utilization by one or two employees may make insurance unaffordable. The costs of workers' compensation and disability insurance are also driven by the claims experience of the company. In addition, the costs of illness are borne by employers as sick time erodes productivity. Therefore, employers have significant financial incentives to screen out potential employees who may be at higher risk for injuries, illness, or disability. Or, in the face of claims of job-related disability, employers may want to use genetic tests to prove that an illness or injury was not employment based. For example, the Burlington Northern Santa Fe Railroad performed DNA testing on employees seeking compensation for work-related carpal tunnel syndrome (New York Times 2001). The purpose of the test was to detect a genetic mutation associated with hereditary neuropathies that predisposed to pressure palsies. The company failed to inform employees of the purpose of the test. After the practice was halted by the Equal Employment Opportunity Commission, the company settled a lawsuit brought by the affected employees.

In the United States, the federal government has not taken action to prohibit or regulate the use of genetic tests by insurers or employers. However, almost every state has enacted some form of legislation preventing discrimination on the basis of genetic information (Clayton 2003). Most frequently, states have restricted the use of genetic tests (and family history information in some instances) in health insurance decisions. Approximately 20% of states have extended some degree of protection to those seeking life insurance. Roughly 60% of states also provide workers protection from discriminatory practices. Employees also receive strong protection from the American With Disabilities Act of 1990, which limits the use of health information in making employment decisions.

New Duties for Physicians

Because genetic tests convey information not only about the tested patient, but also about the patient's relatives, it is not surprising that the question has arisen of whether physicians should have corresponding new duties to affected individuals. The courts have begun to address whether physicians have a duty to warn family members of patients when tests indicate that the relatives may be at risk.

In *Safer v. Pack* (1996), the plaintiff was a woman whose father had died 40 years earlier of colon cancer due to familial adenomatous polyposis, a hereditary disease that results in numerous polyps of the colon and inevitably leads to colon cancer at a young age. Those who are aware of their genetic predisposition can be readily diagnosed by colonoscopy or radiological procedures and can be treated by prophylactic colectomy. Three decades after her father's condition was diagnosed, Ms. Safer, age 36 years, was found to have familial polyposis and metastatic carcinoma of the colon. Apparently, Dr. Pack, her father's physician, had never told the father or his family (Ms. Safer was 10 years old at the time of her father's death) about the underlying condition or its heritability, information known by the medical community at the time of the father's treatment. Ms. Safer, unaware of her high-risk status, took no precautions. The trial court dismissed the suit, stating that as Dr. Pack had no doctor-patient relationship with Ms. Safer, he had no duty to protect her. The New Jersey Superior Court reversed the ruling and held that a physician had a "duty to warn those known to be at risk of avoidable harm from a genetically transmissible condition." Presumably, the duty to warn family members, as articulated in this case, would override the patient's interest in confidentiality. The Florida Supreme Court, in *Pate v. Threlkell* (1995), enunciated a narrower duty—to warn the patient of the risk presented to family members—in a similar case involving a claim brought by the family of a patient with medullary carcinoma of the thyroid.

The *Safer v. Pack* and *Pate v. Threlkell* cases addressed physicians' duty to warn regarding hereditary diseases but did not specifically include consideration of information derived from genetic testing. To date, one court has addressed such a duty, but in circumstances that do not implicate a patient's right to privacy. In *Molloy v. Meier* (2004), the mother of a daughter with fragile X syndrome, a hereditary form of mental retardation, claimed that her child's physicians had failed to inform her (and her second husband) about the possibility that subsequently conceived children would be at risk for mental retardation. The Minnesota Supreme Court allowed the suit to go forward, holding that "a physician's duty regarding genetic testing and diagnosis extends beyond the patient to biological parents who foreseeably may be harmed by a breach of that duty."

Together, these cases suggest that courts are inclined to find that there is a duty to warn and that legal analyses will turn on three factors: 1) the likelihood that family members are at risk, 2) the severity of the potential consequences, and 3) whether effective interventions or actions exist to mitigate the risk. In *Safer v. Pack*, the plaintiff had a 50% chance of inheriting the autosomal dominant disorder, the consequences of untreated familial polyposis were potentially lethal, and an effective and proven intervention was available. Genetic testing for most psychiatric disorders is likely to involve one or more alleles that are associated with a moderate increase in relative risk (fragile X syndrome may be one of the few exceptions), the disorders themselves are treatable to some extent, and preventive measures are not likely to be available in the near future. Therefore, it will be difficult to justify warning family members directly, particularly if doing so would involve a breach of confidentiality. Of course, it would generally be good practice to advise the patient of any increased risk to family members, as this step would allow the patient to decide whether, and how, to share the information with others. This approach appears supported by public attitudes (Lehmann et al. 2000) and in practice by genetic counselors (Dugan et al. 2003) and therefore may evolve into a standard of care.

Ethics in Genetic Research

Research in psychiatric genetics is burgeoning and undoubtedly accounts for a considerable proportion of genetic testing in the mental health arena. Perhaps the most common and difficult ethical issue that arises in the research setting is the question of when subjects should be told the results of the tests they undergo. It is noteworthy that most of the associations of genetic loci with psychiatric disorders have not subsequently been confirmed. Moreover, the incremental increase in absolute risk from a single allele is likely to be small. It is likely that a number of alleles will be found to act together to increase susceptibility. Much research will be necessary to identify alleles, to determine their interactions, and to understand gene–environment interactions. And once valid information is available regarding meaningful genetic susceptibility, further research will be needed to develop and test effective interventions that might reduce the risk of developing the disorder in question.

Institutional review boards are responsible for the protection of research subjects and have the authority to determine whether and under what circumstances they should receive genetic test results obtained for research purposes. Anecdotal reports indicate that institutional review boards generally follow the consensus of ethicists and researchers that results of genetic research should not be revealed to subjects unless the effect on risk is substantial and intervention is possible (Appelbaum 2004). As research findings emerge, it will be necessary to decide how substantial a risk and how effective an intervention justify disclosure. It will also be necessary to determine at what point the weight of research findings reaches a level of reasonable certainty, with respect to both issues (Biesecker and Peay 2003). One might consider whether current research findings regarding the increased risk of depression with stress in individuals with the short allele for the serotonin transporter are sufficient to warrant disclosure. Does the directive to parents to "help your child avoid stress" qualify as an intervention? How should we weigh the absence of research findings regarding the effectiveness of the proposed intervention? Finally, we should consider whether subjects may have an interest in knowing their test results regardless of how substantial the risk is or whether interventions are available. For example, individuals at risk for Alzheimer's disease may make financial and other personal decisions based on risk status. It may be that a narrow focus on medical interventions does not do full justice to individuals' concerns.

Generally, results of genetic testing in psychiatric research will not be disclosed to family members, as their risk is less than that faced by the subjects. However, there is an exception to this general rule that is problematic. Often, when entire families are tested in the course of research, results indicate that specific children are not the progeny of the identified father. The standard practice in clinical settings (e.g., prenatal testing) is to inform the mother but not the father (Lucassen and Parker 2001). In the future, when genetic tests become more useful in defining risk status, disclosure of information may become justified. Failure to inform a father of his nonpaternity may mislead regarding his risk for a disorder and the risk that subsequent children of the couple will be affected. One suggestion is that the issue of nonpaternity be discussed with research participants prior to testing, at which point their preferences regarding whether such information should be disclosed—and to whom—could be ascertained (Lucassen and Parker 2001). Respecting the wishes of the family is probably the most reasonable way to address this issue.

Conclusions

The mental health field faces a range of ethical issues as a result of developments in psychiatric genetics. To a large extent, the ethical problems will be driven by the power of the genetic technologies. As the predictive powers of genetic tests increase, our ethical dilemmas will increase as well. Only time will tell where genetic research will take us.

Psychiatrists and other mental health professionals currently are not well informed about the science of genetics. Although grand rounds programs and continuing medical education schedules increasingly feature experts in the field of genetics, serious deficiencies in knowledge of the field are the rule among practicing psychiatrists. In residency training programs, significant time should be devoted to providing grounding in genetics to the next generation of psychiatrists. Professional organizations have only begun to focus attention on the implications of genetic developments for psychiatric practice. As the science moves into the clinic, it will be important for the professional groups to provide guidance to clinicians.

Educating professionals is a key step in the education of the public. Clinicians play a crucial role in guiding patients and will be in the front lines in applying new genetic technologies. However, it should be noted that the educational process is not a one-way street. An understanding of patients' concerns and interests will be a critical link in the iterative process of generating new professional practice norms in this area. It is critical for psychiatrists and other professionals to act as guides to patients and to advocates for their interests. Ultimately, the legal and ethical norms regarding the use of psychiatric genetics will be largely based on the wisdom distilled from doctor-patient interactions.

References

American Psychiatric Association: Use of apolipoprotein E testing for Alzheimer disease (policy statement approved by the Board of Trustees). Washington, DC, American Psychiatric Association, July 1995

Appelbaum PS: Ethical issues in psychiatric genetics. J Psychiatr Pract 10:343–351, 2004

Beauchamp TL, Childress JF: Principles of Biomedical Ethics. New York, Oxford University Press, 2001

Biesecker BB, Peay HL: Ethical issues in psychiatric genetics research: points to consider. Psychopharmacology (Berl) 171:27–35, 2003

Brakel SJ: Family laws, in The Mentally Disabled and the Law, 3rd ed. Edited by Brakel SJ, Parry J, Weiner BA. Chicago, IL, American Bar Foundation, 1985, pp 507–558

Brosius J, Kreitman M: Eugenics—evolutionary nonsense? Nat Genet 25:253, 2000

Buck v Bell, 274 US 200 (1927)

Burke W, Pinsky LE, Press NA: Categorizing genetic tests to identify their ethical, legal, and social implications. Am J Med Genet 106:233–240, 2001

Caspi A, Sugden K, Moffitt TE, et al: Influence of life stress on depression: moderation by a polymorphism in the 5-HTT gene. Science 301:386–389, 2003

Clark A: The Genetic Testing of Children: Report of a Working Party of the Clinical Genetics Society. London, Clinical Genetics Society, 1994

Clayton EW: Ethical, legal, and social implications of genomic medicine. N Engl J Med 349:562–569, 2003

Dugan RB, Wiesner GL, Juengst ET, et al: Duty to warn at-risk relatives for genetic disease: genetic counselors' clinical experience. Am J Med Genet C Semin Med Genet 119:27–34, 2003

ELSI Research and Evaluation Planning Group: A review and analysis of the Ethical, Legal, and Social Implications (ELSI) research programs at the National Institutes of Health and the Department of Energy (ERPEG Final Report). February 10, 2000. Available at: http://www.genome.gov/10001727. Accessed June 13, 2005.

Faroaone SV, Tsuang MT, Tsuang DW: Clinical applications of psychiatric genetics, in Genetics of Mental Disorders: A Guide for Students, Clinicians, and Researchers. New York, Guilford, 1999, pp 159–195

Finn CT, Wilcox MA, Korf BR, et al: Psychiatric genetics: a survey of psychiatrists' knowledge, opinions, and practice patterns. J Clin Psychiatry 66:821–830, 2005

Freundlich M, Peterson L: Wrongful adoption: litigation/practice issues. May 1999. Available at: http://www.lightlink.com/nysccc/wrongfuladopt/litigat-notes.htm. Accessed October 21, 2005.

Geller G, Tambor ES, Chase GA, et al: Incorporation of genetics in primary care practice: will physicians do the counseling and will they be directive? Arch Fam Med 2:1119–1125, 1993

Genetic testing in adoption. The American Society of Human Genetics Social Issues Committee and American College of Medical Genetics Social, Ethical, and Legal Issues Committee. Am J Hum Genet 66:761–767, 2000

Gollust SE, Hull SC, Wilfond BS: Limitations of direct-to-consumer advertising for clinical genetic testing. JAMA 288:1762–1767, 2002

Hassenfeld IN: Doctor-patient relationships in Nazi Germany and the fate of psychiatric patients. Psychiatr Q 73:183–194, 2002

Hodgkinson KA, Murphy J, O'Neill S, et al: Genetic counseling for schizophrenia in the era of molecular genetics. Can J Psychiatry 46:123–130, 2001

Hofman KJ, Tambor ES, Chase GA, et al: Physicians' knowledge of genetics and genetic tests. Acad Med 68:625–632, 1993

International HapMap Consortium: The International HapMap Project. Nature 426:789–796, 2003

International HapMap Consortium: Integrating ethics and science in the International HapMap Consortium. Nat Rev Genet 5:467–475, 2004

Jamison KR: Touched With Fire: Manic-Depressive Illness and the Artistic Temperament. New York, Free Press, 1993

Jansen LA, Ross LF: The ethics of preadoption genetic testing. Am J Med Genet 104:214–220, 2001

Jones I, Scourfield J, McCandless F, et al: Attitudes towards future testing for bipolar disorder susceptibility genes: a preliminary investigation. J Affect Disord 71:189–193, 2002

Kaplan A: Advances in pharmacogenomics reduce side effects and save lives. Psychiatric Times 32(7). June 2005. Available at: http://www.psychiatrictimes.com/showArticle.jhtml?articleId=164902190. Accessed Nov 8, 2005.

Kass L: Life, Liberty, and the Defense of Dignity: The Challenge for Bioethics. New York, Encounter Books, 2004

Lapham EV, Kozma C, Weiss JO: Genetic discrimination: perspectives of consumers. Science 274:621–624, 1996

Lehmann LS, Weeks JC, Klar N, et al: Disclosure of familial genetic information: perceptions of the duty to inform. Am J Med 109:705–711, 2000

Lucassen A, Parker M: Revealing false paternity: some ethical considerations. Lancet 357:1033–1035, 2001

Marteau TM, Croyle RT: The new genetics: psychological responses to genetic testing. BMJ 316:693–696, 1998

Marteau TM, Drake H, Bobrow M: Counseling following diagnosis of a fetal abnormality: the differing approaches of obstetricians, clinical geneticists, and genetic nurses. J Med Genet 31:864–867, 1994

Meyer J-E: The fate of the mentally ill in Germany during the Third Reich. Psychol Med 18:575–581, 1988

Milner KK, Collins EE, Connors GR, et al: Attitudes of young adults to prenatal screening and genetic correction for human attributes and psychiatric conditions. Am J Med Genet 76:111–119, 1998

Moldrup C: When pharmacogenomics goes public. New Genet Soc 21:29–37, 2002

Molloy v Meier, 679 NW 2d 711 (Minn 2004)

Netzer C, Biller-Andorno N: Pharmacogenetic testing, informed consent and the problem of secondary information. Bioethics 18:344–360, 2004

New York Times: Burlington Northern settles suit over genetic testing. April 19, 2001, p C4

Nickman SL, Rosenfeld AA, Fine P, et al: Children in adoptive families: overview and update. J Am Acad Child Adolesc Psychiatry 44:987–995, 2005

Nuffield Council on Bioethics: Mental Disorders and Genetics: The Ethical Context. West Sussex, UK, RPM Reprographics, 1998

Pate v Threlkell, 661 So 2d 278 (Fla 1995)

Raithatha N, Smith RD: Disclosure of genetic tests for health insurance: is it ethical not to? Lancet 363:395–396, 2004

Safer v Pack, 677 A 2d 1188 (NJ Super Ct 1996)

Smith LB, Sapers B, Reus VI, et al: Attitudes towards bipolar disorder and predictive genetic testing among patients and providers. J Med Genet 33:544–549, 1996

Trippitelli CL, Jamison KR, Folstein MF, et al: Pilot study on patients' and spouses' attitudes toward potential genetic testing for bipolar disorder. Am J Psychiatry 155:899–904, 1998

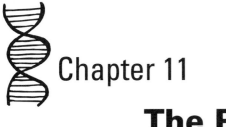

Chapter 11

The Road Ahead

Jordan W. Smoller, M.D., Sc.D.
Bruce R. Korf, M.D., Ph.D.

The interface of genetics and psychiatry has seen both exciting advances and frustrating setbacks. The role of familial and heritable influences on behavior and psychopathology has been recognized for more than a century. However, as reviewed by Hoge and Appelbaum in Chapter 12 ("Ethical, Legal, and Social Implications of Psychiatric Genetics and Genetic Counseling") of this volume, the early twentieth century saw the tragic perversion of genetic principles to justify eugenic policies in the United States and Europe. The merits of eugenics were even debated in mainstream psychiatric journals in the early twentieth century (Joseph 2005). This awful history cast a pall over genetic research and led many people to consider such research inherently suspect or even dangerous. Nevertheless, in the last 50 years, genetic research in psychiatry and other fields has made substantial contributions to our understanding of the etiology of rare and common medical disorders. The successful completion of the Human Genome Project and other recent milestones have facilitated rapid advances in genetic and genomic research that offer the potential to improve treatment and even prevention for a wide range of illness, including psychiatric illness.

Broadly speaking, we can discern three phases of modern psychiatric genetic research. In the first phase genetic epidemiologic studies–family, twin, and adoption studies–established that psychiatric disorders are familial and heritable. Indeed, to our knowledge, all of the modern psychiatric diagnoses for which family and twin studies are available have exhibited evidence of familial and genetic transmission. Spurred by this evidence and the advent of molecular genetic technologies, psychiatric genetics entered a second phase in the 1980s in which genetic linkage studies were undertaken to map the underlying genes. The successful mapping of the Huntington's disease locus in 1983 (Gusella et al. 1983) ushered in a period of optimism that genes for psychiatric disorders would be identified. Early estimates suggested that as few as 8–10 moderate-sized pedigrees might be required to map single major loci underlying psychiatric disorders (Gershon and Goldin 1987). Initial reports of significant linkage in extended pedigrees for schizophrenia and bipolar disorder supported this optimism (Baron et al. 1987; Egeland et al. 1987; Sherrington et al. 1988). Media reports trumpeting the discovery of the "gene for" manic depression or the "gene for" schizophrenia fueled expectations and created a kind of "irrational exuberance." However, replication of early findings proved more difficult than expected, and by 1996, the history of linkage studies for bipolar disorder was itself characterized as "manic depressive" for its cycle of dramatic successes followed by the demoralizing inability to replicate previous results (Risch and Botstein 1996).

In the latter half of the 1990s, a key realization put this pessimistic picture into context: as with most common medical conditions, the genetic basis of psychiatric disorders is likely to be complex. That is, common presentations of psychiatric disorders are likely to reflect the effects of multiple loci of modest effect interacting with other genetic and environmental factors. Rather than single-gene mutations that produce disease in most carriers by dramatic effects on cellular function, genetic variants contributing to psychiatric disorders may have small individual effects on susceptibility by subtly biasing the function of a biological system. Given this characteristic, we would not expect linkage analysis, which is best suited to mapping of single genes of major effect (such as the recessive mutations that cause cystic fibrosis), to provide consistent evidence of where a susceptibility gene is located.

Thus, the third phase of psychiatric genetics research (which is ongoing at this writing) has focused on psychiatric disorders as complex disorders. Association studies (see Chapter 1, "Psychiatric Genetics: A Primer"), which offer more power than linkage studies for studying complex traits, have become a predominant research strategy. This study design is used to examine whether specific variants or alleles of genes are statistically associated with disease risk in populations. Until recently, these studies have been limited by the need to study "candidate genes"—that is, genes that are suspected, a priori, of contributing to a phenotype. Because of our limited understanding of the biology of psychiatric illnesses, selecting appropriate candidate genes has been difficult. In large part, candidate genes have been chosen based on what we know about the targets of drugs that treat mental illness. For example, the serotonin transporter gene, which encodes the target of selective serotonin reuptake inhibitor (SSRI) antidepressants, has become one of the most widely studied candidates. Recently, however, the completion of the International HapMap project, as well as advances in genotyping technology and statistical methods, has made it possible to design and perform whole genome association studies. In these studies, essentially all of the common genetic variants in the genome are tested, directly or indirectly, with up to 1 million markers being used. Because of this approach, researchers are no longer constrained to study a limited set of candidate genes–the so-called usual suspects. Whole genome association analyses in psychiatry are under way as of this writing and are likely to reveal novel genetic influences on psychiatric disorders and medication response.

So, although the field of psychiatric genetics is, in many ways, still nascent, "the road thus far" has provided some information that is relevant for clinicians, patients, and families. As summarized in the previous chapters and in Table 11–1, the familial recurrence risks for first-degree relatives have been estimated from family studies. In addition, a number of "classic" single gene and chromosomal disorders may have psychiatric presentations. Psychiatrists familiar with these conditions may identify patients who would benefit from referral to genetics professionals and from monitoring of or intervention for the underlying genetic disorder.

What about the "the road ahead"? Where is this road likely to lead, and what are some of the issues that psychiatrists, genetic counselors, and others involved in the care of patients with psychiatric illness are likely to face? As Niels Bohr is reputed to have said, "Prediction is very difficult, especially about the future." With this caveat in mind, we suggest that a number of foreseeable themes may emerge as genetic medicine continues along its path to the clinic. In particular, we highlight the potential of genetic research to inform three clinically relevant domains: drug development, personalized medicine, and our understanding of the role of the gene-environment interaction.

Role of Gene Identification and Characterization in Treatment Development

A central goal of psychiatric genetic research has been the identification of susceptibility genes and the elucidation of their role in the development of psychiatric illness. Our understanding of the pathogenesis and neurobiology of mental illnesses remains limited. Reflecting these limitations, the development of psychotropic drugs has focused on a restricted set of fa-

TABLE 11–1. Estimated empiric risks to first-degree relatives for several disorders

Disorder	Risk, %[a]	RRR[b]	References
Autism	2–8	50–100	Muhle et al. 2004
Alzheimer disease (late-onset)	27–44	2	Green et al. 2002
Schizophrenia	5–16	10	NIMH Genetics Workgroup 1998; Tsuang 2000
Bipolar disorder	4–13	10	Smoller and Finn 2003
Major depressive disorder	15–30	3	Smoller and Finn 2003; Sullivan et al. 2000
Panic disorder	8–17	5	Hettema et al. 2001
Phobic disorders	10–31	4	Hettema et al. 2001
Generalized anxiety disorder	9–20	6	Hettema et al. 2001
Obsessive-compulsive disorder	1–12	4	Hettema et al. 2001
Alcoholism	29–37	2–4	Merikangas et al. 1998; Nurnberger et al. 2004
ADHD	16–25	2–8	Faraone et al. 2001, 2005
Anorexia nervosa[c]	1–7	11	NIMH Genetics Workgroup 1998; Strober et al. 2000
Bulimia nervosa[c]	2–10	4	NIMH Genetics Workgroup 1998; Strober et al. 2000

Note.   ADHD=attention-deficit/hyperactivity disorder; RRR=recurrence risk ratio.
[a]Approximate absolute risk to first-degree relatives of affected proband.
[b]Approximate relative risk to first-degree relatives of affected proband.
[c]Risk estimates based on female relatives.

miliar targets. For example, almost all available antidepressant drugs were developed to target monoaminergic receptors and transporters (Berton and Nestler 2006). Since the 1960s, almost all new marketed antidepressant drugs have focused on binding to serotonin and/or norepinephrine transporters and receptors. Most of these drugs have been "me-too" agents that act as serotonin reuptake inhibitors (e.g., SSRIs) and serotonin-norepinephrine reuptake inhibitors. Although these drugs are superior to placebo, remission rates are typically less than 50% in clinical trials (Thase et al. 2005), and there are no clear-cut differences in efficacy for most commonly used antidepressants (Hansen et al. 2005).

There has been a long-standing hope that identification of genes involved in the pathophysiology of psychiatric disorders will reveal novel and more effective targets for drug development. This effort should be facilitated by newer approaches to gene identification that make use of so-called unbiased methods. As noted earlier, genetic association studies in psychiatry have, until recently, focused on a set of "usual suspects"–that is, genes that reflect our limited understanding of the neurobiology of illness and drug mechanisms. As a result, we have a vast number of studies that have examined the serotonin transporter gene (*SLC6A4*), catechol-*O*-methyl transferase gene (*COMT*), and monoamine oxidase A gene (*MAOA*). Although these genes are undoubtedly strong candidates for involvement in a range of psychiatric disorders, they undoubtedly represent only a fraction of the genes involved. In addition, because they were derived largely from our assumptions about the action of known therapeutic agents, they are unlikely to reveal new approaches to treatment, even if unequivocal association can be demonstrated. Fortunately, by making use of available data and advances in laboratory and statistical methods, we are now in a position to move beyond our bias toward this narrow set of genes. At least three approaches illustrate this path along the "road ahead."

The first is the identification of *positional candidate genes*. Although genome scan linkage studies have not conclusively identified the location of susceptibility genes for major psychiatric disorders, the accumulated results of two decades of these studies are providing strong evidence that certain chromosomal regions harbor genes for schizophrenia, bipolar disorder, and other illnesses. For example, with the use of meta-analysis to combine the results of linkage studies, strong signals have emerged for schizophrenia (Levinson et al. 2003) and bipolar disorder (McQueen et al. 2005). With evidence that a chromosomal region contains one or more genes influencing a disorder, one can focus a search on genes in the linked region. These genes are strong candidates based on their chromosomal position and do not require us to have prior evidence of their role in the disorder. By thoroughly examining the region, researchers may uncover association with genes whose involvement had not been suspected. This approach has already borne fruit. Several of the genes that have accrued the strongest evidence of association with schizophrenia were revealed by detailed linkage disequilibrium mapping of chromosomal regions linked to the disorder. These genes include those for neuregulin (*NRG1*) on chromsome 8p (Stefansson et al. 2002), dysbindin (*DTNBP1*) on chromosome 6p (Straub et al. 2002), and *d*-amino acid oxidase activator (*DAOA*) on chromosome 13q (Chumakov et al. 2002). Such findings have stimulated vigorous efforts to characterize the functional effects of these genes. Dissecting these effects may reveal new pathogenetic pathways and, as a result, novel targets for intervention. For example, studies of neuregulin have implicated diverse effects on neuronal migration, neurite growth, and modulation of neurotransmitter receptor expression (Scolnick et al. 2006). Characterizing the effects of the gene for such a protein may reveal an entire network of upstream and downstream molecules that contribute to the biology of schizophrenia and that could be "druggable targets."

A second approach to expanding the search for susceptibility genes has only recently become feasible—*whole genome association analysis*. With advances in high-throughput genotyping technology and bioinformatics as well as statistical methods for handling large amounts of data and statistical tests, it has become possible to examine hundreds of thousands of genetic markers throughout the genome. Completion of the HapMap project has vastly reduced the number of single nucleotide polymorphisms that must be typed to cover the genome, thereby reducing the costs of whole genome studies to realistic levels. By effectively capturing most of the genetic variation among individuals, these methods allow an unbiased search of the entire genome for alleles that influence psychiatric and other complex disorders (de Bakker et al. 2005). This approach has been successfully used to identify susceptibility genes for a growing range of complex medical conditions, including age-related macular degeneration (Klein et al. 2005), obesity (Herbert et al. 2006), type 2 diabetes (Grant et al. 2006), and QT interval prolongation (Grant et al. 2006). Whole genome association studies of psychiatric disorders are ongoing. Again, because they do not require a pre-specified hypothesis about which genes are important, these methods offer the opportunity to uncover novel "players" in the biology of disease risk or response to treatment. However, as in the case of positional candidates, it should be noted that even if association studies clearly implicate a gene, this finding is only a beginning. A great deal of work may be needed to characterize the functional effects of the associated gene, clarify its role in the illness, and determine if and how it might be therapeutically modulated by a drug.

A third resource for "unbiased" approaches to gene discovery and characterization involves *gene expression analysis*. Gene expression studies can be used to quantify and compare relative amounts of mRNAs between two samples—for example, postmortem brain tissue from ill versus non-ill individuals (Bunney et al. 2003). Genes that are over- or underexpressed in a disorder may be candidates for therapeutic modulation by pharmacotherapy. Microarray technologies now enable researchers to examine simultaneously the expression of many thousands of genes. The profile or "signature" of gene expression in a disease state might also be used to define illness subtypes that may respond to specific treatments (as has been done successfully for certain malignancies) (Quackenbush 2006). Gene expression signatures of drugs known to be effective might also be used to predict whether a novel compound is likely to be a good antidepressant, antipsychotic, or mood stabilizer (Gunther et al. 2003).

Although the work of moving psychiatric genetic findings from "bench to bedside" is in its early stages, advances in other areas of medicine provide reason for optimism. The defining of genetic lesions that underlie several malignancies has led to chemotherapeutic drugs that offer greater effectiveness and reduced toxicity (at least for defined subsets of patients). A pioneering example was the development of imatinib, which targets the BCR-ABL tyrosine kinase involved in the pathogenesis of chronic myeloid leukemia (Savage and Antman 2002). In neuropsychiatry, a similar strategy is being used to advance drug treatment based on genetic findings. For example, drug therapies for Alzheimer's disease that act by inhibiting brain acetylcholinesterase have offered only modest benefit. Newer drugs targeting proteins implicated by genetic findings (e.g., amyloid-β) are under development and may offer more specific and effective interventions by more directly targeting the pathophysiology of the disease.

Pharmacogenetics and Personalized Medicine

Arguably, one of the most immediate clinical applications of genetic research may come in the realm of pharmacogenetics. *Pharmacogenetics* refers to "the study of the role of inheritance in inter-individual variation in drug response" (Weinshilboum and Wang 2004). The related domain of pharmacogenomics is concerned with the genome as a source of drug targets or as a resource for stratifying disease for drug-response predictors. The potential benefit of identifying genetic predictors of drug response is clear, given the current state of psychopharmacological treatment. Although clinicians have a range of effective medications for the treatment of psychotic, mood, anxiety, and other disorders, prescribing for an individual patient remains largely a trial-and-error proposition. For example, although the majority of patients with depression may ultimately respond to antidepressant therapy, most will not experience remission of depression with an individual medication trial (Trivedi et al. 2006; Whooley and Simon 2000). At present, clinicians have little a priori basis for identifying the most effective agent for a given patient. The cost of each ineffective medication trial may include weeks of unremitted illness, attendant functional impairment, and possible medication nonadherence. Adverse drug reactions, ranging from minor to life-threatening in severity, limit the use or dosing of many otherwise effective medications. For example, clozapine, recognized to have superior effectiveness, requires hematologic monitoring and is not recommended for first-line use given the risk (~ 1%) of agranulocytosis. The ability to identify patients for whom agranulocytosis risk is negligible might make this agent available to many more patients. (It should be noted, however, that the degree to which agranulocytosis is related to heritable genetic factors has not yet been determined.)

Clinicians in training are often taught that family history can help guide drug selection. For example, in selecting an antidepressant, one might favor fluoxetine if there is a family history of good response to fluoxetine. It is surprising that the evidence base for this widespread teaching is fairly scant. Studies of the familiality of drug response are few and have typically involved small samples. In a study of 45 first-degree relative pairs treated with fluvoxamine for at least 6 weeks, Franchini et al. (1998) found that 30 (67%) were concordant for response, which the authors concluded was greater than the 50% expected by chance. In another small study, unequivocal response to lithium was more common among bipolar disorder patients who were relatives of lithium responders than among a comparison group of bipolar disorder patients (Grof et al. 2002). However, there has been little other direct evidence supporting the familial nature of psychotropic drug response.

In modern pharmacogenetics, an aim is to identify specific genetic variants that could predict drug effectiveness or tolerability for individual patients, a goal that has been called "personalized medicine." Pharmacogenetically relevant genes are often divided into two groups: 1) those that predominantly affect pharmacokinetics, most notably drug-metabolizing enzymes such as the P450 enzymes and 2) those that predominantly affect pharmacodynamics (i.e., genes that encode neurotransmitter transporters, receptors, and other therapeutic drug targets).

Pharmacokinetic Genes

A pharmacogenetic test that is relevant to psychiatry and that has been approved by the U.S. Food and Drug Administration was marketed in 2004. It is used to test two pharmacokinetic genes that are commonly involved in the metabolism of antidepressants and antipsychotics: cytochrome P450

2D6 and 2C19 (Mrazek et al. 2006). These enzymes affect the disposition of a broad range of psychotropics. It has been estimated that 2D6 is the major metabolic pathway for 25% of all prescribed drugs, and four of the most prescribed 2D6-metabolized drugs in 2003 were antidepressants (Phillips and Van Bebber 2005). Individual differences in 2D6 and 2C19 phenotype can result from differences in the number and activity of the genes encoding these enzymes. For example, individuals with two nonfunctional P450 2D6 genes (approximately 7% of Caucasians, and 1%–2% of Asians and African Americans) have a "poor metabolizer" genotype that renders their 2D6 enzymes inactive. Studies of volunteers and patients have documented that plasma levels of several antidepressant and antipsychotic medications are elevated in individuals who carry a poor metabolizer genotype at 2D6 or 2C19 (Desta et al. 2002; Kirchheiner et al. 2004). For example, plasma levels may be 10-fold higher for a given dose of nortriptyline among poor metabolizers, compared with ultra-rapid metabolizers (Ingelman-Sundberg 2004). Plasma levels have similarly been reported to vary by 2D6 genotype for other drugs, including haloperidol (Brockmoller et al. 2002) and paroxetine (Sindrup et al. 1992).

Despite the importance of these enzymes for antidepressant metabolism, data supporting a role for P450 genotype in drug response or adverse drug effects remain limited. For antidepressants, adverse events related to drug-metabolizing enzymes have mainly been limited to case reports and small studies (Bertilsson et al. 1981; Lessard et al. 1999; Spina et al. 1997). In other studies an association between adverse drug reactions and 2D6 genotype has not been observed (Murphy et al. 2003; Roberts RL et al. 2004). For example, in a randomized controlled trial of 246 patients with geriatric depression, 2D6 genotypes were not associated with adverse drug reactions or therapeutic drug response among patients treated with paroxetine or mirtazapine (Murphy et al. 2003).

Several antipsychotics are substrates of P450 2D6, including thioridazine, perphenazine, haloperidol, risperidone, and aripiprazole. In case reports and small studies, clinically significant adverse reactions have been reported among 2D6 poor metabolizers taking typical antipsychotics, including perphenazine and haloperidol (Scordo and Spina 2002), and 2D6 poor metabolizer status is a contraindication for thioridazine because of the potential for increased risk of cardiac arrhythmia and prolongation of the corrected QT interval among these patients. Mixed results have been reported in studies examining the role of P450 genotype on movement-related adverse effects of antipsychotics (Andreassen et al. 1997; Arthur et al. 1995; Bertilsson et al. 2002; Brockmoller et al. 2002; de Leon et al. 2005b; Kapitany et al. 1998; Ohmori et al. 1999; Schillevoort et al. 2002; Tiwari et al. 2005; Vandel et al. 1999). In one naturalistic study of 325 patients in stable condition while taking risperidone and 212 patients with a history of risperidone discontinuation, de Leon et al. (2005a) reported a threefold increased odds of moderate to marked adverse drug reactions in the patients taking risperidone and as much as a sixfold increased odds of risperidone discontinuation due to adverse drug reactions among 2D6 poor metabolizers.

Approximately 1%–10% of Caucasians and 2% of African Americans have an ultra-rapid metabolism genotype at 2D6, resulting from duplicated and/or high-activity 2D6 alleles (de Leon et al. 2006). Pharmacokinetic data and case reports suggest that patients with an ultra-rapid metabolizer genotype who are treated with 2D6 substrates may require higher than usual doses to achieve therapeutic response (Brockmoller et al. 2002; Kawanishi et al. 2004; Kirchheiner et al. 2004).

For many psychotropic agents, however, clear concentration-response relationships have not been established, and more research is needed to determine whether genotype-based alternative drug selection or dose modification alters clinical outcome. Genotype-specific antidepressant and antipsychotic guidelines for dosing or drug selection for poor metabolizers and ultra-rapid metabolizers have been proposed (de Leon et al. 2006; Kirchheiner et al. 2001, 2004). However, because most studies that have examined drug levels or outcomes by genotype have been relatively small and have varied in terms of whether single-dose or repeated dosing was used, definitive recommendations are difficult to derive at present. In addition, the effect of such dose alterations on clinical outcomes has yet to be established.

Pharmacodynamic Genes

Although pharmacogenetic testing of drug-metabolizing enzymes has been the first to reach clinical psychiatry, more research attention has focused on genes involved in pharmacodynamic actions of drugs. The known targets of available drugs suggest compelling candidate genes for drug response and toxicity. One of the most obvious is the gene for the serotonin transporter (*5-HTT*), because the serotonin transporter is the target of SSRI antidepressants. As reviewed in Chapter 6 ("Genetics of Mood and Anxiety Disorders"), the serotonin transporter length polymorphic region (5-HTTLPR) of this gene has a common variation that affects the gene expression and transporter levels. The "short" or "*s*" allele, associated with reduced *5-HTT* expression, has been associated with reduced or delayed response to SSRI treatment in several, although not all studies (Kim et al. 2006). In a combined analysis of six studies, Smits et al. (2004) concluded that results showed substantial heterogeneity across studies but overall supported a reduced response to SSRIs with the *s/s* genotype, compared with other genotypes. Still, the magnitude of this effect was relatively modest: mean decreases in depression scores at week 4 were 35.4%, 46.3%, and 48.0% for patients with the *s/s*, *s/l*, and *l/l* genotypes, respectively. A somewhat larger difference was seen in studies that included only Caucasian patients. A recent meta-analysis of 15 studies found significant evidence of association between 5-HTTLPR genotype and antidepressant treatment outcomes, again with more consistent results in Caucasian samples, compared with Asian samples (Serretti et al. 2007). Overall, the results indicated that individuals carrying the *l/l* genotype have a 2-fold increased odds of favorable response and a 2.57-fold increased odds of favorable response in the first 4 weeks of treatment, compared to those carrying the short allele. The 5-HTTLPR short allele has also been implicated in adverse drug reactions (Murphy et al. 2004), including insomnia/agitation (Perlis et al. 2003) and switching to mania (Masoliver et al. 2006; Mundo et al. 2001; Popp et al. 2006), but this relationship remains to be established. A variety of other genes have been associated with psychotropic drug response in at least some studies (Malhotra et al. 2004). These findings include a reported association between a single nucleotide polymorphism marker in the serotonin 5-HT_{2A} receptor gene and antidepressant response in a large study ($N=1,953$) of patients treated with the SSRI citalopram. In that study, homozygosity for one allele of the associated single nucleotide polymorphism was associated with an 18% lower risk of nonresponse to citalopram, compared with homozygosity for the other allele.

Although there may be differences in drug response by genotype, it remains to be seen whether the available findings will translate into clinically useful tests. Like psychiatric disorders themselves, drug response is a complex trait that reflects the influence of multiple genes and nongenetic factors. Predicting a large share of the variance in treatment response may require simultaneously testing multiple contributing genetic variants. Findings in a study of clozapine response suggest that such an approach could be clinically informative. Arranz and colleagues (Mrazek et al. 2006) reported that a combination of six polymorphisms (from the 5-HT_{2A} and 5-HT_{2C} receptor genes, the 5-HTTLPR variation, and a variant in the H_2 receptor gene) correctly predicted positive response to clozapine in 76% of cases in a sample of 200 treated patients. Although this finding awaits replication, it suggests that a highly predictive test could be assembled by assaying multiple variants. Newer microarray technology, in which a large number of tests can be performed simultaneously, should facilitate such an approach. Perlis et al. (2005) reported that the test described by Arranz and colleagues could be used cost-effectively to triage certain patients to first-line use of clozapine. The estimated additional cost of using the test to identify predicted clozapine responders and treating them with clozapine first was $47,705 per additional quality-adjusted life-year compared with not testing and using clozapine only for treatment-resistant patients. This cost is comparable to that of other medical interventions that are considered cost-effective.

In addition to developing tests that have adequate predictive value and are cost-effective, a third prerequisite for clinical utility is demonstrating that such tests can improve patient outcomes. Such outcomes may include more rapid or robust therapeutic response, fewer adverse drug reactions, and improved quality of life and patient satisfaction. This demonstration will likely require prospective, randomized studies comparing outcomes when clinicians are given pharmacogenetic information versus outcomes with treatment as usual (Kirchheiner et al. 2005).

Genetic Counseling and Genetic Testing

As reviewed in other chapters in this volume, family and genetic studies have already provided clinically relevant information for a range of psychiatric disorders and genetic disorders with psychiatric manifestations. In the years ahead, as specific susceptibility genes involved in psychiatric disorders are identified, genetic counseling for psychiatric disorders may move beyond estimating recurrence risks based only on family study data.

Genetic Counseling

If patients or families request genetic counseling, which clinicians are best suited to provide it? The answer may involve a collaborative approach on the part of at least two groups of practitioners: genetics professionals and psychiatrists. Genetics professionals–including genetic counselors, geneticists, and advanced practice nurses–have advanced training in genetics. They are experts in understanding and relaying information regarding the genetic basis of disease and are trained to facilitate decision making and provide counseling in a nondirective manner. Nevertheless, the complexities of diagnosis in psychiatry can make counseling for these disorders challenging for a clinician with little exposure to or training in psychiatry. Peay and McInerney (2002) surveyed 201 practicing genetic counselors and genetic counseling students regarding their ability to provide genetic counseling for major psychiatric disorders. A substantial proportion reported feeling "somewhat" to "very" unprepared to raise the issue of psychiatric disease with consultands (32% of practicing genetic counselors and 67% of genetic counseling students) or to answer questions regarding psychiatric illness raised by their clients (44% of practicing genetic counselors and 96% of genetic counseling students). When taking a family history, 22% of practicing genetic counselors and 46% of genetic counseling students reported raising issues related to psychiatric illness "seldom to never." This finding may not be surprising, because psychiatric illnesses have not been a traditional component of genetics training.

In contrast, psychiatrists are experienced in psychiatric diagnoses, course of illness, treatment options, and appreciation of psychodynamic issues related to counseling, but may be less experienced with principles of genetics and the communication of probabilistic risk. Findings from the largest survey to date of psychiatrists' genetic knowledge suggested that practicing psychiatrists may be unfamiliar with aspects of medical and psychiatric genetics relevant to genetic counseling (Finn et al. 2005). For a series of questions dealing with general knowledge of genetic principles, psychiatrists answered a median of only 44% correctly, significantly less than a group of genetic counselors and a group of endocrinologists who were administered the same questions. Psychiatrists also correctly answered a median of only 33% of a series of questions dealing specifically with psychiatric genetics. When presented with a hypothetical counseling scenario involving a fetus at high risk for a variety of psychiatric or medical conditions, 33% of psychiatrists said they would counsel in a "directive" manner, advising pregnancy termination or continuation. This result is consistent with other study findings that clinicians without expertise in genetics may be more directive in genetic counseling than are genetics professionals (Geller et al. 1993; Marteau 1999). The majority of psychiatrists responding to the survey thought that they lacked competence in the area of genetic knowledge (77%) and that their medical training had failed to prepare them for conveying genetic information to patients and their families (85%). Nevertheless, more than 80% thought that it was their role to do so, and 93% said that they discuss genetic contributions to illness with at least some of their patients (Finn et al. 2005). If faced with a patient who asks about recurrence risk of mental illness in her child, more than 70% said they would address such questions themselves rather than refer to a genetic counselor. Given that genetic counseling for complex disorders is among the most challenging topics encountered by genetics professionals, gaps in genetic knowledge may become a major limiting factor in psychiatrists' ability to provide counseling.

The results of the studies reviewed in this section suggest that both genetics professionals and psychiatrists could benefit from further education in issues relevant to psychiatric genetics. Ultimately, a multidisciplinary and collaborative approach between psychiatrists and genetics professionals may provide the best outcome for patients and their families. For example, genetics professionals may be particularly well-equipped to evaluate and counsel patients about medical genetic disorders that may underlie psychiatric symptoms, to interpret pedigree-related risks, and to coordinate genetic testing (as that becomes available), whereas the expertise of a psychiatrist may be essential in counseling about the course of, and treatment options for psychiatric illness that may run in families.

Genetic Testing

As reviewed by Finn and Smoller (2006), findings from several studies suggest that patients and families would welcome the availability of genetic counseling and genetic testing for psychiatric disorders (Austin and Honer 2005; Jones et al. 2002; Meiser et al. 2005; Milner et al. 1998, 1999; Quaid et al. 2001; Smith et al. 1996; Trippitelli et al. 1998). For example, in one survey of 45 individuals with bipolar disorder and their spouses (Trippitelli et al. 1998), all of the affected individuals indicated that they would definitely or probably take a genetic test for bipolar disorder. Most spouses (80%) also said they would definitely or probably be tested themselves, and 85% said they would definitely or probably want to know the results of their affected spouse's test. Asked about the potential benefits of testing, the majority of patients and spouses felt that the most important benefit was "to obtain treatment to prevent attacks," and no respondents felt that the potential risks and costs of testing (including psychological and financial ones) outweighed the benefits. A majority of patients and spouses also felt that it would be appropriate to test presymptomatic minors for a gene for bipolar disorder, and nearly half supported prenatal testing. Nevertheless, most respondents said that they would not abort a fetus that tested positive for a gene for bipolar disorder.

Smith et al. (1996) reported similar results in their survey of mental health support group members, medical students, and psychiatry residents who showed substantial interest in the hypothetical use of genetic testing for bipolar disorder for diagnostic, preventive, and reproductive purposes. The predictive value of the test, the course of disorder, and the availability of prophylactic treatment appeared to influence attitudes toward testing. For example, 89% favored testing of presymptomatic children if prophylactic drug treatments were available, but this figure declined to 56% in the absence of such treatment. When the respondents were asked about pregnancy termination, only about 10% indicated they would terminate a pregnancy if a fetus had a 25% risk of developing bipolar disorder, but 40%–60% would do so if the risk of disorder were 100%. Similarly, only 5% said they would terminate if the child was likely to experience a mild course of illness (single episode of mania and depression), whereas 75% would terminate if the expected course of illness was severe (e.g., severe suicide risk, 50% of lifetime hospitalized).

In a survey in the United Kingdom that included individuals with bipolar disorder and a group of psychiatrists, Jones et al. (2002) found that affected individuals were significantly more positive than were psychiatrists about the prospect of presymptomatic testing of adults and children, as well as about prenatal testing (although most respondents in both groups did not favor prenatal testing). In another survey of several hundred psychiatrists, Finn et al. (2005) found that a majority would favor use of an accurate genetic test for schizophrenia or bipolar disorder to clarify diagnosis or as a prenatal test in affected families.

Such surveys must be interpreted cautiously, however, because the testing scenarios implied in these studies usually involved highly predictive single-gene tests. Such tests are not available now, and, given the complex, multifactorial etiology of most psychiatric disorders, they may never be. In addition, estimating demand based on hypothetical testing scenarios may be misleading. Prior to the availability of testing for the Huntington's disease mutation, several surveys indicated that demand for testing would be substantial, but actual utilization of the test has been closer to the 10%–15% range (Kessler et al. 1987; Meiser and Dunn 2000). Nevertheless, advances in psychiatric genetics research raise the prospect that specific variants in susceptibility genes may be established within the foreseeable future. In theory, there are two scenarios in which testing could be applied (Finn and Smoller 2006).

First, and already available, is genetic testing for several highly penetrant single-gene or chromosomal abnormalities that can cause psychiatric symptoms (see Table 11–2). One example, discussed in Chapter 5 ("Genetics of Schizophrenia and Psychotic Disorders"), involves velocardiofacial/ DiGeorge syndrome, which is caused by a microdeletion of chromosome 22q11 that occurs in 1 in 4,000 live births. In addition to a variety of physical features, individuals with velocardiofacial syndrome have elevated risks of psychiatric symptoms. In particular, rates of psychotic disorders have been reported to be as high as 25%–30% (Bassett and Chow 1999; Murphy 2002). It is interesting to note that the features of schizophrenia in patients with velocardiofacial syndrome are not readily distinguishable from the phenotype of schizophrenia in patients without velocardiofacial syndrome (Bassett et al. 2003). The prevalence of unrecognized velocardiofacial syndrome in patients with schizophrenia may be as high as 1 in 50 (Bassett et al. 1999), and the syndrome may be even more common among those with schizophrenia and a history of developmental delay (Bassett et al. 2003). Diagnostic testing for the deletion is available by using a blood sample processed through fluorescence in situ hybridization (FISH) (http://genetests. org) or array comparative genomic hybridization, and such testing may be indicated when other characteristic features accompany psychotic disor-

TABLE 11–2. Available genetic tests for phenotypes relevant to psychiatry

Phenotype	Test	Comments
Velocardiofacial syndrome	Fluorescence in situ hybridization	Also detectable using array comparative genomic hybridization
Fragile X syndrome	Southern analysis and/or polymerase chain reaction for expanded CGG repeat	Premutation female carriers may have increased risk of depression
Huntington's disease	Polymerase chain reaction for expanded CAG repeat	
Acute intermittent porphyria	*HMBS* mutations	Characterized by anxiety, "histrionic personality"; medications that upregulate P450 enzymes may exacerbate symptoms

ders (Murphy and Owen 2001). Other specific single-gene disorders and chromosomal abnormalities have also been associated with psychiatric phenotypes (see Chapter 8, "Neuropsychiatric Aspects of Genetic Disorders," in this volume). Thus, one application of genetic testing in the psychiatric setting would be for rare subtypes of psychiatric disorder that are attributable to specific genetic lesions.

A second, less straightforward use of testing would involve testing for susceptibility variants in the more common, complex, multifactorial forms of psychiatric illness. To date, findings from psychiatric genetics research suggest that individual effects of susceptibility genes for common forms of psychiatric disorders are likely to be modest. As described in Chapter 6, one of the most widely studied genetic variants in psychiatry has been a functional promoter polymorphism (5-HTTLPR) in the serotonin transporter gene (whose protein product is the target of SSRI antidepressants). Although findings have been mixed, several studies have indicated that the short allele of this polymorphism is associated with depression, but only in the setting of stressful life events (Caspi et al. 2003; Eley et al. 2004; Kaufman et al. 2004; Kendler et al. 2005). Even in these studies, however, the allele appears to account for only a small proportion of the risk for depression. Clearly, the small effect size and the importance of gene–environment interactions for the expression of risk make it difficult to conceive of a useful genetic test for such a susceptibility gene. The results of studies of other genes suggest that such small effects are likely to be the rule rather than the exception for common psychiatric disorders. Thus, tests of susceptibility gene variants would yield only probabilistic results, and their positive predictive value is likely to be low. As Ware (2006) recently pointed out, even well-validated risk factors can perform poorly as prognostic factors. Given sufficient sample size, a risk factor (e.g., genetic variant) can be strongly associated with an outcome but not necessarily have an effect size that robustly discriminates affected from unaffected individuals.

The example of Alzheimer's disease provides a useful illustration of the clinical and ethical dilemmas that might be involved in genetic testing for susceptibility variants. Testing is currently available on a clinical basis in the United States for a gene associated with early-onset (prior to age 65 years) familial Alzheimer's disease—namely, the presenilin 1 gene (*PSEN1*), located on chromosome 14q24.3. In addition, testing is available on a research basis or overseas for two other genes associated with early-onset familial Alzheimer's disease: those for amyloid precursor protein (*APP*) and presenilin 2 (*PSEN2*). Early-onset familial Alzheimer's disease is thought to account, however, for fewer than 5% of total Alzheimer's disease cases (Bird et al. 1989). A larger proportion of Alzheimer's disease cases is attributable, in part, to a variant of the apolipoprotein E gene (*APOE*); carriers of one *APOE* ε*4* allele have a 3-fold increased risk of Alzheimer's disease, and those homozygous for the ε*4* allele have an approximately 15-fold increased risk relative to those who have no ε*4* alleles (Bertram and Tanzi 2004). However, given the lack of highly effective preventive or therapeutic interventions for Alzheimer's disease, the potential for stigmatization and discrimination based on test results, and the fact that the *APOE* risk allele is neither necessary nor sufficient for the development of Alzheimer's disease, there continues to be a consensus that *APOE* testing should not, at least for now, be used for predictive purposes (Post et al. 1997; Relkin et al. 1996).

Nevertheless, recent evidence from a randomized clinical trial suggests that there might be substantial demand for *APOE* testing if it were widely offered (Roberts et al. 2004). In the REVEAL (Risk Evaluation and Education for Alzheimer's Disease) study, offspring of parents with Alzheimer's disease were randomly assigned to either an intervention arm in which genetic counseling and risk assessment were based on gender, family history, and *APOE* genotype, or a control arm in which genetic counseling and risk assessment were based only on gender and family history. Randomization to possible APOE testing was accepted by 24% of participants who were systematically contacted through research registries and by 64% of self-referred participants. Roberts et al. (2004) reported that the uptake rate among systematically contacted participants exceeded the uptake rates in similarly ascertained groups for other disorders without effective prevention or treatment options, such as Huntington's disease (10%) or cystic fibrosis (4%–23%), although it is lower than that reported for genetic forms of cancer in which prevention or treatment options exist (30%–85%). They noted that, given the high prevalence of Alzheimer's disease, even the 24% uptake rate could strain available educational and counseling resources; the high prevalence of several psychiatric disorders suggests that similar concerns might apply if susceptibility gene testing was offered.

Because susceptibility genes are, by definition, neither necessary nor sufficient for disease, they are likely to have modest predictive value in many circumstances. In a study of genetic testing for cardiovascular disease, Humphries et al. (2004) pointed out that a predictive genetic test for a disease with complex inheritance would be useful only if it could provide risk information over and above other established, more easily measurable risk factors. One implication for psychiatry is that in many cases, family history by itself may be a better predictor of illness risk (by integrating the effects of multiple genetic and environmental influences) than a susceptibility variant that confers a small increase in risk. For example, having a first-degree relative with bipolar disorder may confer a 7- to 10-fold increased risk of the disorder, whereas the increased risk associated with most genetic variants identified to date by genetic association studies do not exceed 2-fold.

It is conceivable, however, that in the coming years, the ability to simultaneously assay multiple susceptibility genes could substantially improve the predictive value of genetic testing (Evans et al. 2001; Yamada et al. 2002; Yang et al. 2003). Yang et al. (2003) demonstrated that concurrently testing five genes, each of which individually confers a disease risk of only about 10%, could predict the risk of developing a multifactorial disease with a probability exceeding 80%. If it were possible to identify and incorporate the presence of a known environmental risk factor, the predicted probability of developing disease could be further increased (to nearly 90% in their example of an environmental exposure with a prevalence of 15% that raised disease risk twofold). Applying this analysis to the prediction of venous thrombosis, they found that concurrently assaying as few as three known susceptibility genes could yield a positive predictive value exceeding 60%.

More recently, Janssens et al. (2006) used simulations to show that simultaneous testing of multiple susceptibility alleles could be used to produce highly predictive genetic tests for complex diseases. They found that the discriminative accuracy of such tests (an index of the ability to predict risk) is a function of the number of genes involved, the proportion of the variance explained by genes (heritability), the frequency of the risk alleles, and the magnitude of risk associated with risk allele genotypes. Under the assumptions of their simulations (including that all genes involved in the disease and their effects could be quantified), excellent discriminative accuracy could be achieved. For an illness with a prevalence of 1% and a heritability of 23% or higher (schizophrenia would fit this description), discriminative accuracy could exceed 95%.

It is important to note that even if the scientific and statistical limitations of testing can be overcome, the complex ethical issues, coupled with the potential for adverse psychological effects that might accompany genetic testing for psychiatric disorders, would require careful consideration before such tests could be introduced (Austin and Honer 2005; Hodgkinson et al. 2001). The feasibility of testing is different from the desirability or clinical utility of testing, which may depend on the availability of effective interventions for those at increased risk, the adverse psychological and economic impact of false positives and false negatives, and other factors that are not strictly features of test performance.

Gene–Environment Interaction

Although genes play an important role in the etiology of psychiatric disorders, environmental influences are clearly crucial. Even for highly heritable disorders such as schizophrenia, bipolar disorder, and autism, concordance rates for monozygotic twin-pairs are substantially less than 100%, demonstrating that nongenetic factors contribute. For other disorders, such as major depressive disorder and most anxiety disorders, findings from twin studies suggest that nongenetic factors explain most of the variance in risk at a population level (i.e., heritability is less than 50%). And of course, for some disorders, including posttraumatic stress disorder and substance use disorders, specific environmental exposures are prerequisite. Family studies showing that psychiatric disorders run in families cannot distinguish genetic from environmental causes.

Arguments about "nature versus nurture" predate modern psychiatry and have been debated by philosophers, psychologists, policy makers, and the lay public. The pendulum favoring nature or nurture explanations has swung several times over the past century. Recently, there has been concern that the field has been overtaken by a belief in genetic determinism in which genetic contributions are overvalued and nongenetic factors are discounted. Overemphasis on genetic contributions to illness could detract from attention and resources given to important and modifiable environmental roots of psychiatric illness, including socioeconomic inequities, psychosocial stress, and trauma. In fact, however, research findings support neither genetic nor environmental determinism. Genes operate in the inextricable context of environments. Thus, another emerging theme in psychiatric genetic research is the combined and interactive effects of genes and environment. As summarized by Matt Ridley (2003) in his book *Nature via Nurture*, "the more we lift the lid on the genome, the more vulnerable to experience genes appear to be."

In recent years, a series of studies have combined molecular genetic methods and environmental measures to directly examine gene-environment interaction in psychiatry. One of the most obvious applications of the concept of gene-environment interaction is the field of pharmacogenetics (discussed earlier in the section on pharmacogenetics and personalized medicine), whose subject is individual differences in response to environmental exposures (drugs) by genotype. Another line of research has examined gene-environment interaction in the etiology of psychiatric phenotypes. One of the best-known examples has been a reported interaction between variation in the serotonin transporter gene and stressful life events in relation to risk for depression. In their study of a large longitudinal birth cohort, Caspi et al. (2003) first reported that the short allele of the 5-HTTLPR promoter variation was associated with risk for depressive symptoms, major depressive disorder, and suicidality, but only in the presence of a history of stressful life events. In a recent review, seven of nine studies of the interaction of 5-HTTLPR and stress were supportive of an effect on depression or depressive symptoms, although the two largest studies were not (Zammit and Owen 2006). Other studies have implicated an interaction between a variant of *MAOA* and early maltreatment in risk for antisocial behavior among males (Caspi et al. 2002; Kim-Cohen et al. 2006).

From a research standpoint, the appeal of such studies is clear. If we believe that psychiatric disorders are complex and multifactorial, we would expect that studies examining both genetic and environmental factors are more likely to be fruitful than studies that simply look at genes. But beyond their value in illuminating susceptibility factors, such studies may have implications for clinical and policy interventions. A companion fallacy to the idea of genetic determinism is the notion that the stronger the genetic influence on a trait, the less amenable it is to environmental intervention. In reality, even the most heritable phenotypes may be entirely amenable to environmental intervention (an oft-cited example is the recessive genetic disorder phenylketonuria, in which mental retardation can develop but is preventable by limiting dietary phenylalanine intake). The results of studies of gene-environment interactions can highlight environmental and psychosocial influences that may inform treatment and prevention. A growing amount of research now exists clearly demonstrating that early childhood maltreatment interacts with genetic susceptibility to increase risk for psychopathology (Rutter et al. 2006). Kaufman et al. (2004, 2006) have reported that environmental factors can also have protective effects, even in the face of genetic susceptibility. In studies of maltreated children, they found that positive social supports were protective against risk for depressive symptoms among children with genetic (risk alleles of the serotonin transporter and brain-derived neurotrophic factor genes) and environmental (maltreatment) risk factors. Such results underscore the importance of interventions to reduce early adverse experience and improve psychosocial supports for children at risk.

The coming years may see further clarification of how genes and environment interact to confer or modify risk for psychiatric illness. There are many methodological challenges to this research (Moffitt et al. 2005), not the least of which is that measuring environmental factors can be much more difficult than measuring genotypes. Implementing more careful and valid measures of environmental factors will be an important project for the near future if we are to learn more about the interaction of environmental risk and genetic susceptibility.

Conclusions

Psychiatric genetics is a complex and evolving area of research. Despite intense interest and attention to genetics, it is important to acknowledge that clinical applications of genetic knowledge in psychiatry remain limited. Researchers and clinicians should maintain appropriate caution in interpreting the results of the available research. The current volume is intended to inform clinicians both about what is known and what is not known about the role of genetic factors in psychiatric illness. Nevertheless, progress in the field is likely to accelerate in the foreseeable future. An awareness of both the potential and the limitations of genetic research will be increasingly relevant for clinical practice.

References

Andreassen OA, MacEwan T, Gulbrandsen AK, et al: Non-functional CYP2D6 alleles and risk for neuroleptic-induced movement disorders in schizophrenic patients. Psychopharmacology (Berl) 131:174–179, 1997

Arthur H, Dahl ML, Siwers B, et al: Polymorphic drug metabolism in schizophrenic patients with tardive dyskinesia. J Clin Psychopharmacol 15:211–216, 1995

Austin JC, Honer WG: The potential impact of genetic counseling for mental illness. Clin Genet 67:134–142, 2005

Baron M, Risch N, Hamburger R, et al: Genetic linkage between X-chromosome markers and bipolar affective illness. Nature 326:289–292, 1987

Bassett AS, Chow EW: 22q11 deletion syndrome: a genetic subtype of schizophrenia. Biol Psychiatry 46: 882–891, 1999

Bassett AS, Chow EW, AbdelMalik P, et al: The schizophrenia phenotype in 22q11 deletion syndrome. Am J Psychiatry 160:1580–1586, 2003

Bertilsson L, Mellstrom B, Sjokvist F, et al: Slow hydroxylation of nortriptyline and concomitant poor debrisoquine hydroxylation: clinical implications. Lancet 1:560–561, 1981

Bertilsson L, Dahl ML, Dalen P, et al: Molecular genetics of CYP2D6: clinical relevance with focus on psychotropic drugs. Br J Clin Pharmacol 53:111–122, 2002

Berton O, Nestler EJ: New approaches to antidepressant drug discovery: beyond monoamines. Nat Rev Neurosci 7:137–151, 2006

Bertram L, Tanzi RE: The current status of Alzheimer's disease genetics: what do we tell the patients? Pharmacol Res 50:385–396, 2004

Bird TD, Sumi SM, Nemens EJ, et al: Phenotypic heterogeneity in familial Alzheimer's disease: a study of 24 kindreds. Ann Neurol 25:12–25, 1989

Brockmoller J, Kirchheiner J, Schmider J, et al: The impact of the CYP2D6 polymorphism on haloperidol pharmacokinetics and on the outcome of haloperidol treatment. Clin Pharmacol Ther 72:438–452, 2002

Bunney WE, Bunney BG, Vawter MP, et al: Microarray technology: a review of new strategies to discover candidate vulnerability genes in psychiatric disorders. Am J Psychiatry 160:657–666, 2003

Caspi A, McClay J, Moffitt TE, et al: Role of genotype in the cycle of violence in maltreated children. Science 297: 851–854, 2002

Caspi A, Sugden K, Moffitt TE, et al: Influence of life stress on depression: moderation by a polymorphism in the 5-HTT gene. Science 301:386–389, 2003

Chumakov I, Blumenfeld M, Guerassimenko O, et al: Genetic and physiological data implicating the new human gene G72 and the gene for D-amino acid oxidase in schizophrenia. Proc Natl Acad Sci U S A 99:13675–13680, 2002

de Bakker PI, Yelensky R, Pe'er I, et al: Efficiency and power in genetic association studies. Nat Genet 37:1217–1223, 2005

de Leon J, Susce MT, Pan RM, et al: The CYP2D6 poor metabolizer phenotype may be associated with risperidone adverse drug reactions and discontinuation. J Clin Psychiatry 66:15–27, 2005a

de Leon J, Susce MT, Pan RM, et al: Polymorphic variations in GSTM1, GSTT1, PgP, CYP2D6, CYP3A5, and dopamine D2 and D3 receptors and their association with tardive dyskinesia in severe mental illness. J Clin Psychopharmacol 25:448–456, 2005b

de Leon J, Armstrong SC, Cozza KL: Clinical guidelines for psychiatrists for the use of pharmacogenetic testing for CYP450 2D6 and CYP450 2C19. Psychosomatics 47:75–85, 2006

Desta Z, Zhao X, Shin JG, et al: Clinical significance of the cytochrome P450 2C19 genetic polymorphism. Clin Pharmacokinet 41:913–958, 2002

Egeland JA, Gerhard DS, Pauls DL, et al: Bipolar affective disorders linked to DNA markers on chromosome 11. Nature 325:783–787, 1987

Eley TC, Sugden K, Corsico A, et al: Gene-environment interaction analysis of serotonin system markers with adolescent depression. Mol Psychiatry 9:908–915, 2004

Evans JP, Skrzynia C, Burke W: The complexities of predictive genetic testing. BMJ 322:1052–1056, 2001

Faraone SV, Biederman J, Mick E, et al: A family study of psychiatric comorbidity in girls and boys with attention-deficit/hyperactivity disorder. Biol Psychiatry 50:586–592, 2001

Faraone SV, Perlis RH, Doyle AE, et al: Molecular genetics of attention-deficit/hyperactivity disorder. Biol Psychiatry 57:1313–1323, 2005

Finn CT, Smoller JW: Genetic counseling in psychiatry. Harv Rev Psychiatry 14:109–121, 2006

Finn CT, Wilcox MA, Korf BR, et al: Psychiatric genetics: a survey of psychiatrists' knowledge, opinions, and practice patterns. J Clin Psychiatry 66:821–830, 2005

Franchini L, Serretti A, Gasperini M, et al: Familial concordance of fluvoxamine response as a tool for differentiating mood disorder pedigrees. J Psychiatr Res 32:255–259, 1998

Geller G, Tambor ES, Chase GA, et al: Incorporation of genetics in primary care practice. Will physicians do the counseling and will they be directive? Arch Fam Med 2:1119–1125, 1993

Gershon ES, Goldin LR: The outlook for linkage research in psychiatric disorders. J Psychiatr Res 21:541–550, 1987

Grant SF, Thorleifsson G, Reynisdottir I, et al: Variant of transcription factor 7-like 2 (TCF7L2) gene confers risk of type 2 diabetes. Nat Genet 38:320-333, 2006

Green RC, Cupples LA, Go R, et al: Risk of dementia among white and African American relatives of patients with Alzheimer disease. JAMA 287:329–336, 2002

Grof P, Duffy A, Cavazzoni P, et al: Is response to prophylactic lithium a familial trait? J Clin Psychiatry 63:942–947, 2002

Gunther EC, Stone DJ, Gerwien RW, et al: Prediction of clinical drug efficacy by classification of drug-induced genomic expression profiles in vitro. Proc Natl Acad Sci U S A 100:9608–9613, 2003

Gusella JF, Wexler NS, Conneally PM, et al: A polymorphic DNA marker genetically linked to Huntington's disease. Nature 306:234–238, 1983

Hansen RA, Gartlehner G, Lohr KN, et al: Efficacy and safety of second-generation antidepressants in the treatment of major depressive disorder. Ann Intern Med 143:415–426, 2005

Herbert A, Gerry NP, McQueen MB, et al: A common genetic variant is associated with adult and childhood obesity. Science 312:279–283, 2006

Hettema JM, Neale MC, Kendler KS: A review and meta-analysis of the genetic epidemiology of anxiety disorders. Am J Psychiatry 158:1568–1578, 2001

Hodgkinson KA, Murphy J, O'Neill S, et al: Genetic counselling for schizophrenia in the era of molecular genetics. Can J Psychiatry 46:123–130, 2001

Humphries SE, Ridker PM, Talmud PJ: Genetic testing for cardiovascular disease susceptibility: a useful clinical management tool or possible misinformation? Arterioscler Thromb Vasc Biol 24:628–636, 2004

Ingelman-Sundberg M: Pharmacogenetics of cytochrome P450 and its applications in drug therapy: the past, present and future. Trends Pharmacol Sci 25:193–200, 2004

Janssens AC, Aulchenko YS, Elefante S, et al: Predictive testing for complex diseases using multiple genes: fact or fiction? Genet Med 8:395–400, 2006

Jones I, Scourfield J, McCandless F, et al: Attitudes towards future testing for bipolar disorder susceptibility genes: a preliminary investigation. J Affect Disord 71:189–193, 2002

Joseph J: The 1942 "euthanasia" debate in the American Journal of Psychiatry. Hist Psychiatry 16:171–179, 2005

Kapitany T, Meszaros K, Lenzinger E, et al: Genetic polymorphisms for drug metabolism (CYP2D6) and tardive dyskinesia in schizophrenia. Schizophr Res 32:101–106, 1998

Kaufman J, Yang BZ, Douglas-Palumberi H, et al: Social supports and serotonin transporter gene moderate depression in maltreated children. Proc Natl Acad Sci U S A 101:17316–17321, 2004

Kaufman J, Yang BZ, Douglas-Palumberi H, et al: Brain-derived neurotrophic factor-5-HTTLPR gene interactions and environmental modifiers of depression in children. Biol Psychiatry 59:673–680, 2006

Kawanishi C, Lundgren S, Agren H, et al: Increased incidence of CYP2D6 gene duplication in patients with persistent mood disorders: ultrarapid metabolism of antidepressants as a cause of nonresponse. A pilot study. Eur J Clin Pharmacol 59: 803–807, 2004

Kendler KS, Kuhn JW, Vittum J, et al: The interaction of stressful life events and a serotonin transporter polymorphism in the prediction of episodes of major depression: a replication. Arch Gen Psychiatry 62:529–535, 2005

Kessler S, Field T, Worth L, et al: Attitudes of persons at risk for Huntington disease toward predictive testing. Am J Med Genet 26:259–270, 1987

Kim H, Lim SW, Kim S, et al: Monoamine transporter gene polymorphisms and antidepressant response in Koreans with late-life depression. JAMA 296:1609–1618, 2006

Kim-Cohen J, Caspi A, Taylor A, et al: MAOA, maltreatment, and gene-environment interaction predicting children's mental health: new evidence and a meta-analysis. Mol Psychiatry 11:903–913, 2006

Kirchheiner J, Brosen K, Dahl ML, et al: CYP2D6 and CYP2C19 genotype-based dose recommendations for antidepressants: a first step towards subpopulation-specific dosages. Acta Psychiatr Scand 104:173–192, 2001

Kirchheiner J, Nickchen K, Bauer M, et al: Pharmacogenetics of antidepressants and antipsychotics: the contribution of allelic variations to the phenotype of drug response. Mol Psychiatry 9:442–473, 2004

Kirchheiner J, Fuhr U, Brockmoller J: Pharmacogenetics-based therapeutic recommendations—ready for clinical practice? Nat Rev Drug Discov 4:639–647, 2005

Klein RJ, Zeiss C, Chew EY, et al: Complement factor H polymorphism in age-related macular degeneration. Science 308:385–389, 2005

Lessard E, Yessine MA, Hamelin BA, et al: Influence of CYP2D6 activity on the disposition and cardiovascular toxicity of the antidepressant agent venlafaxine in humans. Pharmacogenetics 9:435–443, 1999

Levinson DF, Levinson MD, Segurado R, et al: Genome scan meta-analysis of schizophrenia and bipolar disorder, part I: methods and power analysis. Am J Hum Genet 73:17–33, 2003

Malhotra AK, Murphy GM Jr, Kennedy JL: Pharmacogenetics of psychotropic drug response. Am J Psychiatry 161:780–796, 2004

Marteau TM: Communicating genetic risk information. Br Med Bull 55:414–428, 1999

Masoliver E, Menoyo A, Perez V, et al: Serotonin transporter linked promoter (polymorphism) in the serotonin transporter gene may be associated with antidepressant-induced mania in bipolar disorder. Psychiatr Genet 16:25–29, 2006

McQueen MB, Devlin B, Faraone SV, et al: Combined analysis from eleven linkage studies of bipolar disorder provides strong evidence of susceptibility loci on chromosomes 6q and 8q. Am J Hum Genet 77: 582–595, 2005

Meiser B, Dunn S: Psychological impact of genetic testing for Huntington's disease: an update of the literature. J Neurol Neurosurg Psychiatry 69:574–578, 2000

Meiser B, Mitchell PB, McGirr H, et al: Implications of genetic risk information in families with a high density of bipolar disorder: an exploratory study. Soc Sci Med 60:109–118, 2005

Merikangas KR, Stolar M, Stevens DE, et al: Familial transmission of substance use disorders. Arch Gen Psychiatry 55:973–979, 1998

Milner KK, Collins EE, Connors GR, et al: Attitudes of young adults to prenatal screening and genetic correction for human attributes and psychiatric conditions. Am J Med Genet 76:111–119, 1998

Milner KK, Han T, Petty EM: Support for the availability of prenatal testing for neurological and psychiatric conditions in the psychiatric community. Genet Test 3:279–286, 1999

Moffitt TE, Caspi A, Rutter M: Strategy for investigating interactions between measured genes and measured environments. Arch Gen Psychiatry 62:473–481, 2005

Mrazek D, Smoller JW, de Leon J: Incorporating pharmacogenetics into clinical practice: reality of a new toll in psychiatry. CNS Spectr 11(suppl 3):1–13, 2006

Muhle R, Trentacoste SV, Rapin I: The genetics of autism. Pediatrics 113:e472–e486, 2004

Mundo E, Walker M, Cate T, et al: The role of serotonin transporter protein gene in antidepressant-induced mania in bipolar disorder: preliminary findings. Arch Gen Psychiatry 58:539–544, 2001

Murphy GM Jr, Kremer C, Rodrigues HE, et al: Pharmacogenetics of antidepressant medication intolerance. Am J Psychiatry 160:1830–1835, 2003

Murphy GM Jr, Hollander SB, Rodrigues HE, et al: Effects of the serotonin transporter gene promoter polymorphism on mirtazapine and paroxetine efficacy and adverse events in geriatric major depression. Arch Gen Psychiatry 61:1163–1169, 2004

Murphy KC: Schizophrenia and velo-cardio-facial syndrome. Lancet 359:426–430, 2002

Murphy KC, Owen MJ: Velo-cardio-facial syndrome: a model for understanding the genetics and pathogenesis of schizophrenia. Br J Psychiatry 179:397–402, 2001

NIMH Genetics Workgroup: Genetics and Mental Disorders. Bethesda, MD, National Institute of Mental Health, 1998

Nurnberger JI Jr, Wiegand R, Bucholz K, et al: A family study of alcohol dependence: coaggregation of multiple disorders in relatives of alcohol-dependent probands. Arch Gen Psychiatry 61:1246–1256, 2004

Ohmori O, Kojima H, Shinkai T, et al: Genetic association analysis between CYP2D6*2 allele and tardive dyskinesia in schizophrenic patients. Psychiatry Res 87:239–244, 1999

Peay H, McInerney J: A pilot study on psychiatric genetic counseling: counselors' needs. J Genet Couns 11:485, 2002

Perlis RH, Mischoulon D, Smoller JW, et al: Serotonin transporter polymorphisms and adverse effects with fluoxetine treatment. Biol Psychiatry 54:879–883, 2003

Perlis RH, Ganz DA, Avorn J, et al: Pharmacogenetic testing in the clinical management of schizophrenia: a decision-analytic model. J Clin Psychopharmacol 25:427–434, 2005

Phillips KA, Van Bebber SL: Measuring the value of pharmacogenomics. Nat Rev Drug Discov 4:500–509, 2005

Popp J, Leucht S, Heres S, et al: Serotonin transporter polymorphisms and side effects in antidepressant therapy—a pilot study. Pharmacogenomics 7:159–166, 2006

Post SG, Whitehouse PJ, Binstock RH, et al: The clinical introduction of genetic testing for Alzheimer disease. An ethical perspective. JAMA 277:832–836, 1997

Quackenbush J: Microarray analysis and tumor classification. N Engl J Med 354:2463–2472, 2006

Quaid K, Aschen S, Smiley C, et al: Perceived genetic risks for bipolar disorder in a patient population: an exploratory study. J Genet Couns 10:41–51, 2001

Relkin NR, Kwon YJ, Tsai J, et al: The National Institute on Aging/Alzheimer's Association recommendations on the application of apolipoprotein E genotyping to Alzheimer's disease. Ann N Y Acad Sci 802:149–176, 1996

Ridley M: Nature via Nuture. New York, NY, HarperCollins, 2003

Risch N, Botstein D: A manic depressive history. Nat Genet 12:351–353, 1996

Roberts JS, Barber M, Brown TM, et al: Who seeks genetic susceptibility testing for Alzheimer's disease? Findings from a multisite, randomized clinical trial. Genet Med 6:197–203, 2004

Roberts RL, Mulder RT, Joyce PR, et al: No evidence of increased adverse drug reactions in cytochrome P450 CYP2D6 poor metabolizers treated with fluoxetine or nortriptyline. Hum Psychopharmacol 19:17–23, 2004

Rutter M, Moffitt TE, Caspi A: Gene-environment interplay and psychopathology: multiple varieties but real effects. J Child Psychol Psychiatry 47:226–261, 2006

Savage DG, Antman KH: Imatinib mesylate–a new oral targeted therapy. N Engl J Med 346:683–693, 2002

Schillevoort I, de Boer A, van der Weide J, et al: Antipsychotic-induced extrapyramidal syndromes and cytochrome P450 2D6 genotype: a case-control study. Pharmacogenetics 12: 235–240, 2002

Scolnick EM, Petryshen T, Sklar P: Schizophrenia: do the genetics and neurobiology of neuregulin provide a pathogenesis model? Harv Rev Psychiatry 14:64–77, 2006

Scordo MG, Spina E: Cytochrome P450 polymorphisms and response to antipsychotic therapy. Pharmacogenomics 3:201–218, 2002

Serretti A, Kato M, De Ronchi D, et al: Meta-analysis of serotonin transporter gene promoter polymorphism (5-HTTLPR) association with selective serotonin reuptake inhibitor efficacy in depressed patients. Mol Psychiatry 12:247–257, 2007

Sherrington R, Brynjolfsson J, Petursson H, et al: Localization of a susceptibility locus for schizophrenia on chromosome 5. Nature 336:164–167, 1988

Sindrup SH, Brosen K, Gram LF, et al: The relationship between paroxetine and the sparteine oxidation polymorphism. Clin Pharmacol Ther 51:278–287, 1992

Smith L, Sapers B, Reus V, et al: Attitudes towards bipolar disorder and predictive genetic testing among patients and providers. J Med Genet 33:544–549, 1996

Smits KM, Smits LJ, Schouten JS, et al: Influence of SERTPR and STin2 in the serotonin transporter gene on the effect of selective serotonin reuptake inhibitors in depression: a systematic review. Mol Psychiatry 9:433–441, 2004

Smoller JW, Finn CT: Family, twin, and adoption studies of bipolar disorder. Am J Med Genet C Semin Med Genet 123:48–58, 2003

Spina E, Gitto C, Avenoso A, et al: Relationship between plasma desipramine levels, CYP2D6 phenotype and clinical response to desipramine: a prospective study. Eur J Clin Pharmacol 51:395–398, 1997

Stefansson H, Sigurdsson E, Steinthorsdottir V, et al: Neuregulin 1 and susceptibility to schizophrenia. Am J Hum Genet 71:877–892, 2002

Straub RE, Jiang Y, MacLean CJ, et al: Genetic variation in the 6p22.3 gene DTNBP1, the human ortholog of the mouse dysbindin gene, is associated with schizophrenia. Am J Hum Genet 71:337–348, 2002. Erratum in Am J Hum Genet 72:1007, 2002

Strober M, Freeman R, Lampert C, et al: Controlled family study of anorexia nervosa and bulimia nervosa: evidence of shared liability and transmission of partial syndromes. Am J Psychiatry 157:393–401, 2000

Sullivan PF, Neale MC, Kendler KS: Genetic epidemiology of major depression: review and meta-analysis. Am J Psychiatry 157:1552–1562, 2000

Thase ME, Haight BR, Richard N, et al: Remission rates following antidepressant therapy with bupropion or selective serotonin reuptake inhibitors: a meta-analysis of original data from 7 randomized controlled trials. J Clin Psychiatry 66:974–981, 2005

Tiwari AK, Deshpande SN, Rao AR, et al: Genetic susceptibility to tardive dyskinesia in chronic schizophrenia subjects, III: lack of association of CYP3A4 and CYP2D6 gene polymorphisms. Schizophr Res 75:21–26, 2005

Trippitelli C, Jamison K, Folstein M, et al: Pilot study on patients' and spouses' attitudes toward potential genetic testing for bipolar disorder. Am J Psychiatry 155:899–904, 1998

Trivedi MH, Rush AJ, Wisniewski SR, et al: Evaluation of outcomes with citalopram for depression using measurement-based care in STAR*D: implications for clinical practice. Am J Psychiatry 163:28–40, 2006

Tsuang M: Schizophrenia: genes and environment. Biol Psychiatry 47:210–220, 2000

Vandel P, Haffen E, Vandel S, et al: Drug extrapyramidal side effects. CYP2D6 genotypes and phenotypes. Eur J Clin Pharmacol 55:659–665, 1999

Ware JH: The limitations of risk factors as prognostic tools. N Engl J Med 355:2615–2617, 2006

Weinshilboum R, Wang L: Pharmacogenomics: bench to bedside. Nat Rev Drug Discov 3:739–748, 2004

Whooley MA, Simon GE: Managing depression in medical outpatients. N Engl J Med 343:1942–1950, 2000

Yamada Y, Izawa H, Ichihara S, et al: Prediction of the risk of myocardial infarction from polymorphisms in candidate genes. N Engl J Med 347:1916–1923, 2002

Yang Q, Khoury MJ, Botto L, et al: Improving the prediction of complex diseases by testing for multiple disease-susceptibility genes. Am J Hum Genet 72:636–649, 2003

Zammit S, Owen MJ: Stressful life events, 5-HTT genotype and risk of depression. Br J Psychiatry 188:199–201, 2006

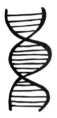

Glossary

allele   One of the alternate forms of DNA present at a particular polymorphic locus.

association   In the context of a case-control genetic study, an overrepresentation of a particular allele, genotype, or haplotype among individuals affected by a disorder, compared with control individuals without the disorder; in the context of a family-based genetic study, an overtransmission of a particular allele or haplotype from parents to their affected children.

chromosome   Tightly condensed strands of DNA that contain the genes of an organism.

concordant   Similar with respect to one or more traits.

crossing-over   Exchange of genetic material between a pair of homologous chromosomes, resulting in recombination.

discordant   Dissimilar with respect to one or more traits.

DNA markers   Identifiable physical locations on a chromosome.

gene   The basic unit of inheritance, a segment of DNA that codes for a functional product, such as a protein.

genetic epidemiology   A science that deals with inherited causes of disease in populations and with etiology, distribution, and control of disease in groups of relatives.

genome   The entire DNA sequence of all chromosomes of an organism.

genotype   The combination of maternally inherited and paternally inherited alleles present at a particular site in the genome.

haplotype   The pattern of alleles of multiple polymorphisms within or across different genes that occur on the same chromosome.

haplotype relative risk   The probability of affected offspring receiving the risk allele relative to the normal allele of a risk gene.

heritability   The degree to which a trait is influenced by genetic factors as opposed to environmental factors; usually expressed as a percentage or proportion.

linkage   The relationship between genes on the same chromosome that causes them to be inherited together; in the context of linkage analysis, an increase in the likelihood of co-inheritance of two genes on the same chromosome.

linkage disequilibrium   Unusually tight linkage between two or more polymorphisms.

locus   The site or position of a gene on a particular chromosome.

lod score   Logarithm of the odds of obtaining the observed pattern of genetic and phenotypic marker similarity, given a particular pedigree structure.

odds ratio   A ratio of the probabilities of a certain event occurring in two groups.

phenotype   The observable properties of an organism that are produced by the interaction of the genotype and the environment.

polymorphism   A site in the genome where more than one alternate pattern of DNA is present.

proband   The first member of a family to be ascertained for a genetic study.

population stratification   Background genetic differences between case and control groups.

syntenic   On the same chromosome.

Index

*Page numbers printed in **boldface** type refer to tables or figures.*

American Academy of Neurology,
262
American College of Obstetricians
and Gynecologists, 236
American College of Medical
Genetics (ACMG), 262, 267–268
American Psychiatric Association,
141, 262
American Society of Human Genetics,
50, 262, 267–268
Americans With Disabilities Act of
1990, 270
d–Amino acid oxidase activator gene
(*DAOA*)
bipolar disorder and, 138–139
schizophrenia and, **111**
Amino acids, and metabolic disorders,
215
Ammonia, and metabolic disorders, **215**
Amniocentesis, and prenatal genetic
testing, 264
Amyloid-β protein precursor gene
(*APP*), and Alzheimer's disease,
181, 182, 293
Animal models, for obsessive-
compulsive disorder, 82
Anorexia nervosa, **22, 280.** *See also*
Eating disorders
Anticipation, and genetic inheritance,
199
Anticipatory guidance, and genetic
counseling, 41–42
Anticonvulsant medications, and
pregnancy, 240–242
Antidepressants. *See also* Tricyclic
antidepressants
adverse reactions to and 2D6
genotypes, 285
genetic research and efficacy of,
281
pregnancy and, 229, 235–238
Antipsychotics. *See also* Atypical
antipsychotics
pharmacokinetic genes and,
285–286

pregnancy and, 242–245
schizophrenia and, 100, **115**
Antisocial personality disorder, **22**
Anxiety disorders
complex genetic boundaries of,
158–161
core features of, **151**
course of during pregnancy,
230–231
DSM-IV-TR and, 150–151
family planning and history of,
228–229
genetic determinants of depression
and, 150
genetic epidemiology of, **155**
treatment of during pregnancy,
231–235, 245–248
Anxiolytic medications, and
pregnancy, 244–245
Apolipoprotein E gene (*APOE*), and
Alzheimer's disease, 28, 181,
184–185, 187, 188, 261–263, 267,
293–294
Aripiprazole, 243, 285
Association analysis
of bipolar disorder, 138–139, 144
history of genetic research and,
278–279
methodology of genetic research
and, 5, 15–19, 21, 23–24
Assortative mating, 38
Attention-deficit/hyperactivity
disorder (ADHD)
clinical phenotype of, 70
early-onset bipolar disorder and,
133, 143
family studies and, **22**
genetic disorders and, **200, 202,
203, 204, 205, 206**
genetic epidemiology of, 70–73
relative risk of, 73–74, **280**
summary of genetic findings for, **76**
Tourette's disorder and, 85
Atypical antipsychotics, 243–244. *See
also* Antipsychotics